MONOCLONAL ANTIBODIES

Hybridomas: A New Dimension in Biological Analyses

MONOCLONAL ANTIBODIES

Hybridomas: A New Dimension in Biological Analyses

Edited by

Roger H. Kennett and
Thomas J. McKearn

University of Pennsylvania School of Medicine
Philadelphia, Pennsylvania

and

Kathleen B. Bechtol

The Wistar Institute
Philadelphia, Pennsylvania

Plenum Press · New York and London

Library of Congress Cataloging in Publication Data

Main entry under title:

Monoclonal antibodies.

Includes index.
1. Immunoglobulins. 2. Gammopathies, Monoclonal. 3. Cell hybridization.
I. Kennett, Roger H. II. McKearn, Thomas J. III. Bechtol, Kathleen B. [DNLM:
1. Antibodies. 2. Clone cells — Immunology. QW575 M751]
QR186.7.M66   599.02'93   80-15118
ISBN 0-306-40408-7

©1980 Plenum Press, New York
A Division of Plenum Publishing Corporation
227 West 17th Street, New York, N.Y. 10011

Printed in the United States of America

In Memoriam

WILLIAM J. MELLMAN

Scientist, Pediatrician, and Friend
May 7, 1928—February 27, 1980

Contributors

C. ABRAMS, Department of Human Genetics, University of Pennsylvania, School of Medicine, Philadelphia, Pennsylvania 19104

KATHLEEN B. BECHTOL, Wistar Institute of Anatomy and Biology, Philadelphia, Pennsylvania 19104

YEHUDIT BERGMAN, Howard Hughes Medical Institute Laboratories and Department of Medicine, Stanford University Medical Center, Stanford, California 94305

IRWIN D. BERNSTEIN, Pediatric Oncology Program of the Fred Hutchinson Cancer Research Center, Seattle, Washington 98104, and Department of Pediatrics, University of Washington, Seattle, Washington 98195

PAUL H. BLACK, Department of Medicine, Harvard Medical School, and Massachusetts General Hospital, Boston, Massachusetts 02114

ROGER J. BRIDEAU, MRC Cellular Immunology Unit, Sir William Dunn School of Pathology, University of Oxford, Oxford OX1 3RE, England

SHERRI BROWN, Howard Hughes Medical Institute Laboratories and Department of Medicine, Stanford University Medical Center, Stanford, California 94305

W. NEAL BURNETTE, Tumor Virology Program of the Fred Hutchinson Cancer Research Center, Seattle, Washington 98104

M.P. CANCRO, Department of Pathology, University of Pennsylvania, School of Medicine, Philadelphia, Pennsylvania 19104

EDWARD A. CLARK, Department of Genetics, University of Washington, Seattle, Washington 98195

BRIAN CLEVINGER, Department of Microbiology and Immunology, Washington University School of Medicine, St. Louis, Missouri 63110

M. C. COSEO, Department of Human Genetics, University of Pennsylvania, School of Medicine, Philadelphia, Pennsylvania 19104

JOSEPH DAVIE, Department of Microbiology and Immunology, Washington University School of Medicine, St. Louis, Missouri 63110

KATHLEEN DENIS, Department of Human Genetics, University of Pennsylvania, School of Medicine, Philadelphia, Pennsylvania 19104

BETTY DIAMOND, Department of Cell Biology, Albert Einstein College of Medicine, Bronx, New York 10461

JEANETTE DILLEY, Howard Hughes Medical Institute Laboratories and Department of Medicine, Stanford University Medical Center, Stanford, California 94305

EDGAR G. ENGLEMAN, Department of Pathology, Stanford University Medical Center, Stanford, California 94305

FRANK W. FITCH, The Committee on Immunology and the Department of Pathology, University of Chicago, Chicago, Illinois 60637

MARK E. FRANKEL, Wistar Institute of Anatomy and Biology, Philadelphia, Pennsylvania 19104

WALTER GERHARD, Wistar Institute of Anatomy and Biology, Philadelphia, Pennsylvania 19104

JAMES W. GODING, Department of Genetics, Stanford University School of Medicine, Stanford, California 94305

RICHARD A. GOLDSBY, Department of Chemistry, University of Maryland, College Park, Maryland 20742

ROGERS GRIFFITH, Department of Microbiology and Immunology, Washington University School of Medicine, St. Louis, Missouri 63110

J. B. HAAS, Department of Human Genetics, University of Pennsylvania, School of Medicine, Philadelphia, Pennsylvania 19104

EDGAR HABER, Department of Medicine, Harvard Medical School, and Massachusetts General Hospital, Boston, Massachusetts 02114

DANIEL HANSBURG, Department of Microbiology and Immunology, Washington University School of Medicine, St. Louis, Missouri 63110

H. HARRIS, Department of Human Genetics, University of Pennsylvania, School of Medicine, Philadelphia, Pennsylvania 19104

HANS HENGARTNER, Basel Institute for Immunology, CH-4005 Basel 5, Switzerland

LEONARD A. HERZENBERG, Department of Genetics, Stanford University School of Medicine, Stanford, California 94305

LEROY HOOD, Division of Biology, California Institute of Technology, Pasadena, California 91125

L.L. HOUSTON, Tumor Virology Program of the Fred Hutchinson Cancer Research Center, Seattle, Washington 98104

J. C. HOWARD, Department of Pathology, University of Pennsylvania, School of Medicine, Philadelphia, Pennsylvania 19104

ZDENKA L. JONAK, Wistar Institute of Anatomy and Biology, Philadelphia, Pennsylvania 19104

E. A. JONES, Genetics Laboratory, Department of Biochemistry, University of Oxford, Oxford OX1 3QU, England. *Present address:* Division of Immunology, Stanford University Medical School, Stanford, California 94305

ROGER H. KENNETT, Department of Human Genetics, University of Pennsylvania, School of Medicine, Philadelphia, Pennsylvania 19104

DENNIS M. KLINMAN, Department of Pathology, University of Pennsylvania, School of Medicine, Philadelphia, Pennsylvania 19104

NORMAN KLINMAN, Department of Cellular and Developmental Immunology, Scripps Clinic and Research Foundation, La Jolla, California 92037

HILARY KOPROWSKI, Wistar Institute of Anatomy and Biology, Philadelphia, Pennsylvania 19104

LOIS A. LAMPSON, Department of Anatomy, University of Pennsylvania, School of Medicine, Philadelphia, Pennsylvania 19104

JEFFREY A. LEDBETTER, Department of Genetics, Stanford University School of Medicine, Stanford, California 94305

RONALD LEVY, Howard Hughes Medical Institute Laboratories and Department of Medicine, Stanford University Medical Center, Stanford, California 94305

A. DWIGHT LOPES, Wistar Institute of Anatomy and Biology, Philadelphia, Pennsylvania 19104

MARK E. LOSTROM, Tumor Virology Program of the Fred Hutchinson Cancer Research Center, Seattle, Washington 98104

THOMAS J. MCKEARN, Department of Pathology, Divisions of Research Immunology and Laboratory Medicine, University of Pennsylvania, School of Medicine, Philadelphia, Pennsylvania 19104

BRIAN MCMASTER, Pediatric Oncology Program of the Fred Hutchinson Cancer Research Center, Seattle, Washington 98104

W. ROBERT MCMASTER, MRC Cellular Immunology Unit, Sir William Dunn School of Pathology, University of Oxford, Oxford OX1 3RE, England

DAVID H. MARGULIES, Department of Cell Biology, Albert Einstein College of Medicine, Bronx, New York 10461

DONALD W. MASON, MRC Cellular Immunology Unit, Sir William Dunn School of Pathology, University of Oxford, Oxford OX1 3RE, England

TOMASO MEO, Basel Institute for Immunology, CH-4005 Basel 5, Switzerland

CHRISTINE MOLINARO, Department of Cellular and Developmental Immunology, Scripps Clinic and Research Foundation, La Jolla, California 92037

EDITH MÜLLER, Basel Institute for Immunology, CH-4005 Basel 5, Switzerland

ROBERT C. NOWINSKI, Tumor Virology Program of the Fred Hutchinson Cancer Research Center, Seattle, Washington 98104, and Department of Microbiology, University of Washington, Seattle, Washington 98195

PAUL V. O'DONNELL, Memorial Sloan-Kettering Cancer Center, New York, New York 10021

BARBARA A. OSBORNE, Department of Genetics, Stanford University Medical Center, Stanford, California 94305

RICHARD A. POLIN, Department of Pediatrics, University of Pennsylvania, School of Medicine, and The Children's Hospital of Philadelphia, Philadelphia, Pennsylvania 19104

MATTHEW D. SCHARFF, Department of Cell Biology, Albert Einstein College of Medicine, Bronx, New York 10461

JAMES SCHILLING, Division of Biology, California Institute of Technology, Pasadena, California 91125

LINDA SHERMAN, Department of Cellular and Developmental Immunology, Scripps Clinic and Research Foundation, La Jolla, California 92037

C. A. SLAUGHTER, Department of Human Genetics, University of Pennsylvania, School of Medicine, Philadelphia, Pennsylvania 19104

DAWN E. SMILEK, Department of Pathology, Division of Research Immunology, University of Pennsylvania, School of Medicine, Philadelphia, Pennsylvania 19104

E. SOLOMON, Genetics Laboratory, Department of Biochemistry, University of Oxford, Oxford OX1 3QU, England. *Present address:* Imperial Cancer Research Fund, P.O. Box 123, Lincoln's Inn Fields, London WC2A 3PX, England

TIMOTHY A. SPRINGER, Pathology Department, Harvard Medical School, Boston, Massachusetts 02115

LOUIS STAUDT, Wistar Institute of Anatomy and Biology, Philadelphia, Pennsylvania 19104

MARY R. STONE, Tumor Virology Program of the Fred Hutchinson Cancer Research Center, Seattle, Washington 98104

MILTON R. TAM, Tumor Virology Program of the Fred Hutchinson Cancer Research Center, Seattle, Washington 98104

TAKESHI TOKUHISA, Department of Genetics, Stanford University School of Medicine, Stanford, California 94305

MICHAEL WEBB, MRC Cellular Immunology Unit, Sir William Dunn School of Pathology, University of Oxford, Oxford OX1 3RE, England

ROBERT A. H. WHITE, MRC Cellular Immunology Unit, Sir William Dunn School of Pathology, University of Oxford, Oxford OX1 3RE, England

TADEUSZ WIKTOR, Wistar Institute of Anatomy and Biology, Philadelphia, Pennsylvania 19104

ALAN F. WILLIAMS, MRC Cellular Immunology Unit, Sir William Dunn School of Pathology, University of Oxford, Oxford OX1 3RE, England

DALE E. YELTON, Department of Cell Biology, Albert Einstein College of Medicine, Bronx, New York 10461

JONATHAN YEWDELL, Wistar Institute of Anatomy and Biology, Philadelphia, Pennsylvania 19104

VINCENT R. ZURAWSKI, JR., Department of Medicine, Harvard Medical School, and Massachusetts General Hospital, Boston, Massachusetts 02114

Preface

On August 7, 1975, Köhler and Milstein published in *Nature* (**256:**495) a report describing "Continuous cultures of fused cells secreting antibody of predefined specificity." Their report has become a classic and has already had a profound effect on basic and applied research in biology and medicine. By the time the first Workshop on Lymphocyte Hybridomas (*Current Topics in Microbiology and Immunology* **81,** 1978) was held on April 3–5, 1978, in Bethesda, Maryland, investigators from many laboratories had made hybrids between plasmacytomas and spleen cells from immunized animals and had obtained monoclonal antibodies reacting with a broad variety of antigenic determinants.

At the time Köhler and Milstein introduced this new technology, the editors of this volume were involved in the production of antisera against differentiation antigens (K.B.B.), histocompatibility antigens (T.J. McK.), and human tumor-associated antigens (R.H.K.). Because of the potential usefulness of monoclonal antibodies in these areas, we each began production of hybridomas and analysis of the resulting monoclonal reagents. One of the most interesting aspects of participation in the early stages of the development and application of hybridoma technology has been observing how the implications of the initial observations gradually spread first among the practitioners of immunology and immunogenetics, and then to other areas of the biological sciences, such as developmental biology, biochemistry, human genetics, and cell and tumor biology.

Besides providing a novel way of obtaining homogeneous antibodies that will be useful in many areas of biology, Köhler and Milstein's achievement also provides a prototype for the use of hybrid cells to "trap" clones of cells performing a specialized function as transformed cell lines producing a specific product or performing a specific function *in vitro*. When one considers that the production of specific immunoglobulins may be only the first of several such functions that could be "immortalized" by cell fusion, then it appears likely that the full implications of Köhler and Milstein's report may still be far from full realization.

This volume is designed to present an overview of the production and uses of monoclonal antibodies and to facilitate their application to other areas of biology. It is intended for advanced undergraduates, graduate students, and scientists in the biological and medical sciences. We do not presume to consider the volume comprehensive, but have attempted to include examples of many of the approaches and applications that have been developed to exploit this technology.

Roger H. Kennett
Thomas J. McKearn
Kathleen B. Bechtol

Philadelphia

Acknowledgments

Roger Kennett acknowledges with thanks his co-editors; his three technicians, Jeannie Haas, Barbara Meyer, and Harriet Davis, who kept his laboratory functioning well while he worked on this volume; Carol, who remained a patient and loving wife; and the Lord Jesus Christ, who blessed him with all of the above.

Tom McKearn acknowledges and thanks his family for their support.

Kathleen Bechtol wishes to thank Dr. Z. Jonak, Kim Holt-Sarra, and Marian Butts for their support in the lab during the preparation of this monograph.

Contents

7 The Use of Hybridomas in Enzyme Genetics

C. A. SLAUGHTER, M. C. COSEO, C. ABRAMS, M. P. CANCRO, AND H. HARRIS

8 Characterization of a Human T-Cell Population Identified and Isolated by a Monoclonal Antibody

RICHARD A. GOLDSBY, BARBARA A. OSBORNE, AND EDGAR G. ENGLEMAN

9 Mouse × Human Hybridomas

RONALD LEVY, JEANETTE DILLEY, SHERRI BROWN, AND YEHUDIT BERGMAN

10 Monoclonal Antibodies against Human Tumor-Associated Antigens

ROGER H. KENNETT, ZDENKA L. JONAK, AND KATHLEEN B. BECHTOL

PART IV   MONOCLONAL ANTIBODIES AS PROBES IN THE STUDY OF
          CELLULAR DIFFERENTIATION AND IMMUNOGENETICS

11   Germ-Cell-Related and Nervous-System-Related Differentiation
     and Tumor Antigens

KATHLEEN B. BECHTOL, ZDENKA L. JONAK, AND ROGER H. KENNETT

12   Cell-Surface Differentiation in the Mouse
     Characterization of "Jumping" and "Lineage" Antigens Using
     Xenogeneic Rat Monoclonal Antibodies

TIMOTHY A. SPRINGER

13   Rat–Mouse Hybridomas and Their Application to Studies of the
     Major Histocompatibility Complex

THOMAS J. MCKEARN, DAWN E. SMILEK, AND FRANK W. FITCH

14 Murine T-Cell Differentiation Antigens Detected by Monoclonal
Antibodies

JEFFREY A. LEDBETTER, JAMES W. GODING, TAKESHI TOKUHISA, AND
LEONARD A. HERZENBERG

15 Monoclonal Antibodies That Define T-Lymphocyte Subsets
in the Rat

DONALD W. MASON, ROGER J. BRIDEAU, W. ROBERT McMASTER,
MICHAEL WEBB, ROBERT A. H. WHITE, AND ALAN F. WILLIAMS

16 Monoclonal Antibody Therapy of Mouse Leukemia

IRWIN D. BERNSTEIN, ROBERT C. NOWINSKI, MILTON R. TAM,
BRIAN McMASTER, L. L. HOUSTON, AND EDWARD A. CLARK

PART V   MONOCLONAL ANTIBODIES TO MICROORGANISMS

Part I

Introduction
Production of Specific Antibodies from Continuous Cell Lines *in Vitro*

1
Plasmacytomas and Hybridomas
Development and Applications

Dale E. Yelton, David H. Margulies,
Betty Diamond, and Matthew D. Scharff

I. Introduction

Köhler and Milstein (1975) launched a new era in immunological research by showing that somatic cell hybridization could be used to generate a continuous "hybridoma" cell line producing a monoclonal antibody. The hybridoma technology has already fulfilled one of the major goals that immunologists have been trying to achieve for years: the routine production of large amounts of homogeneous antibody against a wide variety of antigens. Each of the subsequent chapters in this monograph will illustrate the usefulness of such reagents.

Recently several investigators have shown that cell fusion can also be used to obtain cell lines that produce effector molecules of immunological interest or that respond to immunological regulation. Such hybrids may fulfill a second major goal of immunologists: to obtain homogeneous cell lines that can be used to investigate the genetic, biochemical, and molecular basis of cellular interactions in the immune response.

The development of the hybridoma technology, the approaches used to overcome technical difficulties, and the problems that still persist are reflections of the biochemistry and genetics of cell fusion and of immunoglobulin production. A brief review of some relevant experiments as well as earlier attempts to produce homogeneous antibodies provides a useful perspective. In any case, it will serve to remind us that studies with the most basic goals can lead to findings of great practical importance.

Dale E. Yelton, David H. Margulies, Betty Diamond, and Matthew D. Scharff • Department of Cell Biology, Albert Einstein College of Medicine, Bronx, New York 10461.

II. Experimental Uses of Plasmacytomas

The realization that multiple myeloma is a neoplasm of antibody-producing cells and that each tumor represents the proliferation of a single clone of antibody-forming cells led to the use of paraproteins from patients to study antibody structure. The availability of an analogous tumor in mice that could be experimentally induced and passaged indefinitely provided an unlimited supply of homogeneous mouse immunoglobulins for chemical analysis (Potter, 1972). The usefulness of mouse myelomas is perhaps best appreciated by looking at the Cold Spring Harbor Symposium in 1967 on *Antibodies.* That volume also illustrates the enormous impact of Potter's myeloma induction program at the NIH, and subsequently of the Salk induction program, directed by Cohn and his colleagues. Not only were the tumors themselves important, but their distribution promoted an interchange of ideas and reagents that has played a crucial role in the progress of modern immunology, culminating in the recent explosion of information on the structure of immunoglobulin genes (Seidman *et al.,* 1978; Bernard *et al.,* 1978; Sakano *et al.,* 1978).

Initially the relevance of myelomas and their products to the normal immune response was questioned. This concern has been largely allayed by the finding that many myeloma proteins not only react with a variety of environmental antigens but also are serologically identical to normal antibodies generated against the same antigens (Potter, 1978). Furthermore, it has been possible to generate homogeneous antibodies against certain antigens, especially bacterial polysaccharides (Krause, 1970; Haber, 1970). The amino acid sequences of these antibodies and others have been analyzed, and the conclusions from such studies agree with studies of myeloma proteins (Cebra *et al.,* 1974; Capra *et al.,* 1975a,b; Haber *et al.,* 1977). Even the synthesis and assembly of the immunoglobulin molecules in myeloma cells closely resembles these processes in normal lymphoid cells (Scharff and Laskov, 1970; Kuehl, 1977; Williamson, 1971). In fact the only reproducible difference in the metabolism of immunoglobulin in normal and malignant cells has been the kinetics of secretion, which appears to occur more rapidly and in a more ordered way in normal cells (Helmreich *et al.,* 1961; Baumal and Scharff, 1973).

Mouse myeloma cells have been extremely useful in the study of the biochemistry of immunoglobulin production because they can be introduced into culture, cloned, and maintained as continuously growing, relatively homogeneous cultured lines (Pettengill and Sorenson, 1967; Horibata and Harris, 1970; Laskov and Scharff, 1970). These cell lines also provide an excellent somatic-cell genetic system. Variants in immunoglobulin production and structure can be obtained with relative ease (Scharff, 1974; Margulies *et al.,* 1977), and cells producing different types of normal or variant molecules can be fused to study the interactions of genes and gene products (Margulies *et al.,* 1977; Milstein *et al.,* 1977). In fact the cultured myeloma cell system is unique in that the variant cells can be injected back into mice and hundreds of milligrams of the mutant gene product can be purified from the serum or the ascites of the recipient animals and sequenced (Adetugbo *et al.,* 1977; Francus and Birshtein, 1978).

In spite of all of these benefits the myeloma system has been disappointing as a source of antibodies against most antigens. It has not been possible to immunize animals and then generate mouse myelomas making antibody against the immunizing antigen. Of thousands of mouse myeloma tumors induced only a few produce immunoglobulins that react with known antigens (Potter et al., 1977). These antigen-binding paraproteins have been identified by brute force screening against a battery of potential antigens (Cohn, 1967). Such an approach clearly does not have the capability of providing a source of homogeneous antibody against the wide variety of haptens and antigens of interest to biologists.

In the past many investigators have attempted to overcome these difficulties by transforming heterogeneous populations of immunized lymphoid cells with a wide variety of viruses. In most cases these experiments have not resulted in continuous cell lines producing antibody against the immunizing antigen. For example, some years ago Baumal et al. (1971) took peripheral blood cells from sensitized individuals, stimulated them in vitro with antigen and transformed with Epstein–Barr (EB) virus to produce continuous lymphoblastoid cell lines. Under the conditions used the generation of a cell line required antigen, i.e., when cells were incubated with an antigen against which the cell donor was sensitive a continuous cell line was generated, while no cell lines arose either in the absence of antigen or when cells were incubated with an antigen to which the donor was not sensitive. All of the cell lines produced rather large amounts of immunoglobulin, but none of 10 cell lines produced detectable antibody against the stimulating antigen. Similar experiments have been carried out by others using mouse cells and Abelson virus, and variations on this theme have no doubt been attempted in many laboratories. There have, however, been a few successes. For example, Stosberg et al. (1974) use SV40 virus to transform rabbit cells from an animal making large amounts of homogeneous antibody against pneumococcal type III polysaccharide and obtained a cell line that produced small amounts of this homogeneous antibody. More recently Zurawski et al. (1978) have obtained continuous human lymphoblastoid cell lines producing antibody against tetanus toxoid (see Zurawski, Black, and Haber, this volume). Steinitz et al. (1977) have also obtained EB-transformed cell lines producing antibody against the hapten 4-hydroxy-3,5-dinitrophenacetic acid (NNP). This approach, however, has generated antibody against few antigens, and the amounts of antibody produced by the cells have been small.

Studies on the fusion of mouse myeloma cell lines were originally undertaken to gain insights into the regulation of expression of immunoglobulin genes. Most of the early attempts to fuse myeloma cells employed inactivated Sendai virus to increase the very low spontaneous frequency of myeloma myeloma hybrids. This was not successful presumably because most, if not all, mouse myeloma cells do not contain receptors for Sendai (P. Mauces and M. Cohn, personal communication). However, Cotton and Milstein (1973) were able to obtain hybrids between mouse and rat myeloma cells. These hybrids continued to produce mouse heavy and light chains and rat light chains. Subsequently Köhler and Milstein (1975) and our own laboratory (Margulies et al., 1976) were able to obtain a low frequency of fusion between drug-marked mouse myeloma cell lines and to demonstrate that true hybrids had been formed. In our own experience, the frequency of spontaneous hybrids was about $1/10^6$–10^7 cells and was not significantly increased by the addition of Sendai, lysolecithin, or other agents that had been shown to increase the fusion frequency of other types of cells. However, enough hybrids were obtained to analyze the expression of immunoglobulin genes. These experiments, which are relevant to understanding the success of the hybridoma technology, have shown that (1) hybrids can be formed between different mouse myeloma cells; (2) the expression of immunoglobulin chains is codominant, i.e., the hybrids continue to synthesize all of the immunoglobulin chains produced by both parental cell lines; and (3) the total number of chromosomes in the hybrids is less than the sum of the parental complement, indicating chromosome loss. This loss is sometimes associated with the loss of expression of one or more immunoglobulin polypeptide chains.

By way of illustration Table I describes a sample fusion between the P3 cell line P326BU4 (P3), which produces IgG1(κ) immunoglobulin, and 45.6.TG1.7 (45.6), which produces IgG2b(κ). The first two lines of the table describe the chromosomal characteristics of the parent cell lines. The heavy and light chains were distinguished electrophoretically, and the heavy chains were also identified with subclass-specific antisera. Hybrids were obtained by mixing the two cell lines together and growing the cells in selective medium containing hypoxanthine, aminopterin, and thymidine (HAT), which killed both parental cells but allowed hybrids to survive (Littlefield, 1964). Aside from immunoglobulin production, the hybrid nature of the clones was deduced from the facts that (1) they grew in the selective medium due to complementation of the defect present in each parental cell line; (2) the total chromosome number of the hybrids exceeded that

TABLE I

Immunoglobulin Expression and Chromosomes in a Hybrid between 45.6.TG1.7 and P326BU4[a]

| | Chromosomes | | | Immunoglobulins | | | |
| | | | | Heavy chains | | Light chains | |
Cell line	Mean ± SD	Range	Mean biarmed	P3	45.6	P3	45.6
Parents							
45.6.TG1.7	62.4 ± 2.2	58–66	0.9	−	+	−	+
P326BU4	61.7 ± 2.7	55–66	3.9	+	−	+	−
Hybrids							
10.3				+	+	+	+
10.3.2	112.4 ± 7.0	93–123	2.7	+	+	+	+
10.3.2.3	107.4 ± 6.9	98–124	4.1	+	+	+	+
10.3.2.4	105.7 ± 4.3	99–111	4.3	+	+	+	+
10.3.2.5	105.1 ± 2.9	101–109	2.9	+	+	+	+
10.3.2.6	104.8 ± 6.7	87–119	2.7	−	+	+	+
10.3.2.7	102.1 ± 7.9	86–129	6.0	+	−	+	+

[a]Hybrids were isolated following HAT selection. One initial hybrid, 10.3, was recloned, and a subclone of it, 10.3.2, was again recloned to provide clones 10.3.2.3–7. Chromosome analysis was done 31 weeks after the initial fusion by analyzing 15–20 metaphase spreads. Heavy chains were identified serologically and electrophoretically, and light chains were identified electrophoretically, as described by Margulies et al. (1976).

of either parent, and marker chromosomes were present in the hybrids; and (3) in other fusions H-2 surface markers that distinguished the parents were present in the hybrids (Margulies *et al.*, 1976). The crucial observation is that most of the hybrids continue to produce all of the immunoglobulin polypeptide chains that are synthesized by each of the parent cell lines. Studies from both Milstein's laboratory and our own (Milstein *et al.*, 1977; Margulies *et al.*, 1977) showed that this was true irrespective of the class or subclass of the immunoglobulin produced by the parental myeloma. Furthermore, studies of Milstein and Köhler (1977) revealed that there were no new immunoglobulins synthesized. All of these observations led to the conclusion that the expression of the immunoglobulin genes in hybrids is codominant, indicating that soluble repressors and/or activators are not involved in the regulation of expression of the immunoglobulin genes in myeloma cells. Furthermore, if a nonproducing variant of a myeloma line is fused to an immunoglobulin-producing line it does not extinguish immunoglobulin production. The hybrid synthesizes the immunoglobulin of only the producing parent (Köhler *et al.*, 1976).

Detailed studies of the immunoglobulins secreted by these myeloma × myeloma hybrids revealed another phenomenon that was important in refinement of the hybridoma technology. Many of the secreted immunoglobulins are mixed molecules consisting of heavy and/or light chains synthesized by both parental cells. This is illustrated in Fig. 1. The radiolabeled secretion from a hybrid between the IgG1(κ)-producing P3 and IgG2b(κ)-producing 45.6 cell lines was chromatographed on DEAE–cellulose (dashed lines) along with a mixture of the secreted immunoglobulin from each of the parental cell lines (solid line). A large amount of material chromatographed between the two markers. These mole-

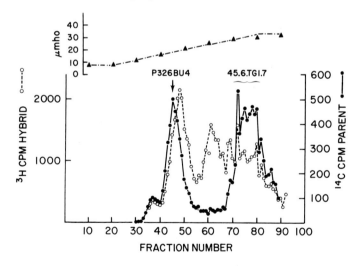

FIGURE 1. Hybrid cells were incubated with [¹⁴C]valine for 3 hr and each of the parental cell lines was incubated separately with [³H]valine for the same amount of time. The media from these incubations were mixed and purified as a single peak from DEAE–cellulose, using discontinuous elution. This peak was then rechromatographed, using a linear gradient. [For details of methods see Margulies *et al.* (1977).]

cules contain heavy and light chains from both parents. In addition electrophoretic analysis of the individual fractions revealed that molecules secreted by the hybrid which chromatographed slightly differently from the parent P3 contained P3 heavy chains and 45.6 light chains. On the other hand, very few P3 light chains were found associated with 45.6 heavy chains. Subsequent studies with other hybrids revealed varying quantities of mixed molecules (Margulies et al., 1977).

All of the above studies of myeloma × myeloma hybrids were complicated by the low frequency of hybrids. When it was reported that polyethylene glycol (PEG) increased the fusion frequency of attached cell lines (Davidson and Gerald, 1976) this technique was modified for use with suspended myeloma (Margulies et al., 1977) and spleen (Kohler and Milstein, 1976) cells. Gefter et al. (1977) showed that the concentration and time of exposure to PEG are important and that fusion frequencies can be increased appreciably under appropriate conditions.

III. The Fusion of Mouse Myeloma to Immune Spleen Cells

While all of the results described in the previous sections provided useful fundamental information, they achieved broader significance when Köhler and Milstein (1975) fused cultured mouse myeloma cells to normal spleen cells from an immunized mouse and showed that some of the resulting hybrids produced homogeneous antibodies against the immunizing antigen. These hybridomas grew continuously in culture, thus "immortalizing" a particular antibody, and formed tumors when injected into syngeneic mice. A high titer of the homogeneous antibody was present in the serum and ascites fluid of the tumor-bearing mice. This spectacular finding has now been extended to many types of antigens. It seems inevitable that this technology will become the standard method of producing serological reagents that will be of much higher quality and reliability than those used in the past.

As could be anticipated from studies with myeloma × myeloma hybrids, several technical problems had to be solved to realize the full potential of the hybridoma technology. The first of these, illustrated in Fig. 1, is the presence of immunoglobulin molecules composed of both myeloma and spleen polypeptide chains. If associations were completely random, only 1 out of 10 of the H_2L_2 molecules produced would contain only the spleen-derived (antigen-binding) polypeptide chains. This not only reduces the titer of the antibody, but may even result in new antigenic specification (Köhler and Milstein, 1976). In fact in many combinations the homologous chains associate preferentially with each other, but even then mixed molecules do occur.

The problem of mixed molecules was overcome by using as one parent variant myeloma cell lines that do not express either the myeloma light or heavy chain. Such variants had been described previously by both Milstein and our laboratory (Cotton et al., 1973; Scharff, 1974). They arise frequently and can easily be obtained by cloning cells in soft agar and overlaying the clones with antisera specific for the heavy and light chains (Coffino *et al.*, 1972). The wild-type cells are surrounded by antigen–antibody precipitates that can be visualized with a low-power microscope. Variants are not surrounded by a precipitate and can be recovered and grown to mass culture. Such nonproducing variants do not extinguish immunoglobulin production when they are fused to other myeloma cells or to spleen cells. Some of these variants have not given large numbers of hybrids, but there are now a number of variant lines that have been used effectively (Schulman *et al.*, 1978; Kearney *et al.*, 1979).

A second and continuing problem has been the relatively low frequency of fusion. Using PEG and unfractionated spleen cells, it has generally been possible to obtain 1 hybrid for every 2×10^5 spleen cells. This results in 500 hybrids/spleen, which is adequate if good immunogens are being used, but is a serious problem for weak immunogens. This is illustrated in Table II. Sheep red blood cells (SRBC) are an excellent immunogen, and it is quite easy to immunize animals so that 1 out of every 100 spleen cells is secreting antibody. If the frequency of fusion is 1 hybrid for every 2×10^5 spleen cells, then one would expect to obtain at least 5 antibody-forming hybrids/10^8 spleen cells. In fact, as originally reported by Köhler and Milstein (1975), fusion produces an apparent enrichment with respect to plaque-forming cells (PFC), and we routinely obtain more positive hybrids than might be expected. This may result from the selective fusion of myeloma cells to replicating spleen B cells, from the generation of antibody-producing hybrids through the fusion of non-plaque-forming precursor cells, or from some unknown factors. Whatever the explanation, apparent enrichment is almost always observed and welcomed. When a poor immunogen is used the lower frequency of antibody-forming cells presents a serious problem. This is also illustrated in Table II with specificity 33 of the *H-2^b* haplotype. Here we have determined the frequency of antibody-secreting cells to be approximately 1/10,000 spleen cells. The immunized spleen therefore contains only 10^4 antibody-secreting cells. Even with the expected enrichment we would anticipate generating only one hybrid from each three to five spleens. We have in fact been unable to generate a stable anti-33 hybrid, although others have obtained hybrids producing homogeneous antibodies against other H-2 specificities (*Current Topics in Microbiology and Immunology* **81**, 1978).

There are two potential solutions to this problem. One is to increase the

TABLE II
Frequency of Hybrids[a]

Per spleen	Anti-SRBC	Anti-H-2.33
PFC	10^6	10^4
Hybrids		
Calculated	5	0.05
Actual	20–30	0.2–0.3

[a] 1 spleen = 10^8 cells; fusion frequency = 1 hybrid/2×10^5 spleen cells (500 hybrids/spleen).

fusion frequency. Various investigators have explored the use of different molecular weight PEG, the importance of pH during fusion (J. Sharon and S. L. Morrison, personal communication), the ratio of spleen to myeloma cells (between 10/1 and 1/1 have been used successfully), different batches of serum and types of medium, thymocytes and other feeders, and different methods of plating the fused cells (*Current Topics in Microbiology and Immunology* **81**, 1978). Care with each of these variables probably produces more reproducible results, but none has resulted in a significant increase in the absolute yield of recoverable hybrids per immunized spleen.

A second approach is to increase the frequency of antibody-forming cells. Most investigators routinely do this by immunizing a number of animals and using spleen cells from those mice with the highest antibody titer. It should also be possible to enrich for antibody-forming or antigen-binding cells. However, it is not yet clear which type of spleen cell actually fuses with the myeloma cell to produce antibody-forming hybrids. Because of the low fusion frequency, any enrichment procedure must also give good absolute yields of the appropriate spleen population. These and other problems have so far frustrated most attempts to improve the technology through the manipulation of the spleen cells used in the fusion.

A third major technical problem is the instability of some, but not all, hybridomas. The reasons for this instability are not completely clear. This instability is no doubt due in part to the loss of heavy- or light-chain synthesis associated with chromosome loss and/or to overgrowth by contaminating clones or variants that arise during the propagation of the hybridomas. It is not clear which of these factors is most important or if others play a role. Overgrowth by simultaneously generated non-antibody-producing hybrids can be minimized either by plating the fused cells at low population densities in small volumes in microtiter dishes or by cloning immediately after fusion in soft agar (Sharon *et al.*, 1979). Even then some cloned hybrids are very unstable, while others need to be recloned only occasionally. If many hybrids making the desired homogeneous antibody can be generated it is, in our experience, easier to discard unstable hybrids than to try to maintain them. When a newly generated hybridoma has a unique specificity and must be preserved it is possible to maintain it by repeated cloning or enriching for antigen-binding cells by any of a variety of methods (Haas and Von Boehmer, 1978).

In addition to these obvious technical problems, many aspects of the hybridoma technology are still poorly understood. It is generally assumed that the phenotype of the malignant cell partners in a fusion should closely resemble that of the cell line one wishes to generate. For example, it has been shown that when fibroblasts or epithelial cells are fused to myeloma cells the expression of the heavy- and light-chain genes is extinguished (Coffino *et al.*, 1971). However, there are very few experimental data on how similar the two cells participating in a fusion have to be to allow continued antibody production. It is possible that nonmyeloma B-cell lines or some as yet untested lymphoma would give a higher frequency of fusion or more stable hybrids than the myeloma lines currently being used.

The hybridoma technology has been applied successfully to only a few species. Hybridomas between mouse myeloma and mouse spleen cells are most frequently generated, but a number of investigators have fused rat spleen cells to either mouse (Galfre *et al.*, 1977) or rat myeloma (Galfre *et al.*, 1979). In xenogeneic fusions the hybridomas can be injected into irradiated or nude mice to generate high-titer antibody in serum or ascites. It is more difficult to maintain antibody production in mouse myeloma × rabbit spleen or mouse myeloma × human blood cell hybrids presumably because of the rapid loss of rabbit and human chromosomes from the hybrids. The potential of other types of fusions has (to our knowledge) not yet been extensively studied.

IV. Applications of Monoclonal Antibodies

The potential uses of monoclonal antibodies are legion, and many will be described in detail in following chapters. The attractions of the hybridoma approach to serology have been aptly described by Milstein *et al.* (1979):

> The major interest of this technique derives from two fundamental points. First, the monoclonal antibody produced by an isolated clone is a well defined chemical and not an undefined heterogeneous mixture which changes with each immunized animal and even with each bleed of the same animal. The permanent cultures are capable of unlimited supply of exactly the same chemical structure. Second, the technique is ideally suited for the preparation of pure antibodies using non-purified antigens.

These benefits have fired the imagination of investigators in many areas of biology. Among the applications are the production of large amounts of high-affinity antibody specific for (1) immunogenic histocompatibility or differentiation antigens; (2) differentiation, tumor- or other cell-surface antigens that lack polymorphism and are not immunogenic in allogeneic systems but are recognized in xenogeneic immunization; (3) viral and bacterial antigens; and (4) single antigenic determinants on a wide variety of proteins, nucleic acids, and sugars. Such antibodies will allow the definition and separation of subpopulations of cells, the discrimination of different stages in development, more accurate tissue typing, the purification of minor surface antigens, a more refined identification of microorganisms for both diagnosis and epidemiology, and more reliable radioimmunoassays and other immunologic assays for biologically important macromolecules.

The hybridoma technology has also provided a new approach to the study of antibody-forming clones of normal B cells to examine the repertoire of antibodies made in response to antigenic challenge. This technique has the advantage of generating amounts of antibody from each clone that can be studied chemically. In essence it has all of the benefits of the myeloma systems plus the advantage that the investigators decide which antibodies they wish to study.

With all of these benefits, it is important to remember that a monoclonal antibody is very different from a well-absorbed high-titer antiserum. It will have a fixed affinity which, if low, may present problems. Since it is homogeneous, it cannot be further absorbed to refine its specificity. Since each cell line synthesizes only a single class or subclass of immunoglobulin, each monoclonal antibody will have only a portion of the biological activities found in a heterogeneous antiserum, i.e., it may or may not fix complement, be cytotoxic, or bind *Staphylococcus aureus* protein A. Some monoclonal antibodies do not hemagglutinate presumably because of a lack of flexibility in the hinge region or a low epitope density on the red cells. Aside from these obvious problems, there will no doubt be some surprises as well. For example, Howard *et al.* (1978) have described a monoclonal antibody that binds to a cell-surface antigen more readily if a second monoclonal antibody has already reacted with another site on the same antigen. Myelomas frequently generate variant immunoglobulins with changes in sequences (Cotton *et al.*, 1973; Scharff, 1974; Cook and Scharff, 1977). Not surprisingly, we have identified similar variants in hybridomas (D. E. Yelton, unpublished). If this is a general phenomenon it will be necessary to recheck periodically the affinity and specificity of hybridomas or to return to frozen stocks frequently.

V. The Use of Cell Fusion to Obtain Functional Cell Lines

As noted in the Introduction, a second long-standing goal of cellular immunologists has been to obtain continuous cell lines that would carry out and respond to normal immunoregulatory functions. Just as tumors and virally transformed cells were used in attempt to produce homogeneous antibodies similar approaches have been employed in the past with the hope of generating cell lines that could be regulated. Such tumors and transformed cell lines have been useful for studying specific surface markers that are present at different stages in lymphoid cell differentiation. In some cases such cells continue to carry out the differentiated functions of the presumed parental cell population. Myelomas are, of course, one example. Tumor cells with macrophagelike properties continue to make lysozyme, have Fc receptors, and phagocytize in much the same way that normal macrophages do (Ralph *et al.*, 1975). Some mouse and human lymphomas can be induced to secrete immunoglobulin when stimulated with mitogens (Slavin and Strober, 1978; Fu *et al.*, 1978). Continuous human lymphoblastoid cell lines have also been reported to be regulated by normal T cells or T-cell factors (Kishimoto *et al.*, 1978), and recently even plasmacytomas themselves have been shown to respond to signals from normal cells (Abbas and Klaus, 1977; Rohrer *et al.*, 1979). Nevertheless, such cell lines are relatively rare and their range of function is limited. It seemed possible that hybrids between normal and malignant cells might retain more of the functions of the normal parental cell and be more subject to normal regulatory function. With this in mind, many laboratories have attempted to fuse a variety of malignant cells with lymphoid cells from sensitized animals.

Many attempts have been made to fuse T-cell lymphomas to spleen cells with the hope of obtaining continuous lines of helper, suppressor, or killer T cells. The few successes that have been reported suggest this approach will be very useful (*Current Topics in Microbiology and Immunology* **81,** 1978; Melchers, 1978). T-cell hybrids which secrete immunoregulatory molecules (Taussig and Holliman, 1979; Neauport-Sautes *et al.,* 1979; Taniguchi *et al.,* 1979) could provide material for structural characterization of T-cell factors just as myelo mas did for immunoglobulin over a decade ago.

Our own experience with a presumptive macrophage hybrid and a B-cell hybridoma also suggest the potential of this approach. In the course of cloning a hybridoma-producing antibody against SRBC, one of us (BD) noticed that some of the clones resembled macrophages rather than myelomas. When these two cell types were separated the amount of antibody produced by the B-cell hybrid-oma (UN2) increased. When medium from the macrophagelike hybrids (FC1) was added to the UN2 cells, the amount of antibody decreased (Table III), even though cell division and macromolecular synthesis were not affected. We have recently begun to characterize both types of cells more carefully. The macro-phagelike cell line arose during the fusion of a myeloma to spleen cells. It contains many more (90) chromosomes than the myeloma, and, although we cannot prove this presently, it is assumed to be a hybrid between a spleen macro-phage and the myeloma. It has many characteristics of an activated macrophage not found in other macrophagelike tumor lines such as J774 (Table IV). In addition, the supernatant of the FC1 cell line suppresses the mitogenic effect of phytohemagglutinin PHA and LPS on normal mouse spleen cells (Diamond, unpublished). These findings suggest that the presumptive hybrid FC1 can carry out some biological activities that resemble those of normal suppressor macro-phages and that the B-cell hybridoma can be regulated in its production of antibody. Additional experiments are being carried out to determine the rela-tionship of these phenomena to normal regulatory events.

TABLE III

Suppression of Antibody Production by FC1[a]

	Treatment	Antibody titer (hemagglutination)
UN2 hybrid cell line		1/8192
	FC1	1/1024
	J774.2	1/8192
	MPC11	1/8192
UN2 medium		1/2048
	FC1	1/2048

[a]Cells were grown in medium alone or with 15% FC1, J774.2, or MPC11 supernatant that had been extensively dialyzed against normal medium. Cells were washed at 24 hr and reincubated in the same medium for 48 hr, at which time the supernatants were assayed for hemagglutination titer.

TABLE IV
Characteristics of FC1 and J774[a]

Macrophage properties	FC1	J774.2
Fc receptors	+	+
phagocytosis	+	+
Complement receptors	+	−
Lysozyme secretion	+	+
Plasminogen activator secretion	+	+
Migration	+	−
Response to MIF	+	−
Interferon production	−	−

[a]The presence of Fc receptors and complement receptors was
determined by rosette formation and phagocytosis of opson-
ized SRBC was assayed visually. Lysozyme and plasminogen
activator secretion were determined by breakdown of *Micro-
coccus lysodeikticus* and of radiolabeled fibrin, respectively. The
FC1 cells migrate from capillary chambers and are inhibited in
migration by MIF. Methods for these assays are reported in
Diamond *et al.* (1978) and Bloom *et al.* (1978).

VI. Conclusions

There is no doubt that the hybridoma technology is a powerful new tool in
immunology. As will be described in the following chapters, it has already begun
to revolutionize the serological analysis of immunological phenomena and has
provided a powerful tool in studying viruses and microorganisms. It also seems
likely that hybrids between malignant cells and normal lymphoid cells will provide homogeneous cell lines that can carry out a wide variety of normal immunoregulatory functions.

ACKNOWLEDGMENTS

This work was supported in part by NIH training grant number
5T32GM7288 from NIGMS and by grants from the National Institutes of
Health (AI 10702 and AI 5231) and the National Science Foundation
(PCM75-13609).

References

Abbas, A. K., and Klaus, G. G. B., 1977, Inhibition of antibody production in plasmacytoma cells by
    antigen, *Eur. J. Immunol.* **7:**667.
Adetugbo, K., Milstein, C., and Secher, D. S., 1977, Molecular analysis of spontaneous somatic
    mutants, *Nature* **265:**299.

Baumal, R. and Scharff, M. D., 1973, Synthesis, assembly and secretion of mouse immunoglobulin, *Transplant. Rev.* **14:**163.

Baumal, R., Bloom, B., and Scharff, M. D., 1971, Induction of long-term lymphocyte lines from delayed hypersensitive human donors using specific antigen plus Epstein–Barr virus, *Nature [New Biol.]* **230:**20.

Bernard, O., Nobumichi, H., and Tonegawa, S., 1978, Sequences of mouse immunoglobulin light chain genes before and after somatic changes, *Cell* **15:**1133.

Bloom, B. R., Diamond, B., Muschel, R., Rosen, N., Schneck, J., Damiani, G., Rosen, O., and Scharff, M. D., 1978, Genetic approaches to the mechanism of macrophage functions, *Fed. Proc.* **37:**2765.

Capra, J. D., Tung, A. S., and Nisonoff, A., 1975a, Structural studies on induced antibodies with defined idiotypic specificities. I. The heavy chains of anti-*p*-azophenylarsonate antibodies from A/J mice bearing a cross-reactive idiotype, *J. Immunol.* **114:**1548.

Capra, J. D., Tung, A. S., and Nisonoff, A., 1975b, Structural studies on induced antibodies with defined idiotypic specificities, *J. Immunol.* **115:**414.

Cebra, J. J., Koo, P. H., and Ray, A., 1974, Specificity of antibodies: Primary structural basis of hapten binding, *Science* **186:**263.

Coffino, P., Knowles, B., Nathenson, S., and Scharff, M. D., 1971, Suppression of immunoglobulin synthesis by cellular hybridization. *Nature [New Biol.]* **231:**87.

Coffino, P., Baumal, R., Laskov, R., and Scharff, M. D., 1972, Cloning of mouse myeloma cells and detection of rare variants, *J. Cell. Physiol.* **79:**429.

Cohn, M., 1967, Natural history of the myeloma, *Cold Spring Harbor Symp. Quant. Biol.* **32:**211.

Cold Spring Harbor Symposia on Quantitative Biology, 1967, Vol. 32, *Antibodies.*

Cook, W. D., and Scharff, M. D., 1977, Antigen-binding mutants of mouse myeloma cells, *Proc. Natl. Acad. Sci. USA* **74:**5687.

Cotton, R. G. H., and Milstein, C., 1973, Fusion of two immunoglobulin-producing myeloma cells, *Nature* **244:**42.

Cotton, R. G. H., Secher, D. S., and Milstein, C., 1973, Somatic mutation and the origin of antibody diversity. Clonal variability of the immunoglobulin produced by MOPC 21 cells in culture, *Eur. J. Immunol.* **3:**135.

Current Topics in Microbiology and Immunology, 1978, Vol. 81, *Lymphocyte Hybridomas* (F.Melchers, M. Potter, and N. Warner, eds.), Springer-Verlag, Berlin, Heidelberg, New York.

Davidson, R. L., and Gerald, P. S., 1976, Improved techniques for induction of mammalian cell hybridization by polyethylene glycol, *Somat. Cell Genet.* **2:**165.

Diamond, B., Bloom, B. R., and Scharff, M. D., 1978, The Fc receptors of primary and cultured phagocytic cells studied with homogeneous antibodies, *J. Immunol.* **121:**1329.

Francus, T., and Birshtein, B. K., 1978, An IgG2a-producing variant of an IgG2b-producing mouse myeloma cell line. Structural studies on the Fc region of parent and variant heavy chains, *Biochemistry* **17:**4324.

Fu, S. M., Chiorazzi, N., Kunkel, H. G., Halper, J. P., and Harris, S. R., 1978, Induction of in vitro differentiation and immunoglobulin synthesis of human leukemic B lymphocytes, *J. Exp. Med.* **148:**1570.

Galfre, G., Howe, S. C., Milstein, C., Butcher, G. W., and Howard, J. C., 1977, Antibodies to major histocompatibility antigens produced by hybrid cell lines, *Nature* **266:**550.

Galfre, G., Milstein, C., and Wright, B., 1979, R × rat hybrid myelomas and a monoclonal anti-Fd portion of mouse IgG, *Nature* **277:**131.

Gefter, M. L., Margulies, D. H., and Scharff, M. D., 1977, A simple method for polyethylene glycol-promoted hybridization of mouse myeloma cells, *Somat. Cell Genet.* **2:**231.

Haas, W., and von Boehmer, H., 1978, Techniques for separation and selection of antigen specific lymphocytes, *Curr. Top. Microbiol. Immunol.* **84.**

Haber, E., 1970, Antibodies of restricted heterogeneity for structural study, *Fed. Proc.* **29:**66.

Haber, E., Margolies, M. N., and Cannon, L. E., 1977, Structure of the framework and complementarity regions of elicited antibodies, in: *Antibodies in Human Diagnosis and Therapy* (E. Haber and R. M. Krause, eds.), Raven Press, New York, pp. 45–78.

Helmreich, E., Kern, M., and Eisen, H. N., 1961, The secretion of antibody by isolated lymph node cells, *J. Biol. Chem.* **236:**464.

Horibata, K., and Harris, A. W., 1970, Mouse myelomas and lymphomas in culture, *Exp. Cell Res.* **60:**61.

Howard, J. C., Butcher, G. W., Galfre, G., and Milstein, C., 1978, Monoclonal anti-rat MHC (H-1) alloantibodies, *Curr. Top. Microbiol. Immunol.* **81:**54.

Kearney, J. F., Radbruch, A., Liesegang, B., and Rajewsky, K., 1980, A new mouse myeloma cell line which has lost immunoglobulin expression but permits the construction of antibody secreting hybrid cells lines, *J. Immunol.* **123:**1548.

Kishimoto, T., Hirano, T., Kuritani, T., Yamamura, Y., Ralph, P., and Good, R. A., 1978, Induction of IgG production in human B lymphoblastoid cell lines with normal human T cells, *Nature* **271:**756.

Köhler, G., and Milstein, C., 1975, Continuous cultures of fused cells secreting antibody of predefined specificity, *Nature* **256:**495.

Köhler, G., and Milstein, C., 1976, Derivation of specific antibody-producing tissue culture and tumor lines by cell fusion, *Eur. J. Immunol.* **6:**511.

Köhler, G., Howe, S. C., and Milstein, C., 1976, Fusion between immunoglobulin-secreting and nonsecreting myeloma cell lines, *Eur. J. Immunol.* **6:**292.

Krause, R. M., 1970, The search for antibodies with molecular uniformity, *Adv. Immunol.* **12:**1.

Kuehl, W. M., 1977, Synthesis of immunoglobulin in myeloma cells, *Curr. Top. Microbiol. Immunol.* **76:**1.

Laskov, R., and Scharff, M. D., 1970, Synthesis, assembly and secretion of gamma globulin by mouse myeloma cells, *J. Exp. Med.* **131:**515.

Littlefield, J. W., 1964, Selection of hybrids from matings of fibroblasts in vitro and their presumed recombinants, *Science* **145:**709.

Margulies, D. H., Kuehl, W. M., and Scharff, M. D., 1976, Somatic cell hybridization of mouse myeloma cells, *Cell* **8:**405.

Margulies, D. H., Cieplinski, W., Dharmgrongartama, B., Gefter, M. L., Morrison, S. L., Kelly, T., and Scharff, M. D., 1977, Regulation of immunoglobulin expression in mouse myeloma cells, *Cold Spring Harbor Symp. Quant. Biol.* **41:**781.

Melchers, F., 1978, T cell hybrids: Shortcut or dead end?, *Nature* **271:**9.

Milstein, C., and Köhler, G., 1977, Cell fusion and the derivation of cell lines producing specific antibody, in: *Antibodies in Human Diagnosis and Therapy* (E. Haber and R. M. Krause, eds.), Raven Press, New York, pp. 271–286.

Milstein, C., Adetugbo, K., Cowan, N. J., Kohler, G., Secher, D. S., and Wilde, C. D., 1977, Somatic cell genetics of antibody-secreting cells: Studies of clonal diversification and analysis by cell fusion, *Cold Spring Harbor Symp. Quant. Biol.* **41:**793.

Milstein, C., Galfre, G., Secher, D. S., and·Springer, T., 1979, Monoclonal antibodies and cell surface antigens, *Cell Biol. Int. Rep.* **3**(1):1.

Neauport-Sautes, C., Rabourdin-Combe, C., and Fridman, W. H., 1979, T-cell hybrids bear Fc receptors and secrete suppressor immunoglobulin binding factor, *Nature* **277:**656.

Pettengill, G. S., and Sorensen, G. D., 1967, Murine myeloma cells in suspension culture, *Exp. Cell Res.* **47:**608.

Potter, M., 1972, Immunoglobulin-producing tumors and myeloma proteins of mice, *Physiol. Rev.* **52:**631.

Potter, M., 1978, Antigen-binding myeloma proteins of mice, *Adv. Immunol.* **25:**141.

Potter M., Rudikoff, S., Radlan, E. A., and Vrana, M., 1977, Covalent structure of the antigen binding site: Antigen-binding myeloma proteins of the BALB/c mouse, in: *Antibodies in Human Diagnosis and Therapy* (E. Haber and R. M. Krause, eds.), Raven Press, New York, pp. 9–28.

Ralph, P., Richard, J., and Cohn, M., 1975, Reticulum cell sarcoma: An effector cell in antibody-dependent cell-mediated immunity, *J. Immunol.* **114:**898.

Rohrer, J. W., Odermatt, B., and Lynch R. G., 1979, Immunoregulation of murine myeloma: Isologous immunization with M315 induces idiotype-specific T cells that suppress IgA secretion by MOP-315 cells in vivo, *J. Immunol.* **122:**2011.

Sakano, H., Rogers, J. H., Huppi, K., Brack, C., Traunecker, A., Maki, R., Wall, R., and Tonegawa S., 1978, Domains and the hinge region of an immunoglobulin heavy chain are encoded in separate DNA segments, *Nature* **277:**627.

Scharff, M. D., 1974, The synthesis, assembly and secretion of immunoglobulin: A biochemical and genetic approach, *Harvey Lect.* **69**:125.

Scharff, M. D., and Laskov, R., 1970, Synthesis and assembly of immunoglobulin polypeptide chains, *Prog. Allergy* **14**:37.

Schulman, M., Wilde, C. D., and Köhler, G., 1978, A better cell line for making hybridomas secreting specific antibodies, *Nature* **276**:269.

Seidman, J. G., Leder, A., Nau, M., Norman, B., and Leder, P., 1978, Antibody diversity: The structure of cloned immunoglobulin gene suggests a mechanism for generating new sequences, *Science* **202**:11.

Sharon, J., Morrison, S. L., and Kabat, E. A., 1979, Detection of specific hybridoma clones by replica immunoadsorption of their secreted antibodies, *Proc. Natl. Acad. Sci. USA* **76**:1420.

Slavin, S., and Strober, S., 1978, Spontaneous muring B-cell leukemia, *Nature* **272**:624.

Steinitz, M., Klein, G., Koskimies, S., and Makela, O., 1977, EB virus-induced B lymphocyte cell lines producing specific antibody, *Nature* **269**:420.

Strosberg, A. D., Collins, J. J., Black, P. H., Malamud, D., Wilbert, S., Block, K. J., and Haber, E., 1974, Transformation by simian virus 40 of spleen cells from a hyperimmune rabbit: Demonstration of production of specific antibody to the immunizing antigen, *Proc. Natl. Acad. Sci. USA* **71**:263.

Taniguchi, M., Saito, T., and Tada, T., 1979, Antigen-specific suppressive factor produced by a transplantable I-J bearing T-cell hybridoma, *Nature* **278**:555.

Taussig, M. J., and Holliman, A., 1979, Structure of an antigen-specific suppressor factor produced by a hybrid T-cell line, *Nature* **277**:308.

Williamson, A., 1971, Biosynthesis of antibodies, *Nature* **231**:359.

Zurawski, V. R. Jr., Haber, E., and Black, P. H., 1978, Production of antibody to tetanus toxoid by continuous human lymphoblastoid cell lines, *Science* **199**:1439.

2
Continuously Proliferating Human Cell Lines Synthesizing Antibody of Predetermined Specificity

VINCENT R. ZURAWSKI, JR., PAUL H. BLACK, AND EDGAR HABER

I. Introduction

The explosive growth in the number of laboratories involved in the production of murine monoclonal antibodies *in vitro* using hybridoma technology (Köhler and Milstein, 1975) is a testimony to the utility of monoclonal antibodies as research tools. It is also clear that monoclonal antibodies produced *in vitro* are unique reagents which might provide the clinician with an exciting new means of diagnosing and treating human disorders. Xenogeneic-elicited antibodies have already been used in the reversal of drug toxicity in man (Smith *et al.*, 1976), the scintigraphic imaging of myocardial infarcts (Khaw *et al.*, 1978a,b), and the imaging of tumors in man (Ghose *et al.*, 1975; Goldenberg *et al.*, 1978). Especially in the case where utilization *in vivo* of antibody in humans is contemplated, human monoclonal antibodies would be ideal reagents. Administration of human, instead of xenogeneic, antibodies to patients would eliminate the risk of serum sickness, anaphylactic reaction, or other allergic sequelae often associated with the administration of nonhuman protein to patients.

VINCENT R. ZURAWSKI, JR., PAUL H. BLACK, AND EDGAR HABER • Department of Medicine, Harvard Medical School and Massachusetts General Hospital, Boston, Massachusetts 02114.

Passive immunization against toxins or infectious organisms could be achieved with standard preparations of human antibodies. Modulation of immune response with antibodies directed against transplant antigens or idiotypic sites on other antibody or cell-surface receptor molecules would be facilitated by monoclonal antibodies of high specificity. Monospecific reagents against tumor-associated antigens might allow for both treatment and localization of neoplastic cells through radioimmunoscintigraphy. Modulation or neutralization of drug or hormone effects could also be achieved at minimum risk with appropriate human monoclonal antibody preparations. Moreover, since continuously proliferating cell lines can be frozen and stored practically indefinitely, the source of well-characterized, optimal immunoreagents would not be lost, and the problems associated with constant immunization of animals would be eliminated. Many such applications of antibodies to diagnosis and therapy have been recently reviewed (Haber and Krause, 1977).

Routine methods for establishing cell lines producing human antibody in large quantities would also be useful in the basic research laboratory, for example, in examining human antibody idiotypes (Geha and Weinberg, 1978). Studies of the genetics and regulation of human antibody production might also be facilitated.

Historically, immunoglobulin-producing human cell lines have been established. Most of these have been lymphoblastoid in nature (Fahey et al., 1971) rather than plasmacytoid, although long-term culture of human plasmacytes has been achieved (Jobin et al., 1974) with difficulty. Most of the human lymphoblastoid cell lines established, which synthesize immunoglobulin, have contained the Epstein–Barr virus nuclear antigen (EBNA) (Reedman and Klein, 1973) indicative of the presence of Epstein–Barr virus (EBV).

The potential for establishing cell lines secreting human immunoglobulin through the use of somatic cell hybridization techniques also has not been ignored. Schwaber and his co-workers (Schwaber, 1977; Schwaber and Cohen, 1973; Schwaber and Rosen, 1978) have demonstrated that mouse myeloma–human lymphocyte somatic cell hybrids that secrete human immunoglobulin can be formed.

Recently, it has been demonstrated (Levy and Dilley, 1978; Levy et al., this volume) that the murine myeloma NS1 of Köhler and Milstein can be fused to human chronic lymphocytic leukemia cells to yield somatic cell hybrids which produce large amounts of human immunoglobulin. Clones of these lines have been isolated that secrete only human immunoglobulin, even after several months in tissue culture (R. Levy, personal communication). Moreover, this immunoglobulin bears idiotypic markers associated with the surface immunoglobulin found on the human leukemia cell used for fusion (Levy, this volume). Therefore, despite the known preferential loss of human chromosomes from mouse–human hybrids (Ruddle, 1973), clones can be established from such hybrids that retain their ability to synthesize and secrete human immunoglobulin. This result may have implications for the ultimate attainment of stable cell lines synthesizing large quantities of human immunoglobulin.

II. Specific Antibody-Producing Cell Lines

A. Cell Lines Producing Antibody to Tetanus Toxoid

We have reported (Zurawski et al., 1978a) the establishment of cell lines and clones (Zurawski et al., 1978b) of those lines which produce human antibody to tetanus toxoid and toxin. This was accomplished by in vitro B95-8 infection (Miller and Lipman, 1973) of peripheral blood mononuclear cells from individuals recently given secondary (booster) tetanus toxoid immunizations. Transformed or immortalized (Miller, 1974) lymphoblastoid cultures resulted.

While little or no tetanus-specific antibody was secreted by peripheral mononuclear cells of individuals remotely immunized with tetanus toxoid, a booster immunization led to increased amounts of released antibody into culture supernatants (Zurawski et al., 1978a). The antibody secretion in vitro by the peripheral mononuclear cells is illustrated in Table I, utilizing data from a solid-phase radioimmunometric assay (Zurawski et al., 1978a; Rosenthal et al., 1973). Table I also demonstrates that the amount of antibody released by peripheral mononuclear cells into culture fluids is related to the interval following immunization. In general we have found that peripheral mononuclear cells collected between 7 and 14 days after a toxoid booster immunization release maximal quantities of antibody to tetanus toxoid in vitro, even though serum titers did not peak until after 14 days. In general the longer the interval between booster immunizations, the greater the in vitro release of antibody to tetanus toxoid by the cultured mononuclear cells. This result is similar to that of Stevens and Saxon (1978, 1979), although in their experiments pokeweed mitogen was required to stimulate specific antibody production in vitro. Lymphocyte cultures established from boosted individuals, and depleted of T cells by sheep erythrocyte rosetting or nylon wool absorption, failed to release antibody to tetanus toxoid into culture fluids. This is in agreement with observations of Strelkauskas et al. (1977), who showed diminished synthesis of immunoglobulin in vitro by human peripheral blood lymphocytes depleted of T cells.

In our initial experiments, 44 cell lines were established by EBV infection of cultures of human mononuclear cells in vitro. All the viable cells in these cell lines contained EBNA (Reedman and Klein, 1973). Seven lines produced tetanus-specific antibody, but only two of these produced the antibody for sufficient time to enable them to be studied in some detail.

In each of these lines (4LP-B4 and 3GC-C2) a decline in the quantity of antibody released into the cell-culture supernatant accompanied succeeding passage of these cells (Table II). The amount of antibody secreted could often be increased to levels found at early passage by subculturing the cells on monolayers of human foreskin fibroblasts (Zurawski et al., 1978a,b).

We postulated that at least a part of the reason for the decline in antibody production was due to the overgrowth of antibody-producing cells by other

TABLE I

[^{125}I]Rabbit Anti-Human F(ab')$_2$ Antibody Bound in Solid Phase Radioimmunoassay for Volunteer DC[a]

Culture[b]	Days in culture	Antibody bound (cpm)	Antibody bound[c] with 0.5 μg/ml tetanus toxoid present (cpm)	Antibody bound[c] with 5.0 μg/ml tetanus toxoid present (cpm)
1GM	3	47	—	—
	8	17	—	—
	22	15	—	—
1DC	0	100 + 32	—	—
	2	7301 ± 525	674	88
	10	9137 ± 679	605	479
	16	9851 ± 651	751	263
	22	8499 ± 176	627	54
	29	7569 ± 588	233	28
	51	4125 ± 563	109	0
3DC	0	58	—	—
	5	1764 ± 283	31	4
	8	1925 ± 332	0	0
	16	1711 ± 345	38	19
	21	432 ± 375	18	0

[a]Assay performed according to method outlined in Zurawski et al. (1978a). Binding of labeled antihuman F(ab')$_2$ reflects the presence of specific antibody for tetanus toxoid. Backgrounds of approximately 100 cpm have been subtracted in each case. All samples were run in quadruplicate.

[b]Peripheral mononuclear cells were cultured at 5×10^6 cells/ml in 24-well culture plates. Cultures were initiated at day zero. Cells were washed 3 times with RPMI 1640 medium, incubated for 30 min, washed again, and placed in medium with fetal calf serum and other additives (Zurawski et al., 1978a). Medium was exchanged in cultures twice weekly after 7 days. These cultures had EBV added to them. Antibody was secreted in the absence of virus as well. Donor 1GM had not been recently immunized with tetanus toxoid. Donor DC was boosted 8 days (1DC) and 16 days (3DC) prior to initiation of culture.

[c]Duplicate samples were assayed simultaneously in the presence of soluble toxoid as indicated. Inhibition of antibody binding to microtiter wells was virtually complete at 5.0 μg/ml of tetanus toxoid.

clones better adapted to tissue culture. Other explanations include alterations in chromosomes or loss of differentiated function on account of changes in regulatory mechanisms. That overgrowth by nonsecretory cells was not the sole explanation for the loss of antibody production within passage was confirmed by the observation that even a cloned line also showed a decrease in antibody production with time. Hence the loss of antibody production with passage was not a trivial problem.

Limiting dilution clones of cell line 4LB-B4 were established (Zurawski et al., 1978b). Clone 2F11 maintained stable production of antibody which bound both tetanus toxoid and tetanus toxin for more than 6 months, though the amount of antibody released into the culture medium never exceeded 20 ng/ml. After 7 months, clone 2F11 lost its ability to produce antibody.

Cytoplasmic staining of the parent 4LP-B4 line after acetone fixation with

TABLE II

Production of Antibody to Tetanus Toxoid by Two Cell Lines[a]

Passage	Time in culture (months)	Human γ-globulin[b] (ng/ml)	Antibody[c] (ng/ml)
		Cell Line 3GC-C2	
0	1.0		300
1	1.5		225
2	1.7	1630	200
3	2.1	1530	164
5	2.5	2220	25
6	3.1	1060	15[d]
9	4.0	1960	9[d]
15	4.2	1050	5[d]
24	5.3	930	2–3[d]
		Cell Line 4LP-B4	
0	1.0		150
1	1.2		105
3	1.8		75
5	2.5		15[e]
7	2.7	446	20[e]
8	2.8	515	15[e]
9	3.0	348	18[e]
16	4.0	272	8[e]
18	4.4	271	2[e]
21	4.8	242	2[e]
27	5.6	198	1[e]
40	7.2	259	0.1[e]

[a]Reprinted by permission from Zurawski *et al.* (1978a).
[b]Detected by binding with ^{125}I-labeled protein A. Values represent averages of triplicate samples.
[c]Values represent averages of 6 to 10 samples. Values below 25 ng/ml were determined with undiluted and 10 times concentrated media.
[d]The range of error about the mean is 10 to 20%.
[e]The range of error about the mean is 10 to 50%.

immunospecific fluorescein-conjugated antibodies revealed that the majority of cells contained γ and λ chains with a smaller number containing κ, μ, and α chains. A minority of cells did not contain immunoglobulin. Clone 2F11, in contrast, contained only cells positive for γ and λ chains, or cells which did not stain. Therefore, we concluded that the 2F11 antibody to tetanus toxoid must be of the IgG(λ) isotype. A fraction of the 2F11 cells also showed surface staining for γ and λ chains only.

A more recent series of transformation experiments *in vitro* established new cell lines producing specific antibody. All these new lines also lost the ability to synthesize specific antibody after several passages in tissue culture. To date a line producing tetanus-specific antibody longer than several months has not been established.

Steinitz *et al.* (1977, 1978, 1979) utilized a similar approach to establish cell

TABLE III

Production of Antibody to Toxoid by Various 3GC Cell Lines at Passage 3[a]

Cell line	Human γ-globulin[b] (ng/ml)	Antibody[c] to tetanus toxoid (ng/ml)
3GC-B1	3	0
3GC-B2	35	0
3CC B3	23	0
3GC-B4	120	0
3GC-B5	5820	0
3GC-C1	3960	18
3GC-C2	1530	164
3GC-C3	2680	0
3GC-C4	209	14
3GC-C5	1600	19

[a]Reprinted by permission from Zurawski et al. (1978a).
[b]Detected by binding with ^{125}I-labeled protein A, which does not detect subgroup 3 IgG; values are averages of triplicate samples.
[c]Values of antibody production below 20 ng/ml were determined with triplicate undiluted and 10 times concentrated samples of media; zero indicates <0.1 ng/ml.

lines synthesizing antibody to 4-hydroxy-3,5-dinitrophenacetic acid (NNP). In their experiment cells destined for transformation were selected with antigen-coated erythrocyte rosetting and separation by density centrifugation. These results prompted us to attempt to preselect cells from tetanus-boosted individuals prior to EBV infection by rosetting with tetanus toxoid or toxin-coated sheep erythrocytes. Tetanus toxoid, or highly purified tetanus toxin, was coupled to erythrocytes in piperazine buffer, using the chromium chloride technique (Goding, 1976). The coated erythrocytes bound both rabbit antibodies and monoclonal murine antibodies to tetanus toxoid (Zurawski et al., 1979b) as demonstrated by direct binding experiments using ^{125}I-labeled antiimmunoglobulin, and by hemagglutination at high antiserum dilution, and lysis in the presence of antiserum and complement. These cells did not, however, rosette with lymphocytes from individuals recently boosted with tetanus toxoid, nor were we able to increase the frequency of cell lines synthesizing antibody to toxoid if these coated erythrocytes were used to preselect lymphocytes prior to EBV infection.

Neither direct nor indirect hemolytic plaques were formed with toxoid or toxin-coated erythrocytes in the presence of cell lines 4LP-B4, 3GC-C2, or their clones, or with cells from two murine hybridoma clones demonstrated to secrete large amounts of toxoid-specific antibody. The failure to form hemolytic plaques may be accounted for by random orientation of tetanus molecules on the cell surface leading to a sparse surface distribution of antigenic determinants toward which the monoclonal antibodies are directed. Consequently, monoclonal antibodies produced by individual cells might have bound to erythrocytes at too low a density to fix complement.

Because murine somatic-cell hybrids are generally more stable producers of antibody we attempted fusion of human EBV-transformed cells with two HAT (hypoxanthine–aminopterin–thymidine medium)-sensitive murine myelomas, the NS1 line of Milstein (Köhler and Milstein, 1975), and the 4T.001 ouabain-resistant line of Scharff and co-workers (Gefter *et al.*, 1977). In preliminary experiments using the 4T.001 cell line hybrids were obtained by using HAT–ouabain selection (EBV lines are exceedingly sensitive to ouabain), but none was demonstrated to synthesize either human immunoglobulin or human antibody to tetanus toxoid.

B. Cell Lines Producing Human Antibody to Haptenic Antigens

Steinitz *et al.* (1977) reported establishing EBV-transformed cell lines that synthesized specific antibody to NNP. The three donors for the peripheral blood lymphocytes utilized in the transformation experiment were individuals that had relatively high serum titers against NNP by virtue of previous laboratory exposure.

Prior to EBV transformation, a fraction of the lymphocytes was rosetted with NNP-coated autologous human erythrocytes. Those lymphocytes that bound to the erythrocytes could be transformed with EBV to yield cell lines synthesizing human anti-NNP antibodies. Antibody-producing cell lines could not be established without preselection of lymphocytes. This may indicate that the frequency of NNP-specific cells in their mononuclear cell preparation was lower than that of tetanus-toxoid-specific lymphocytes in our preparation. An examination of other systems will be required before the general requirement for concentration of antibody-producing cells prior to transformation are established; however, it is likely that in most instances concentration of antigen-specific cells will be required (see Section III).

In contrast to the antitetanus-producing cell lines, the anti-NNP lines contained cells which rosetted NNP-coated erythrocytes and formed hemolytic plaques in a direct plaque assay. The antibody isotype in this case was μ,κ.

A common feature of both NNP (M. Steinitz, personal communication) and antitetanus lines was decline in specific antibody production with cell passage. The NNP lines secreted more antibody initially (up to 16.5 μg/ml) than did the antitetanus-producing cells. The transformed cell lines were also readily subject to rosetting with NNP-coated erythrocytes, which permitted a more selective approach to cloning of desirable lines.

Rosetting of transformed cell lines was utilized to great advantage (Kozbor *et al.*, 1979) in establishing an EBV-transformed cell line producing antibody to the trinitrophenyl hapten (TNP). After three successive rosettings of a cell line in the course of a 12-week period following exposure to the virus, a culture demonstrating 75% rosette formation with TNP-erythrocytes was obtained. The anti-TNP antibodies secreted were isotypes as μ,κ,λ, indicating that the line was still polyclonal.

C. Cell Lines Producing Human Antibody to Other Antigens

Koskimies (1979) has recently extended the EBV transformation approach to establish continuously proliferating cell lines that synthesized antibody to the human red blood cell D antigen (anti-Rh antibody). An Rh⁻ donor was immunized several times with D-positive (Rh⁺) erythrocytes. Lymphocytes were isolated and rosetted with A Rh⁺ (Dce/dce) erythrocytes. The rosette-forming cells were selected and transformed with EBV and rerosetted three times to produce a cell line that released substantial amounts of antibody to the Rh D antigen into culture fluids. The D-specific antibody was of the IgG1 isotype.

III. Preselection of Antibody-Producing Cells

Preselection of a population of normal cells secreting an antibody of desired specificity may facilitate the establishment of a continuously proliferating line either by viral transformation or somatic cell fusion. It should be noted that even after immunization *in vivo*, only a small fraction of the B lymphocytes obtained from an individual donor would likely be producing the antibody of choice. Either EBV infection or somatic-cell fusion must then result in a mixed culture of both antibody and non-antibody-producing cells (Köhler and Milstein, 1975; Bechet *et al.*, 1974). Preselection is not needed when the precursor cell culture is monoclonal. For example, the mouse–human fusion by Levy and Dilley (1978), which led to the establishment of a hybrid synthesizing human antibody of a predetermined idiotype, the target human cells for fusion were monoclonal human leukemia cells. Preselection may also not be needed when specific antibody-producing cells occur at high frequency, such as in tetanus toxoid immunization described in Section II.A, or in murine myeloma fusions where it appears that the fusion event is favored with antigen-stimulated cells. Concentration of desired cells is likely to be required in human studies, however, with antigens of low potency or where immunization occurred at a remote time.

The rosetting of cells with antigen-coated erythrocytes pioneered by Klein and his co-workers (Steinitz *et al.*, 1977) has certainly proven to be useful in preselection of human antibody-producing cells (Kozbor *et al.*, 1979; Koskimies, 1979). This method may be limited however, because of the inability of certain antigen-coated erythrocytes to form stable rosettes. Several other methods for separating antigen-specific lymphocytes have been reported, which rely on the binding of lymphocytes to antigen via surface receptors. Some of these may prove useful in particular applications, although none has yet to achieve widespread usage. Binding to antigen-coated supports or cells (Rutishauser *et al.*, 1972; Kiefer, 1975; Haas, 1975; Haas and Layton, 1975; Nossal and Pike, 1978; Kenny *et al.*, 1978) or use of fluorescent-labeled antigen in conjunction with the fluorescence-activated cell sorter (Julius *et al.*, 1972; Julius and Herzenberg, 1974; Parks *et al.*, 1979) are examples of such methods.

Preselection methods which do not rely directly on surface receptors for antigen might also prove valuable. For example, Walker *et al.* (1977) have demonstrated that, following removal of surface immunoglobulin by capping with antigen, B lymphocytes can be separated into fractions by rosetting with antiimmunoglobulin-coated erythrocytes and buoyant density centrifugation. In this case the nonrosetting fraction was enriched for cells synthesizing antibody to the antigen used for capping.

One might also postulate that, following capping of surface immunoglobulin or following immune stimulation, the surface of the involved B lymphocyte would be altered antigenically in such a fashion as to allow separation. We have recently found (Zurawski *et al.*, 1979a; Zurawski, manuscript in preparation) that, following capping of surface immunoglobulin from human B lymphocytes with antiimmunoglobulin antibody or F(ab')₂ fragments of this antibody that the lymphocytes formed rosettes with rhesus monkey erythrocytes (RhMRBC) (Fig. 1). This phenomenon could also be demonstrated following polyclonal pokeweed mitogen activation. Table IV compares the properties of two fractions of both monocyte and T-cell-depleted human lymphocytes after exposure to pokeweed mitogen. One fraction rosetted RhMRBC, the other did not. The rosetting fraction appeared to contain a set of stimulated B lymphocytes, since nearly all the cells containing surface immunoglobulin and complement were in the rosetting fraction. Also in the rosetting fraction were all the large cells (blast transformed) and all of the cells synthesizing large amounts of DNA as measured by [³H]thymidine uptake. RhMRBC have been demonstrated to form rosettes with

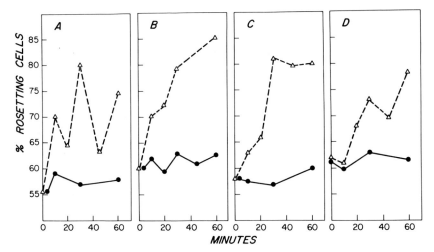

FIGURE 1. Induction of RhMRBC rosetting in peripheral blood lymphocytes *in vitro* by F(ab')₂ fragments of anti-Ig antibody. Percent RhMRBC rosette-forming lymphocytes vs. minutes of incubation. ●—●, RhMRBC rosettes with no added reagent; ∆—∆, RhMRBC rosettes with 20 μg/ml purified F(ab')₂ fragments of rabbit antihuman F(ab')₂ antibody. No increase in SRBC rosetting was observed, nor was any increase in RhMRBC rosetting observed using 20 μg/ml of rabbit antitetanus toxoid antibody. Panel A: donor, SW. Panel B: donor, DD. Panel C: donor, SG. Panel D: donor, ER.

Table IV

Fractionation of Pokeweed-Mitogen-Stimulated T-Cell-Depleted Lymphocytes by Preparative RhMRBC Rosetting[a]

Marker[b]	RhMRBC rosetting fraction	Non-RhMRBC rosetting fraction
RhMRBC rosettes (%)	89	10
SRBC rosettes (%)	1	2
[³H]thymidine uptake (cpm)	21428±2275	580±84
IgG (pg)		
Culture fluid	=10	=10
IgM (¹⁴C cpm)		
Culture fluid	446±27	46±15
Cell lysate	2220±255	433±18
Large cells (%)	25±5.7	0
Small cells (%)	75±5.7	100±0.52
Complement receptors (%)		
Total	30	1
Large cells	0	—
Small cells	39	1
Surface Ig (%)		
Total	12	2
Large cells	6	—
Small cells	23	2

[a]Monocyte and T-cell-depleted lymphocytes were exposed to 5 μg/ml of pokeweed mitogen for 72 hr. This procedure routinely induces 30–70% RhMRBC rosetting cells in a cell population where RhMRBC rosetting was not found. Cells were then rosetted with RhMRBC and centrifuged over a Ficoll–Hypaque cushion. Rosetting and nonrosetting fractions were collected and examined.

[b]Rosetting experiments with RhMRBC and sheep erythrocytes (SRBC) were performed. Uptake of [³H]thymidine in 4 hr was examined. Synthesis of IgG and release into the medium was examined. Synthesis of IgM was followed by intrinsic labeling of cells with [¹⁴C]leucine and examining IgM immunoprecipitates; large cells (blasts) and small cells (lymphocytes) in the two fractions were counted. The cells with complement receptors (via complement–zymosan rosetting) and surface immunoglobulin (via immunofluorescence) were enumerated. B cells (complement receptor positive; surface immunoglobulin positive; SRBC rosette negative) were found in the RhMRBC rosetting fraction.

T lymphocytes (Lohrmann and Novikovs, 1974) and with a subpopulation of human null cells (Chiao *et al.*, 1978) but not with normal peripheral blood B cells. Subsequent to stimulation by antiimmunoglobulin or by a mitogen, the surface of the human B cell appears to be altered in such a fashion that RhMRBC may be bound. If specific stimulation by antigen were to uncover this new surface marker as well, it might lead to a more refined fractionation procedure.

IV. In Vitro Immunization of Human B Lymphocytes

Although a number of reports have appeared which describe methods for antigenically stimulating human B lymphocytes *in vitro* (e.g., Fauci and Pratt, 1976; Dosch and Gelfand, 1977; Delfraissy *et al.*, 1977), no general method has emerged, which might provide the immunologist with a means of immunizing human cells *in vitro* with any antigen of choice.

Fauci and co-workers have developed a system (Fauci and Pratt, 1976) for examining the polyclonal response to pokeweed mitogen generated in human peripheral blood mononuclear cells. They measure a portion of the response to the mitogen utilizing a direct sheep-erythrocyte plaque-forming assay. They have used this system to examine cooperation among immunocytes involved in the immune response (Haynes and Fauci, 1978a,b). Callard has suggested (Callard, 1979) that this system might be adapted to obtain a specific immune response to influenza virus *in vitro*.

Delfraissy *et al.* (1977) have reported that a primary response could be produced in human peripheral blood lymphocytes *in vitro* with antigens attached to polyacrylamide beads. They utilized TNP–polyacrylamide beads to generate an antibody response. This substance has been reported to be a T-cell-independent antigen in mouse spleen cell cultures (Galanaud *et al.*, 1976).

Dosch and Gelfand (1977) have reported generating responses *in vitro* with human tonsillar, bone marrow, and spleen cells, and Geha *et al.* (1973), in studies of lymphocyte mitogenic factor, have generated antibody synthesis *in vitro* in human tonsillar and peripheral blood B cells. Antigens used in these studies were sheep erythrocytes, ovalbumin (Dosch and Gelfand, 1977), and tetanus toxoid (Geha *et al.*, 1973). Because human peripheral blood B lymphocytes may be an immature subpopulation of B lymphocytes (e.g., Ault and Unanue, 1977) the use of tonsillar or splenic lymphocytes to generate an immune response *in vitro* may be efficacious. In any case because of the complex nature of the immune system, future progress in this area may require more sophisticated methods of cell fractionation as well as the reconstitution of cell cooperativity *in vitro*.

V. *Conclusions*

Klein and co-workers (Steinitz *et al.*, 1977), our laboratory (Zurawski *et al.*, 1978a,b), and Koskimies (1979) have demonstrated that human antibodies of predetermined specificity can be produced by continuously proliferating cell lines. These lines were all established as a result of infection of peripheral blood lymphocytes with EBV. The utility of this approach may be limited, since all EBV-transformed lines reported thus far lose antibody production with time. Levy and Dilley (1978) have demonstrated that a specific human immunoglobulin molecule can be produced by a clone of a murine–human hybrid cell line. These results suggest that a general approach to the establishment of human antibody-secreting lines may be affected by somatic-cell fusion of previously transformed cell lines with a myeloma cell line. The availability of appropriate human myeloma lines would undoubtedly facilitate further progress in fusion experiments, whether virally transformed or untransformed cells were used as partners, since repression of human chromosome function or loss of human chromosomes would be eliminated.

Two principal problems will likely need to be solved before production of human antibodies *in vitro* by cell lines becomes a widespread reality. First, a general method for preselecting antigen-specific B cells or plasma cells from among the many clones not of interest would be desirable. The work of Steinitz *et al.* (1977) certainly underscores the idea that enrichment of appropriate cells as targets for infection can increase the probability of obtaining a cell line with desired characteristics. It would be desirable to develop a general method for selecting activated B cells utilizing differences in the antigenic characteristics of the cell surface of resting and stimulated human B cells. A monoclonal antibody to a human B-cell differentiation antigen would be the best tool for separating subpopulations of B lymphocytes. Once such an antibody is available a variety of separation techniques can be applied. The fluorescence-activated cell sorter has been successfully used in similar applications (e.g., Kreth and Herzenberg, 1974).

Second, a reliable method for providing both primary and secondary antigen stimulation of B cells *in vitro* will be required, since it is not feasible to immunize humans *in vivo* with many antigens. The fractionation of various subpopulations of human lymphocytes and macrophages and their subsequent recombination in appropriate mixtures will provide cell cultures capable of being immunized *in vitro* by virtually any antigen. It is likely that specific cell fractionation will utilize murine monoclonal antibodies to cell-surface differentiation antigens. As an example, Reinherz *et al.* (1979) have recently reported the production of a monoclonal antibody (OKT4) which may have specificity to human T helper cells (see also chapter in this text by Goldsby, Osborne, and Engleman).

The ultimate union of the *in vitro* immunization, preselection, and fusion or virus transformation techniques will undoubtedly provide the clinician with a supply of highly specific, nontoxic, and potent therapeutic agents.

Acknowledgments

The authors wish to thank Drs. Klein and Koskimies for providing unpublished manuscripts. Dr. Zurawski is a Fellow of the Medical Foundation. This work was supported in part by USPHS Grants HL 19259 and CA 24432.

References

Ault, K., and Unanue, E., 1977, Failure of B lymphocytes in human blood to regenerate surface immunoglobulin after its removal by antibody, *J. Immunol.* **119:**327.

Bechet, J. M., Fialkow, P. J., Nilsson, K., and Klein, G., 1974, Immunoglobulin synthesis and glucose-6-phosphate dehydrogenase as cell markers in human lymphoblastoid cell lines, *Exp. Cell Res.* **89:**175.

Callard, R. E., 1979, Specific in vitro antibody response to influenza virus by human blood lymphocytes, *Nature* **282**:734.

Chiao, J. W., Dowling, M., and Good, R. A., 1978, Rosette formation of human null lymphocytes with rhesus monkey erythrocytes, *Clin. Exp. Immunol.* **32**:498.

Delfraissy, J.-F., Galanaud, P., Dormont, J., and Wallon, C., 1977, Primary in vitro antibody response from human peripheral blood lymphocytes, *J. Immunol.* **118**:630.

Dosch, H.-M., and Gelfand, E. W., 1977, Generation of human plaque-forming cells in culture: Tissue distribution, antigenic and cellular requirements, *J. Immunol.* **118**:302.

Fahey, J. L., Buell, D. N., and Sox, H. C., 1971, Proliferation of lymphoid cells: Studies with human lymphoid cell lines and immunoglobulin synthesis, *Ann. NY Acad. Sci.* **190**:221.

Fauci, A. S., and Pratt, K. R., 1976, Activation of human B lymphocytes. I. Direct plaque forming cell assay for the measurement of polyclonal activation and antigenic stimulation of human B lymphocytes, *J. Exp. Med.* **144**:674.

Galanaud, P., Crevon, M. C., Evard, D., Wallen, C., and Dormant, J., 1976, Two processes for B cell triggering by T-independent antigens as evidenced by the effect of azothioprine, *Cell. Immunol.* **22**:83.

Gefter, M. L., Margulies, D. H., and Scharff, M. D., 1977, A simple method for polyethylene glycol-promoted hybridization of mouse myeloma cells, *Somat. Cell Genet.* **3**:231.

Geha, R., and Weinberg, R. P., 1978, Anti-idiotypic antisera in man. I. Production and immunochemical characterization of anti-idiotypic antisera to human anti-tetanus antibodies, *J. Immunol.* **121**:1518.

Geha, R. S., Schneeberger, E., Rosen, F. S., and Merler, E., 1973, Interaction of human thymus derived and non-thymus derived lymphocytes in vitro. Induction of proliferation and antibody synthesis in B lymphocytes by a soluble factor released from antigen-stimulated T lymphocytes, *J. Exp. Med.* **138**:1230.

Ghose, T., Guclu, A., Tai, J., MacDonald, A. S., Norvell, S. T., and Aquino, J., 1975, Antibody as carrier of ^{131}I in cancer diagnosis and treatment, *Cancer* **36**:1646.

Goding, J. W., 1976, The chromic chloride method of coupling antigens to erythrocytes: Definition of some important parameters, *J. Immunol. Methods* **10**:61.

Goldenberg, D. M., DeLand, F., Kim, E., Bennett, S., Primus, F. J., van Nagell, J. R., Estes, N., DiSimone, P., and Rayburn, P., 1978, Use of radiolabeled antibodies to carcinoembryonic antigen for the detection and localization of diverse cancers by external photoscanning, *N. Engl. J. Med.* **298**:1384.

Haas, W., 1975, Separation of antigen-specific lymphocytes. II. Enrichment of hapten specific antibody-forming cell precursors, *J. Exp. Med.* **141**:1015.

Haas, W., and Layton, J. E., 1975, Separation of antigen-specific lymphocytes. I. Enrichment of antigen binding cells, *J. Exp. Med.* **141**:1004.

Haber, E., and Krause, R. M. (eds.), 1977, *Antibodies in Human Diagnosis and Therapy*, Raven Press, New York.

Haynes, B. F., and Fauci, A. S., 1978a, Activation of human B lymphocytes. V. Kinetics and mechanisms of suppression of plaque-forming cell responses by concanavalin A-generated suppressor cells, *J. Immunol.* **120**:700.

Haynes, B. F., and Fauci, A. S., 1978b, Activation of human B lymphocytes. X. Heterogeneity of concanavalin A-generated suppressor cells of the pokeweed mitogen-induced plaque-forming cell response of human peripheral blood lymphocytes, *J. Immunol.* **121**:559.

Jobin, M. E., Fahey, J. L., and Price, Z., 1974, Long-term establishment of a human plasmacyte cell line derived from a patient with IgD multiple myeloma. I. Requirement of a plasmacyte-stimulating factor for the proliferation of myeloma cells in tissue culture, *J. Exp. Med.* **140**:494.

Julius, M. H., and Herzenberg, L. A., 1974, Isolation of antigen-binding cells from unprimed mice. Demonstration of antibody-forming cell precursor activity and correlation between precursor and secreted antibody activities, *J. Exp. Med.* **140**:904.

Julius, M. H., Masuda, T., and Herzenberg, L. A., 1972, Demonstration that antigen-binding cells are precursors of antibody-producing cells after purification with a fluorescence-activated cell sorter, *Proc. Natl. Acad. Sci. USA* **69**:1934.

Kenny, J. J., Merrill, J. E., and Ashman, R. F., 1978, A two-step centrifugation procedure for the purification of sheep erythrocyte antigen-binding cell, *J. Immunol.* **120:**1233.

Khaw, B. A., Beller, G. A., and Haber, E., 1978a, Experimental myocardial infarct imaging following intravenous administration of iodine-131 labeled antibody (Fab')$_2$ fragments specific for cardiac myosin, *Circulation* **57:**743.

Khaw, B. A., Gold, H. K., Leinbach, R. C., Fallon, J. T., Strauss, W., Pohost, G. M., and Haber, E., 1978b, Early imaging of experimental myocardial infarction by intracoronary administration of ^{131}I-labeled anticardiac myosin (Fab')$_2$ fragments, *Circulation* **58:**1137.

Kiefer, H., 1975, Separation of antigen specific lymphocytes. A new general method of releasing cells bound to nylon mesh, *Eur. J. Immunol.* **5:**624.

Köhler, G., and Milstein, C., 1975, Continuous cultures of fused cells secreting antibody of predefined specificity, *Nature* **256:**495.

Koskimies, S., 1979, Human lymphoblastoid cell line producing specific antibody against Rh-antigen D, *Scand. J. Immunol.* **10:**371.

Kozbor, D., Steinitz, M., Klein, G., Koskimies, S., and Mäkelä, O., 1979, Establishment of anti-TNP antibody producing human lymphoid lines by preselection for hapten binding followed by EBV-transformation, *Scand. J. Immunol.* **10:**181.

Kreth, H. W., and Herzenberg, L. A., 1974, Fluorescence-activated cell sorting of human T and B lymphocytes. I. Direct evidence that lymphocytes with a high density of membrane bound immunoglobulin are precursors of plasmacytes, *Cell. Immunol.* **12:**396.

Levy, R., and Dilley, J., 1978, Rescue of immunoglobulin secretion from human neoplastic lymphoid cells by somatic cell hybridization, *Proc. Natl. Acad. Sci. USA* **75:**2411.

Lohrmann, H.-P., and Novikovs, L., 1974, Rosette formation between human T-lymphocytes and unsensitized rhesus monkey erythrocytes, *Clin. Immunol. Immunopathol.* **3:**99.

Miller, G., 1974, The oncogenicity of Epstein–Barr virus, *J. Infect. Dis.* **130:**187.

Miller, G., and Lipman, M., 1973, Release of infectious Epstein–Barr virus by transformed marmoset leukocytes, *Proc. Natl. Acad. Sci. USA* **70:**190.

Nossal, G. J. V., and Pike, B. L., 1978, Improved procedures for the fractionation and in vitro stimulation of hapten specific B lymphocytes, *J. Immunol.* **120:**145.

Parks, D. R., Bryan, V. M., Oi, V. T., and Herzenberg, L. A., 1979, Antigen-specific identification and cloning of hybridomas with a fluorescence activated cell sorter, *Proc. Natl. Acad. Sci. USA* **76:**1962.

Reedman, B. M., and Klein, G., 1973, Cellular localization of an Epstein–Barr virus (EBV)-associated complement-fixing antigen in producer and non-producer lymphoblastid cell lines, *Int. J. Cancer* **11:**499.

Reinherz, E. L., King, P. C., Goldstein, G., and Schlossman, S. F., 1979, Separation of functional subsets of human T cells by a monoclonal antibody, *Proc. Natl. Acad. Sci. USA* **76:**4061.

Rosenthal, J. D., Hayashi, K., and Notkins, A. L., 1973, Comparison of direct and indirect solid-phase microradioimmunoassays for the detection of viral antigens and antiviral antibody, *Appl. Microbiol.* **25:**567.

Ruddle, F. H., 1973, Linkage analysis in man by somatic cell genetics, *Nature* **242:**165.

Rutishauser, U., Millette, C. F., and Edelman, G. M., 1972, Specific fractionation of immune cell populations, *Proc. Natl. Acad. Sci. USA* **69:**1596.

Schwaber, J., 1977, Human lymphocyte–mouse myeloma somatic cell hybrids: Selective hybrid formation, *Somat. Cell Genet.* **3:**295.

Schwaber, J., and Cohen, E. P., 1973, Human × mouse somatic cell hybrid clone secreting immunoglobulins of both parental types, *Nature* **244:**444.

Schwaber, J. F., and Rosen, F. S., 1978, Induction of human immunoglobulin synthesis and secretion in somatic cell hybrids of mouse myeloma and human B lymphocytes from patients with agamma globulinemia, *J. Exp. Med.* **148:**974.

Smith, T. W., Haber, E., Yeatman, L., and Butler, V. P., Jr., 1976, Reversal of advanced digoxin intoxication with Fab fragments of digoxin-specific antibodies, *N. Engl. J. Med.* **294:**797.

Steinitz, M., Klein, G., Koskimies, S., and Mäkelä, O., 1977, EB virus-induced B lymphocyte cell lines producing specific antibody, *Nature* **269:**420.

Steinitz, M., Koskimies, S., Klein, G., and Mäkelä, O., 1978, Establishment of specific antibody producing human lines by antigen preselection and EBV-transformation, in: *Current Topics in Microbiology and Immunology*, Vol. 81 (F. Melchers, M. Potter, and N. L. Warner, eds.), Springer-Verlag, Berlin, p. 156.

Steinitz, M., Koskimies, S., Klein, G., and Mäkelä, O., 1979, Establishment of specific antibody producing human lines by antigen preselection and Epstein–Barr virus (EBV) transformation, *J. Clin. Lab. Immunol.* **2**:1.

Stevens, R. H., and Saxon, A., 1978, Immunoregulation in humans. Control of antitetanus toxoid antibody production after booster immunization, *J. Clin. Invest.* **62**:1154.

Stevens, R. H., and Saxon, A., 1979, Reduced in vitro production of anti-tetanus toxoid antibody after repeated in vivo immunization with tetanus toxoid, *J. Immunol.* **122**:592.

Strelkauskas, A. J., Wilson, B. S., Callery, R. T., Chess, L., and Schlossman, S. F., 1977, T-cell regulation of human peripheral blood B-cell responsiveness, *J. Exp. Med.* **146**:1765.

Walker, S. M., Meinke, G. C., and Weigle, W. O., 1977, Enrichment of antigen-specific B lymphocytes by the direct removal of B cells not bearing specificity for the antigen, *J. Exp. Med.* **146**:445.

Zurawski, V. R., Jr., Haber, E., and Black, P. H., 1978a, Production of antibody to tetanus toxoid by continuous human lymphoblastoid cell lines, *Science* **199**:1439.

Zurawski, V. R., Jr., Spedden, S. E., Black, P. H., and Haber, E., 1978b, Clones of human lymphoblastoid cell lines producing antibody to tetanus toxoid, in: *Current Topics in Microbiology and Immunology*, Vol. 81 (F. Melchers, M. Potter, and N. L. Warner, eds.), Springer-Verlag, Berlin, p. 152.

Zurawski, V. R., Jr., Leskowitz, A. J., Black, P. H., and Haber, E., 1979a, Induction of rhesus monkey erythrocyte rosetting in human B lymphocytes, *Fed. Proc.* **38**:1082.

Zurawski, V. R., Jr., Spedden, S. E., Latham, W. C., Haber, E., and Black, P. H., 1979b, In vivo protection against toxification, by monoclonal antibodies to tetanus toxin produced by murine hybridoma clones, Abstracts of 13th International Leucocyte Culture Conference, Ottawa, p. 98.

PART II
ANALYSIS OF IMMUNOGLOBULIN STRUCTURE AND GENETICS

3

Antibody Diversity Patterns and Structure of Idiotypic Determinants on Murine Anti-α(1$\rightarrow$3) Dextran Antibodies

BRIAN CLEVINGER, JAMES SCHILLING, ROGERS GRIFFITH, DANIEL HANSBURG, LEROY HOOD, AND JOSEPH DAVIE

I. Introduction

Idiotypic (variable-region) antigenic determinants have been extremely important to the study of immunoglobulins. These antigenic determinants have been widely used to examine variable-region expression in immunoglobulin populations because they offer a simple, sensitive, serological approach to variable-region structure. There are many different categories of idiotypic determinants: ligand-modifiable (binding site determinants), ligand-nonmodifiable (framework determinants), V_L-specific, V_H-specific, and those requiring both V_L and V_H. In addition, determinants shared by variable regions known to be structurally different are called IdX, cross-reactive, or public idiotypes, while those apparently restricted to identical variable regions are IdI, individual, or private idiotypes.

Because each immunoglobulin may possess several different idiotypic determinants and therefore antiidiotypic reagents may be multispecific, the possibility for confusion and variable results between laboratories is great. Therefore, hybridoma production provides great promise for definition of idiotypic determi-

BRIAN CLEVINGER, ROGERS GRIFFITH, DANIEL HANSBURG, AND JOSEPH DAVIE • Department of Microbiology and Immunology, Washington University School of Medicine, St. Louis, Missouri, 63110. JAMES SCHILLING AND LEROY HOOD • Division of Biology, California Institute of Technology, Pasadena, California 91125.

nants by providing large amounts of monoclonal antibodies for comparison of structure with idiotypic reactivity and by providing monospecific antiidiotypic reagents that can be shared between laboratories. We would like to summarize here our experience with monoclonal antibodies in clarifying idiotypic determinants on mouse antibodies specific for $\alpha(1\rightarrow3)$ dextran.

II. Mouse Anti-α (1→3) Dextran Serum Antibodies

Blomberg et al. (1972) were the first to point out that mouse anti-$\alpha(1\rightarrow3)$ dextran antibodies were exceptionally restricted in heterogeneity. The majority of dextran-specific antibodies which appeared after immunization of mice of the IgCH^a allogroup with B1355 dextran had λ light chains and shared idiotypic determinants with dextran-binding myeloma protein, J558. Our laboratories have confirmed and extended these findings. As we will show here, however, antidextran immunoglobulins are paradoxically both highly homogeneous and highly heterogeneous.

The concept that dextran-binding domains have both common and unique structural features became apparent early in a study of the idiotypic determinants on three dextran-binding myeloma proteins, M104, J558, and U102, derived from BALB/c mice. The idiotypic determinants on the myeloma proteins are summarized in Table I and Fig. 1. It can be seen that four separate determinants are defined: one, IdX, which is shared equally by all three dextran-binding proteins, but absent from other non-dextran-binding proteins, and three determinants unique to each myeloma protein, IdI(M104), IdI(J558), and IdI(U102) (Hansburg et al., 1977). All three myeloma proteins possess λ light chains, and two, M104 and J558, have extensive heavy-chain sequence homology (Barstad et al., 1978) and yet bind dextran differently (Leon et al., 1970; Lundblad et al., 1972).

All of the idiotypic determinants are found among serum antidextran antibodies, but with different relative expressions (Table II; Hansburg et al., 1977). In addition, antidextran antibodies lacking these idiotypes are present. The IdX positive and negative populations are present in about equal proportions, while the individual idiotypic determinants are found in much smaller amounts. If antisera from individual mice are selected for unusually high or low IdX expres-

TABLE I
Idiotypic Determinants on Dextran-Binding Myeloma Proteins

Protein	Class	Specificity	IdX	IdI(M104)	IdI(J558)	IdI(U102)
M104	IgM(λ)	$\alpha(1\rightarrow3)$ dextran	+ +	+ +	—	—
J558	IgA(λ)	$\alpha(1\rightarrow3)$ dextran	+ +	—	+ +	—
U102	IgA(λ)	$\alpha(1\rightarrow3)$ dextran	+ +	—	—	+ +
HOPC-1	IgG$_{2a}$(λ)	?	—	—	—	—
T183	IgM(κ)	?	—	—	—	—

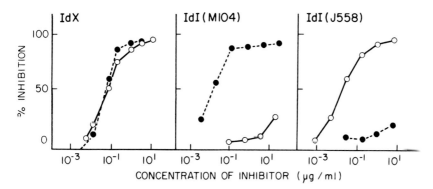

FIGURE 1. Specificity of idiotypic antisera. The relative inhibitory pattern of M104 (●—●) and J558 (○—○) proteins for anti-IdX, anti-IdI(M104), and anti-IdI(J558) reagents is shown. [Adapted from Hansburg *et al.*, 1977.]

sion the IdI determinants seemed associated with the IdX-positive population, a distribution similar to that found with the myeloma proteins studied (Hansburg *et al.*, 1978). The fact that the sum of the expression of individual idiotypes does not equal that of the common idiotype suggests that the IdX population is composed of more than three IdI components.

Support for the multiplicity of clonotypes comes from isoelectric focus analysis of serum IgG antidextran antibodies. By this technique, subtle differences in charged amino acids can be detected by differences in the pI of the protein. Since the antidextran antibodies have λ light chains and 7 S antibodies are predominantly IgG3, differences in pI should reflect differences in the V_H region. Focusing patterns of 7 S antidextran antibodies show simple but multiclonal banding patterns with considerable sharing of spectrotypes between sera from different animals (Hansburg *et al.*, 1976, 1978). While less than 10 different spectrotypes are found, it is likely that this does not delineate the limits of the clonal repertoire, since only charge differences are measured and the discriminatory capacity of this technique for intact immunoglobulins is not yet established.

TABLE II
Idiotypic Distribution of Induced Antidextran Antibodies

Idiotypic determinant	Relative expression of idiotypic determinants[a]	
	19 S	7 S
IdX	63	43
IdX-negative	37	57
IdI (M104)	9.4	5.7
IdI (J558)	1.4	3.7
IdI (U102)	0.3	0.1

[a]Hyperimmune anti-α(1→3) dextran sera from 8 individual BALB/c mice were analyzed for idiotypic determinants after separation into 19 S and 7 S fractions. [Modified from Hansburg *et al.* (1977).]

In spite of the idiotypic differences between the IdX-positive and negative antibodies, the antibodies are clearly related in that both use λ light chains which by isoelectric focusing were indistinguishable. In addition, considerable support for the idea that all dextran-binding antibodies are structurally related came from amino acid sequence analysis of heavy chains from pooled antidextran sera (Table III). Induced antidextran antibodies were pooled into two fractions, one completely IdX-positive and the second primarily IdX-negative. The heavy chains from both the IdX-positive and the IdX-negative pools were identical in sequence for at least 27–53 residues and appeared to be homogeneous. Similarly, the myeloma proteins M104 and J558 are identical to each other and to the antibody heavy chains through the second hypervariable region. All other V_H regions which have been sequenced through this region differ by 43–50% from the dextran-binding proteins. This again indicates that heavy chains of the majority of and possibly all antidextran antibodies are uniform in their N-terminal regions.

Thus extensive analysis of induced antidextran antibodies by isoelectric focusing of whole antibodies and isolated light chains, idiotypic comparison to myeloma proteins, and N-terminal amino acid sequence of V_H regions has led to the concept of a polyclonal family of antibodies composed of identical light chains paired with heavy chains, which probably vary only in the C-terminal portion of the V_H region. It also was evident that additional study of the diversity patterns of these proteins would be difficult because of variability in clonal representation among different animals, the uncertainty of monoclonality of even highly purified serum antibody, and the problem of producing sufficient quantities of antibodies in mice for further analysis. For these reasons, an extensive, coordinated approach was instituted to characterize monoclonal antidextran antibodies from somatic cell hybrids.

TABLE III

N-Terminal Sequence of V_H Regions from M104, J558, and Pooled Serum Antibodies[a]

		Position					
		1	10	20	30	40	50
Protein	IdX				hv1		hv2
M104μ	100.	EVQLQQSGP ELVKPGASUK MSCKASGYTF TD YYMK WVKQSHGKSLEWIGDINP N					
J558 α	100.	———————					
γ Ab	173.	———————— ? ? ?					
μ Ab	108.	———————— ? ? ?					
γ Ab	20.	————————					
μ Ab	37.	————————					

[a] BALB/c mice were immunized with dextran B1355 and *E. coli*, and serum pools were constructed from individuals expressing high or low levels of IdX determinants. Anti-α(1→3) dextran antibodies were isolated, separated into 19 S and 7 S components, and then to heavy and light chains. Amino acid sequences of the heavy chains are shown here (modified from Schilling *et al.*, 1979). Solid lines indicate identity with M104μ.

III. Monoclonal Antidextran Antibodies from Somatic Cell Hybrids

Somatic cell hybrids were prepared essentially as described by Galfre *et al.* (1977). Spleens from dextran immune animals were fused with the HGPRT-deficient MPC-11 line, 45.6TG1.7 or a nonsecreting variant of MOPC-21, NSI/1-Ag4-1, which synthesizes but does not secrete κ chains. Antidextran secreting hybrids were detected by direct binding of ^{125}I-labeled dextran by culture supernatants. Hybrids were cloned in soft agar and grown in large amounts as ascites tumors. More than 18 different hybrids derived from 15 different animals have been produced so far, and structural and serologic characterization have begun. The hybrid proteins are representative of serum antibodies; all possess λ light chains, most are IgM and a few are IgG3. In addition, both idiotype-positive and negative proteins have been found. These proteins thus provide an opportunity to explore the structural diversity patterns of a family of antibodies directed to a single antigenic determinant.

IV. Structure of V_H Regions from Antidextran Antibodies

The complete amino acid sequences of the V_H regions of eight IgM(λ) hybrid proteins and two myeloma proteins specific for dextran are graphically

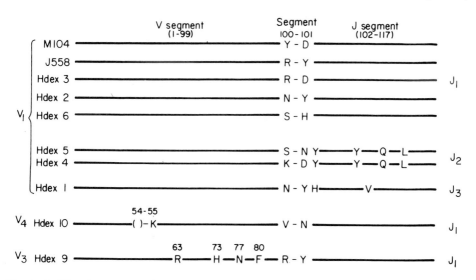

FIGURE 2. Diversity patterns of V_H regions of $a(1\rightarrow3)$ dextran-binding myeloma and hybridoma proteins. The complete amino sequences of the V_H regions of these 10 proteins are presented elsewhere (Schilling *et al.*, 1980). Protein M104 is used for comparison; solid lines for the V segments (1–99) and J segments (102–117) denote identity with M104. Differences are indicated in one-letter code. The D segment (100–101) sequences are given for each protein.

depicted in Fig. 2 (Schilling *et al.*, 1980). The first five proteins in the figure differ by only one or two amino acids at precisely the same positions, 100 and 101, in the third hypervariable region. This pattern of two highly conserved regions separated by a hypervariable region is found in all 10 proteins. The different segments are labeled V segment (positions 1–99), D segment (positions 100 and 101), and J segment (positions 102–117). It is clear from the diversity patterns of these proteins that there are three V segments and three J segments and that these segments segregate independently.

We have interpreted these data in analogy to the current understanding of gene organization for light-chain variable regions (Seidman and Leder, 1978; Brack *et al.*, 1978). It is likely that V and J segments are encoded by separate germline gene segments which, through joining in various combinations, can generate variable region diversity. The origin of the highly variable D segment is less clear and could have several explanations. One of the more likely ideas is that there is a third V-region gene segment. A more detailed consideration of the origin of the D segment is presented elsewhere (Schilling *et al.*, 1980).

V. Structural Correlates of Idiotypic Determinants

The λ light chains of the hybridoma proteins, like those of serum antidextran antibodies, are indistinguishable by isoelectric focusing from those of M104 and J558. Thus within the limits of this assay, we feel confident that most of the idiotypic determinants will reflect changes in the V_H regions of the molecules. Therefore comparison of the amino acid sequence of the V_H regions and the relative idiotypic composition of each protein should allow location of the idiotypic determinants (Clevinger *et al.*, 1980).

As shown in Fig. 3, 9 of 10 proteins are essentially identical in expression of IdX determinants. Hdex 10 is an IdX-negative protein composed of V_4 segment paired with J_1 and D segment residues, valine and asparagine. Neither this D segment nor J_1 is correlated with IdX reactivity, so that the IdX determinant(s) must reside in the V segments. It can be seen in Fig. 3 that V_4 differs from V_1 and V_3 by two and six residues, respectively. Clearly, IdX is only correlated with residues 54 and 55. All nine IdX-positive proteins have two asparagine residues at these positions with a carbohydrate side chain at position 55, while the IdX-negative protein has lysine residues at 54 and 55 and lacks a carbohydrate moiety. This raises the interesting possibility that IdX may be a carbohydrate determinant.

Similarly, the IdI idiotypes can be localized to two amino acids (Table IV). Here the relative IdI(J558) and IdI(M104) expression of each protein is compared to its structure. Four of the ten proteins have IdI(J558) determinants; J558 and Hdex 9 fully express the determinant, whereas Hdex 1 and 2 only partially express the determinant. These four proteins are constructed from two different V segments and two different J segments. Full expression of the IdI (J558) determinant requires arginine–tyrosine residues at position 100 and 101,

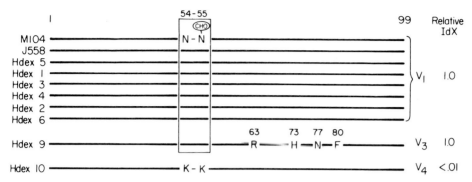

FIGURE 3. Location of IdX determinant. V segment structure is compared to relative IdX expression. Probable location of the IdX determinant is indicated by the box.

whereas the change of arginine to asparagine at position 100 leads to partial expression of the IdI(J558) determinant. The IdI(M104) determinant is also located in the D segment (Table IV). This is clearly demonstrated by comparing M104 with the other V_1J_1 proteins, all of which are negative for the IdI(M104) determinant. Thus either tyrosine at 100 by itself or this residue and adjacent amino acids is the IdI(M104) determinant. It should be noted that expression of idiotypic determinants may be dependent on other parts of the variable region(s) for proper conformation.

VI. Implications from These Studies

1. *Heavy-chain variable regions of anti-α(1→3) dextran antibodies are formed from the combinational association of at least two germline gene segments, V_H and J_H.* The existence of V and J gene segments is established at the DNA level for both κ (Seidman and Leder, 1978) and λ (Brack et al., 1978) light chains. In embryonic DNA these genes are separated by intervening DNA; upon immunological commitment, the V and J gene segments are somatically joined to generate a complete variable region gene. We have demonstrated that V_H and J_H gene segments probably exist for heavy-chain variable regions as well (Schilling et al., 1980). In addition, individual V_H gene segments can pair with several J_H gene segments and vice versa to generate a diverse population of products. Weigert et al. (1978) have recently demonstrated similar combinational association of V_K and J_K gene segments.

2. *Additional diversity is generated at the junction of V_H and J_H gene segments.* A second mechanism for generating variable region diversity is evident by examining the junctional residues between V_H and J_H segments in the antidextran proteins (Fig. 2). Eight different junctional segments are found in 10 V_H regions.

In addition, most heavy chains that have been sequenced have junctional regions that are analogous to those of the antidextran heavy chains (Schilling et

TABLE IV
Structural Localization of IdI(J558) and IdI(M104) Determinants[a]

Protein	V segment 1–99	D segment 100–101		J segment 102–117	Relative idiotypes	
					IdI (J558)	IdI (M104)
J558	V₁	R	Y	J₁	1.0	0.01
Hdex 9	V₃	R	Y	J₁	1.0	0.01
Hdex 1	V₁	N	Y	J₃	0.1	0.01
Hdex 2	V₁	N	Y	J₁	0.1	0.01
Hdex 5	V₁	S	N	J₂	0.01	0.01
Hdex 4	V₁	K	D	J₂	0.01	0.01
Hdex 10	V₄	V	N	J₁	0.01	0.01
Hdex 3	V₁	R	D	J₁	0.01	0.01
Hdex 6	V₁	S	H	J₁	0.01	0.01
M104	V₁	Y	D	J₁	0.01	1.0

[a]Modified from Clevinger et al. (1980).

al., 1980). These junctional segments, which we call D segments, vary in size from zero to seven residues and are highly variable in sequence. It is conceivable that these residues arise because of a third gene segment for the variable region combining with the V_H and J_H gene segments at immunologic commitment.

3. *J_H gene segments that pair with dextran-specific V_H gene segments can also pair with other V_H gene segments.* The most frequent J segment in dextran-binding proteins also occurs in the phosphocholine-binding proteins, T15, M603, and M511 (Schilling et al., 1980). The V segments from these latter proteins differ from the dextran V segments by about 50%. Thus, widely different V segments may share common J segments.

4. *Idiotypes are found on both V segments and D segments in dextran-binding proteins.* Figure 4 summarizes the location of the cross-reactive IdX determinant and the two individual determinants on dextran-binding proteins (Clevinger et al., 1980). All three determinants are located in hypervariable regions and are therefore binding-site idiotypes. IdX is encoded by V segment genes and

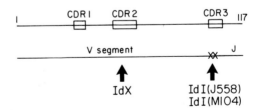

FIGURE 4. Location of IdX and IdI determinants in the V_H region. The upper line shows the position of the complementarity-determining regions (hypervariable regions) of V_H. The lower line shows V segment, J segment, and the D segment between V and J (XX) and the location of IdX, IdI(J558), and IdI(M104).

IdI(J558) and IdI(M104) are both found on D segments. These are important findings. First, they constitute evidence that a highly specific antigenic determinant (IdX) is found on products of more than one germline gene (both V_1 and V_3 express IdX). Second, some individual idiotypes may possibly be encoded by gene segments not found in the germline.

VII. Discussion

The importance of somatic cell hybridization to studies of antibody diversity and to structural identification of idiotypes cannot be overemphasized. Only rarely will sufficient quantities of monoclonal antibodies be available from serum for complete structural characterization. Indeed, judging from some of the subtle sequence differences found in the dextran-binding proteins, one may wonder how frequently truly monoclonal antibody responses occur. Perhaps what in the past has passed for a truly monoclonal response is generally a polyclonal response, whose individual components would be very difficult to purify from one another.

There are several families of immunoglobulins which have been characterized idiotypically. Williams et al. (1968), in a study of human IgM cold agglutinins, were the first to show that both common and unique antigenic determinants could be demonstrated on proteins with similar specificities. Similarly, induced antibodies, myeloma or hybridoma proteins to levan (Lieberman et al., 1975), galactan (Mushinski and Potter, 1977), and poly($Glu^{60}Ala^{30}Tyr^{10}$) (GAT) (Ju et al., 1979), in particular, have been extensively characterized. In each system, common IdX determinants and rare IdI determinants have been described. In spite of the idiotypic similarities of these systems, amino acid sequence data will be required to determine whether the IdX and IdI determinants are localized in V segments and D segments in analogy to the dextran system. As an example of the possible complexities which may be encountered, Lieberman et al. (1977) demonstrated that two separate IdX determinants were found on inulin-binding myeloma proteins, one on V_H and the other on V_L, while the IdI determinants were present on V_L. Furthermore, structural correlates of several of these determinants show complex patterns which seem inconsistent with those found on the dextran-binding proteins (Vrana et al., 1979).

In fact the highly specific nature of the IdX determinant on dextran-binding proteins is surprising. It should be recalled that heterologous antisera to M104 are absorbed only with normal mouse serum and with myeloma proteins to remove μ and λ reactivity (Hansburg et al., 1977). Yet these antisera, when exposed to other proteins sharing the N-terminal 99 residues of the V_H region, react specifically with a determinant dependent on two residues and/or a carbohydrate side group in the second hypervariable region. This may indicate that non-dextran-specific V_H regions may share other potential determinants with the dextran-binding proteins or that the IdX determinant is most immunogenic in that V segment. It is not surprising that the most variable portion of the dextran-binding proteins defines the IdI determinants. Again, however, it does not follow that IdI determinants must always involve the D segments.

The crucial issue is that both IdX and IdI determinants are highly specific and dependent on only one or two amino acids and/or carbohydrate side groups. This must be remembered when idiotypic determinants are used to compare molecules. Idiotypic identity could be shared between two molecules that are very different except for the idiotypic determinant. There are many examples of immunoglobulins with different specificities that share idiotypic determinants (Oudin and Cazenave, 1971), including some like T15 (Sigal, 1977) and A5A (Eichmann et al., 1977), which have been used widely to map variable region gene organization and expression (Eichmann, 1972; Lieberman et al., 1974; Claflin and Davie, 1974) and to compare B- and T-cell antigen-specific receptors (Black et al., 1976; Julius et al., 1977). It should be obvious from a consideration of the idiotypes of dextran-binding proteins that results from the use of idiotypes may vary greatly depending on the specific determinants measured and on the genetic origin of those determinants.

VIII. Summary

Somatic cell hybridization has been used to dissect the murine antibody response directed to a simple antigenic determinant, $\alpha(1\rightarrow3)$ dextran, into individual clonotypes. Amino acid sequence analysis of the V_H regions of these proteins has allowed us to propose two mechanisms for the generation of antibody diversity: (1) combinatorial association of multiple V_H with multiple J_H gene segments, and (2) additional diversity between the V and J segments from possibly a third variable-region gene segment.

Idiotypic determinants have been localized to two amino acids in the second hypervariable region (cross-reactive idiotype) and the third hypervariable region (individual idiotypes).

ACKNOWLEDGMENTS

This work was supported by NIH grants AI-10781, AI-15353, AI-11635, AI-05599, CA-09118, and GM-07616, NSF grant PCM 76-09719, and by Special Postdoctoral Fellowship SPF-13 from the American Cancer Society.

References

Barstad, P., Hubert, J., Hunkapiller, M., Goetze, A., Schilling, J., Black, B., Eaton, B., Richards, J., Weigert, M., and Hood, L., 1978, Immunoglobulins with hapten-binding activity: Structure–function correlations and genetic implications, Eur. J. Immunol. 8:497.

Black, S. J., Hammerling G. J., Berek, C., Rajewsky, K., and Eichmann, K., 1976, Idiotypic analysis of lymphocytes in vitro. I. Specificity and heterogeneity of B and T lymphocytes reactive with anti-idiotypic antibody, *J. Exp. Med.* **143**:846.

Blomberg, B., Geckeler, W. R., and Weigert, M., 1972, Genetics of the antibody response to dextran in mice, *Science* **177**:178.

Brack, C., Hirama, M., Lenhard-Schuller, R., and Tonegawa, S., 1978, A complete immunoglobulin gene is created by somatic recombination, *Cell* **15**:1.

Claflin, J. L., and Davie, J. M., 1974, Clonal nature of the immune response to phosphorylcholine. IV. Idiotypic uniformity of binding site associated antigenic determinants among mouse anti-phosphorylcholine antibodies, *J. Exp. Med.* **140**:673.

Clevinger, B., Schilling, J., Hood, L., and Davie, J. M., 1980, Structural correlates of cross-reactive and individual idiotypic determinants on murine antibodies to $\alpha(1\rightarrow3)$ dextran, *J. Exp. Med.* **151**:1059.

Eichmann, K., 1972, Idiotypic identity of antibodies to streptococcal carbohydrate in inbred mice, *Eur. J. Immunol.* **2**:301.

Eichmann, K., Coutinho, A., and Melchers, F., 1977, Absolute frequencies of lipopolysaccharide-reactive B cells producing A5A idiotype in unprimed, sterptococcal A carbohydrate-primed, anti-A5A idiotype-sensitized and anti-A5A idiotype-suppressed A/J mice, *J. Exp. Med.* **146**:1436.

Galfré, G., Howe, S. C., Milstein, C., Butcher, G. W., and Howard, J. C., 1977, Antibodies to major histocompatibility antigen produced by hybrid cell lines, *Nature* **266**:550.

Hansburg, D., Briles, D. E., and Davie, J. M., 1976, Analysis of the diversity of murine antibodies to dextran B1355. I. Generation of a large, pauci-clonal response by a bacterial vaccine, *J. Immunol.* **117**:569.

Hansburg, D., Briles, D. E., and Davie, J. M., 1977, Analysis of the diversity of murine antibodies to dextran B1355. II. Demonstration of multiple idiotypes with variable expression in several strains, *J. Immunol.* **119**:1406.

Hansburg, D., Perlmutter, R. M., Briles, D. E., and Davie, J. M., 1978, Analysis of the diversity of murine antibodies to dextran B1355. III. Idiotypic and spectrotypic correlations, *Eur. J. Immunol.* **8**:352.

Ju. S.-T., Pierres, M., Waltenbaugh, C., Germain, R. N., Benacerraf, B., and Dorf, M. E., 1979, Idiotypic analysis of monoclonal antibodies to poly (Glu^{60}Ala^{30}Tyr^{10}), *Proc. Natl. Acad. Sci. USA* **76**:2942.

Julius, M. H., Cosenza, H., and Augustin, A. A., 1977, Parallel expression of new idiotypes on T and B cells, *Nature* **267**:437.

Leon, M.A., Young, N. M., and McIntire, K. R., 1970, Immunochemical studies of the reaction between a mouse myeloma macroglobulin and dextrans, *Biochemistry* **9**:1023.

Lieberman, R., Potter, M., Mushinski, E. B., Humphrey, W., and Rudikoff, S., 1974, Genetics of a new IgV$_H$ (T15 idiotype) marker in the mouse regulating natural antibody to phosphorylcholine, *J. Exp. Med.* **139**:983.

Lieberman, R., Potter, M., Humphrey, W., Mushinski, E. B., and Vrana, M., 1975, Multiple individual cross-specific idiotypes on 13 levan-binding myeloma proteins of BALB/c mice, *J. Exp. Med.* **142**:106.

Lieberman, R., Vrana, M., Humphrey, W., Chien, C. C., and Potter, M., 1977, Idiotypes of inulin-binding myeloma proteins localized to variable region light and heavy chains: Genetic significance, *J. Exp. Med.* **146**:1294.

Lundblad, A., Steller, R., Kabat, E. A., Hirst, J. W., Weigert, M. G., and Cohn, M., 1972, Immunochemical studies on mouse myeloma proteins with specificity for dextran or for levan, *Immunochemistry* **9**:535.

Mushinski, E. B., and Potter, M., 1977, Idiotypes on galactan binding myeloma proteins and anti-galactan antibodies in mice, *J. Immunol.* **119**:1888.

Oudin, J., and Cazenave, P. A., 1971, Similar idiotypic specificities in immunoglobulin fractions with different antibody functions or even without detectable antibody function, *Proc. Natl. Acad. Sci. USA* **68**:2616.

Schilling, J., Hansburg, D., Davie, J. M., and Hood, L., 1979, Analysis of the diversity of murine antibodies to dextran B1355: N-terminal amino acid sequences of heavy chains from serum antibodies, *J. Immunol.* **123**:384.

Schilling, J., Clevinger, B., Davie, J. M., and Hood, L., 1980, Amino-acid sequence of homogeneous antibodies to dextran and DNA rearrangements in heavy chain V region segments, *Nature* **283**:35.

Seidman, J. G., and Leder, P., 1978, The arrangement and rearrangement of antibody genes. *Nature* **276**:790.

Sigal, N. H., 1977, Novel idiotypic and antigen-binding characteristics in two anti-dinitrophenyl monoclonal antibodies, *J. Exp. Med.* **146**:282.

Vrana, M., Rudikoff, S., and Potter, M., 1979, The structural basis of a hapten-inhibitable K-chain idiotype, *J. Immunol.* **122**:1905.

Weigert, M., Gatmaitan, L., Loh, E., Schilling, J., and Hood, L., 1978. Rearrangement of genetic information may produce immunoglobulin diversity, *Nature* **276**:785.

Williams, R. C., Kunkel, H. G., and Capra, J. D., 1968, Antigenic specificities related to the cold agglutinin activity of gamma M globulins, *Science* **161**:379.

4

Defining the B-Cell Repertoire with Hybridomas Derived from Monoclonal Fragment Cultures

Kathleen Denis, Roger H. Kennett,
Norman Klinman, Christine Molinaro, and
Linda Sherman

I. Introduction

Despite a decade of intense study, the mechanism responsible for generation of the enormous array of antibody specificities remains an intriguing problem. Our current knowledge of these questions has in large measure been obtained by the analysis of a small set of defined antibodies. These have been obtained either fortuitously from among the array of murine myeloma proteins shown to be identical to naturally derived antibodies (Leon and Young, 1971; Sher and Cohn, 1972; Cohn *et al.*, 1974; Lieberman *et al.*, 1976) or from a rare set of immune responses which are dominated by a single antibody specificity or clonotype (Cohn *et al.*, 1974; Lieberman *et al.*, 1976; Consenza and Köhler, 1972; Gearhart *et al.*, 1975; Eichmann, 1975; Makela and Karjalainen, 1977; Imanishi and Makela, 1975; Nisonoff and Bangasser, 1975). Extensive use of these systems has provided evidence of a large degree of sharing of antibody repertoire among individuals of an inbred strain. This would indicate a significant genetic component in the expression of antibody repertoire. At the same time, since such specificities appear to be largely restricted to mice of a given heavy- or light-chain allotype (Cohn *et al.*, 1974; Eichmann, 1975; Makela and Karjalainen,

Kathleen Denis and Roger H. Kennett • Department of Human Genetics, University of Pennsylvania, School of Medicine, Philadelphia, Pennsylvania 19104. Norman Klinman, Christine Molinaro, and Linda Sherman • Department of Cellular and Developmental Immunology, Scripps Clinic and Research Foundation, La Jolla, California 92037.

49

1977; Laskin et al., 1977), these studies also imply significant polymorphism among the expressed repertoires of murine strains.

Recent studies, however, have indicated that the dominance of a given clonotype within a strain may be the result of influences that are not linked to the heavy- or light-chain allotype locus and that nonexpression may be due to non-allotype-linked influences (Cancro et al., 1978a; Gearhart and Cebra, 1978). More importantly, the clonotypes that have been available for study because of the above-stated fortuitous circumstances represent a minute proportion of the total repertoire, and the control of their expression may not be truly representative of the controls involved in the expression of the total antibody repertoire. It is also not yet known whether significant proportions of the expressed antibodies are determined directly by the heritable genetic information possessed by the individual or, alternatively, generated by random events. Finally, the role of environmental influences on the B lymphocyte, such as tolerance to self antigens, immunoregulatory events, and suppressive phenomena, remains undefined.

II. The Use of Hybridomas in Defining the B-Cell Repertoire

With the development of hybridoma technology (Köhler and Milstein, 1975, 1976) has come the possibility of obtaining unlimited amounts of homogeneous immunoglobulins to use in exploring the extent and the origins of antibody diversity. Most of the studies to date have relied on hybridoma antibodies to better characterize and clarify previously studied systems based on myeloma proteins (Claflin and Williams, 1978; Clevinger et al., 1978) or predominant clonotype responses (Reth et al., 1978; Pierres et al., 1979). However, hybridomas can also provide antibodies which are representative of clonotypes present in the repertoire at much lower frequencies (Köhler and Milstein, 1976; Ju et al., 1979; Gerhard, 1976; Reth et al., 1978). While analyses with such antibodies are still preliminary, the findings indicate that any such individual clonotype is so rarely represented in the repertoire that the demonstration of repeats of a given specificity is experimentally impractical. This finding is consistent with those obtained by analyses of monoclonal antibodies derived by standard stimulation protocols of nondominant clonotypes (Sigal and Klinman, 1978; Ju et al., 1977) and supports the conclusion that the repertoire of an individual mouse or murine strain is extremely diverse. Comparative analyses based upon examination of the total repertoire are therefore logistically unattractive and unlikely to answer the basic questions stated above (Klinman and Press, 1975a; Kreth and Williamson, 1973; Köhler, 1976; Cancro et al., 1978b).

However, it should be possible to conduct a definitive analysis using a subset of the entire repertoire. The interpretations of this analysis must take into account the experimental procedures used as well as the mode of selection of this subset of antibodies in order to make inferences on the repertoire as a whole. For example, while standard hybridoma technology may be adequate for the analysis of the antibodies that are expressed in the serum of an animal after repeated antigenic stimulation, the derived hybridomas would represent those clonotypes which dominate the *in vivo* response to that antigen and escape *in vivo* suppressive mechanisms. In addition the choice of the subpopulation to be analyzed must be made with great care, since (1) its biological relevance should be obvious; (2) it should be reproducibly present in all individuals analyzed; and (3) it should be minimally subject to random environmental influences which are impossible for the investigator to control.

III. The Neonatal B-Cell Repertoire

One subpopulation which meets the above criteria is that present in inbred murine strains during their early neonatal development. Since the immune system arises relatively late in ontogeny, late fetal and early neonatal mice have very few immunocytes. Since any given lymphocyte is essentially unipotential, neonates must therefore have a far smaller repertoire than that available to adults. While the degree of this restriction within individuals and within an entire strain is still controversial (D'Eustachio *et al.*, 1976; Goidl *et al.*, 1976), many studies have now verified the restricted nature of the neonatal repertoire (Klinman and Press, 1975b; Sigal *et al.*, 1976; Marshall-Clarke and Playfair, 1978; Silverstein *et al.*, 1963). Since the developing repertoire has obvious biological significance and the fetal and neonatal environment are relatively well controlled, it may be argued that the neonatal repertoire fulfills the above-stated requirements and should provide a restricted subset of specificities which may be amenable to comprehensive and detailed analysis.

An extensive analysis of the neonatal B-cell anti-dinitrophenyl (DNP) and -trinitrophenyl (TNP) response has been performed previously *in vitro* using the splenic fragment system (Klinman and Press, 1975a,b). Fetal or neonatal lymphoid cells adoptively transferred to syngeneic, irradiated, carrier-primed recipient mice are able to produce antihapten antibody when exposed to hapten–carrier conjugates in an organ culture system *in vitro*. The stimulation of neonatal B cells is similar to that of adult B cells by the criteria of antigen dose and the specificity of response. However, due to the smaller number of lymphocytes present in the neonate, a detailed analysis of the clonotypes responsive to an antigen is possible. Using isoelectric focusing to identify individual clonotypes, the neonatal response to DNP and TNP was found to be very restricted (Klinman and Press, 1975b). Three clonotypes specific for each of these haptens were seen in the response for the first two days after birth; after this time the antibody response becomes more diverse and individual clonotypes are difficult to identify (Klinman and Press, 1975a). Other major findings from the stimulation of neonatal B cells in the splenic fragment culture system can be summarized as follows: (1) in the first few days after birth, neonates display disproportionately high frequencies of responsive cells to certain antigens and low frequencies of responsive cells to other antigens when compared to adult frequencies (Sigal and Klinman, 1978); (2) since each individual expresses from 100 to 400 B cells of each of the neonatal clonotypes and there are approximately 10^6 B cells in the neonatal mouse, the responsive repertoire is dominated by approximately 10,000 clonotypes for the first few days of life (Sigal and Klinman, 1978); (3) after four days of postnatal life the repertoire begins to show considerable diversification and reactivity to antigens which was absent in the first few days of life, such as to phosphorylcholine, begins to appear (Sigal et al., 1976); and (4) even as late as two weeks after birth when the repertoire is considerably more diverse than that found earlier in neonatal development, representing as many as 10^6 specificities, the repertoire among individuals appears shared and also demonstrably more restricted than found in adults (Cancro et al., 1979).

While these findings indicate that the neonatal and developing repertoire is sufficiently restricted and reproducible to enable careful assessment of the genetic and environmental influences on repertoire expression, the methods available for detailed analysis have been inadequate to enable firm conclusions. Experimental approaches to defining the neonatal antibody repertoire have, in the past, been largely restricted to analyses by isoelectric focusing, immunoglobulin antigenicity, such as idiotype, and fine specificity of the antibody-combining site (Goidl et al., 1976; Klinman and Press, 1975b; Sigal et al., 1976; Marshall-Clarke and Playfair, 1978; Cancro et al., 1979; Montgomery and Williamson, 1972). While such approaches are adequate for general estimates of the repertoire and provide evidence for sharing of repertoire among individuals, they are not adequate to provide definitive evidence that antibody specificities are shared among individuals at the amino acid sequence level. Furthermore, for many of the neonatal antibodies that have thus far been identified only isoelectric focusing spectra have been available, and these are not useful in comparing variable-region specificities among strains where isoelectric points may differ due to strain-related differences in amino acid sequences in immunoglobulin constant regions. Thus progress in the area of ascertaining the control of neonatal repertoire expression has been precluded by the inability to obtain large amounts of antibodies from selected subpopulations of B cells, such as neonatal B cells responsive to a given antigenic determinant. For this reason it has seemed appropriate to adapt the hybridoma technology to provide antibody-forming cell lines for this purpose. The antigenic stimulation of neonatal B cells in vivo or in a single cell suspension has proven extremely difficult; therefore we have chosen to use neonatal B cells stimulated in vitro in splenic fragment cultures as the antibody-producing cell parent for hybridization. This also permits us to capitalize on the extensive body of knowledge pertinent to the neonatal repertoire of BALB/c mice examined at the monoclonal level.

We will describe here the methods used to obtain hybridomas with antibody-secreting neonatal cells in fragment culture. For the initial studies, the antibody response in the neonate to the hapten DNP was chosen. Responses to this haptenic determinant in fragment culture have been well defined and are sufficiently vigorous to provide an adequate number of large clones for fusion. In addition, screening assays for anti-DNP antibodies are readily available, and monoclonal antibodies obtained from hybridomas can be compared with clonotypes previously identified in the splenic fragment system.

IV. Hybridomas Obtained from Neonatal Splenic Fragment Cultures

The procedures for obtaining monoclonal antibody responses in splenic fragment cultures have been extensively described elsewhere (Klinman and Press, 1975a,b; Klinman, 1972). Briefly, limiting numbers (2–4×10^6) of spleen cells from mice at different stages of postnatal development are injected intraveneously to lethally irradiated (1300 rad), hemocyanin-primed syngeneic adult mice. After 16 to 18 hr, the recipient spleen is removed and chopped into approximately 50 fragments, which are individually placed into microtiter wells and stimulated with DNP–hemocyanin for three days. The culture fluid is then changed every 2 to 3 days and the collected fluids from day 8 to day 9 cultures are assayed for the presence of anti-DNP antibody by radioimmunoassay. The antibody-producing cells in these fragments have been shown to be of donor origin and monoclonal in nature by several criteria. The solid phase radioimmunoassay used is relatively affinity-independent, hapten-specific, and capable of detecting as little as 0.1 ng of antibody (Klinman, 1972; Pierce and Klinman, 1977). Fragments producing anti-DNP antibody can be used for fusion as early as 8 days after stimulation *in vitro,* or as late as 12 days. However, the earlier a fragment is used for fusion, the better the chances of obtaining hybridomas. Cell suspensions are obtained from individual fragments by teasing the fragments with 26-gauge needles in 0.1 ml of Dulbecco's Modified Eagle's Medium (DMEM) supplemented with HEPES buffer (Kennett *et al.,* 1978). The cells from a single fragment are then mixed with the HAT selectable myeloma cells in a 12 × 75-mm tube and washed in DMEM. Successful fusions have been obtained with either the 45.6TG1.7 (Laskov and Scharff, 1970) or the SP2/0-Ag14 (Schulman *et al.,* 1978) cell lines. Currently, fusions are being carried out exclusively with the SP2/0 line, since it is a total nonproducer of immunoglobulin. We have used 2×10^5 to 2×10^6 myeloma cells for fusion and observed a greater efficiency with the highest number of myeloma cells. Thus, in a typical fusion, the cells from a single fragment are added to 2×10^6 washed SP2/0 cells, and the suspension is washed once in DMEM without HEPES or serum and pelleted. After carefully removing all excess culture fluid, the cells are resuspended in 0.2 ml of 30% polyethylene glycol (MW 1000) in DMEM. The cells are exposed to this solution for a total time of 8 min, during which they are subjected to centrifugation at 800 rpm at room temperature for 3 min. After the 8-min incubation, 4 ml of DMEM is added and the cells are washed two times. Following the final wash, cells are suspended in 4 ml of medium containing 10% fetal calf serum. The actual volume used for this incubation is dependent on the number of tumor cells used for fusion, and lesser volumes are used when fewer cells are used. After 24 hrs in a 10% CO_2 atmosphere, the cells are pelleted and resuspended in media containing hypoxanthine–aminopterin–thymidine (HAT). While it is possible to aliquot the cell mixture at this stage into microtiter wells, we have recently found that fusion is optimized by allowing the cells to incubate in 4 ml of medium for 3 to 7 days. After this time, the cells are aliquoted into 8 to 20 microtiter wells. Wells containing growing cells after 10–14 days are tested by radioimmunoassay for anti-DNP antibody. Positive colonies are cloned in semi-solid agarose or by limiting dilution over UV-irradiated feeder cells.

The success rate of this procedure varies with several parameters. As mentioned above, successful fusions appear to be more frequent with day 8 or 9 fragment cultures than those fused at later times. In addition, success seems to be greater with fragments producing higher quantities of antibody presumably indicating that these reflect larger clones of antibody-producing cells. When conditions are maximized and the fragments used for fusion are producing greater than 1 ng of antibody per day on day 8 or 9 of culture, hybridomas are obtained from approximately 50% of the fragments. These fused cell lines appear to be extremely stable and have been successfully cloned and passed in syngeneic animals to obtain ascitic fluid. There appears to be an enormous variance in the rate of antibody production among the fused cell lines. Some produce antibody at a rate comparable to myelomas in that as much as 4 mg/ml can be obtained from ascites. However, the majority of cell lines appear to produce antibody at a significantly lower rate, often yielding less than 0.5 mg antibody/ml ascitic fluid.

Several of the anti-DNP hybridoma antibodies obtained from neonatal fragment cultures have been grown to yield large quantities of antibody, and a few have been studied extensively. Of the four clones most carefully studied, three appear to consist of κ and μ chains and one appears to consist of κ and $\gamma 1$ (Table I). This reflects the immunoglobulin class of the fragment cultures prior to fusion and approximates of the frequency of these classes in neonatal responses. The two κ, μ antibodies which have been studied most extensively were derived from B cells of day 4–5 BALB/c neonates, and the fusions were carried out with the 45.6TG1.7 cell line (Denis et al., 1979). After agar cloning, the secreted products of the two hybridomas were analyzed by sodium dodecyl sulfate–polyacrylamide gel electrophoresis (SDS–PAGE). Intrinsically labeled culture supernatants demonstrated the presence of the MPC11 heavy and light chain [IgG2b,(κ)] as well as the unique IgM heavy chain and κ light chain of each hybridoma (Fig. 1).

The hybridomas were grown intraperitoneally in pristane-primed BALB/c mice, and the ascites fluid collected contained over 1 mg/ml of anti-DNP antibody. A sodium sulfate precipitation of the ascites was carried out, and the dialyzed precipitate was analyzed for antibody affinity by equilibrium dialysis

TABLE I
Neonatal Hybridomas

Hybridoma	Age of neonatal B-cell donor	Myeloma parent	Immunoglobulin class	K_0 23° (liters/mole)
415-26	Day 4–5	45.6TG1.7	μ, κ	6.9×10^4
432-10	Day 4–5	45.6TG1.7	μ, κ	4.8×10^4
FF8-6g	Day 4–5	SP2/0Ag14	γ_1, κ	1.8×10^5
FF12-13b	Day 4–5	SP2/0Ag14	μ, κ	ND

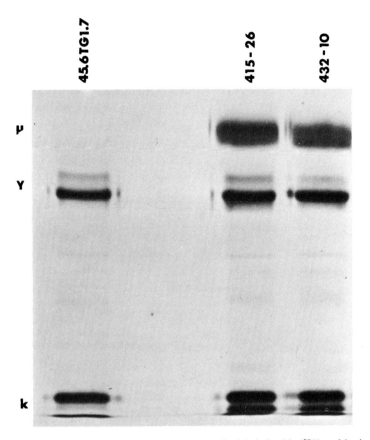

FIGURE 1. SDS–Page. Culture supernatants metabolically labeled with [^{35}S]methionine for 18 hr were reduced and applied to a 10% SDS–polyacrylamide slab gel crosslinked with DATD (N,N'-diallyltartardiamide). Shown is a 24-hr autoradiograph of 415-26 and 432-10 and the myeloma parent line 45.6TG1.7. The myeloma secretes a γ2b chain and a κ chain. Both of the hybridomas secrete these two chains in addition to an anti-DNP μ and κ chain.

(Klinman, 1971). Both IgM hybridomas displayed a relatively low association constant at 23°C, approximately 7 and 5 × 10^4 liters/mole (Table I). Subsequent studies on one of the IgG1 hybridomas showed its association constant to be 2 × 10^5 at 23°C.

The anti-DNP antibody from ascites was purified by affinity chromotography using TNP–BSA (bovine serum albumin) Sepharose with subsequent elution with 0.1 M 2,4-dinitrophenol. The dialyzed antibody was subjected to gel electrophoresis in urea and displayed a single heavy chain and two light chains, one presumably derived from the myeloma parent (Denis *et al.*, 1979). Amino acid sequence analysis of both the heavy and light chains is currently being carried out in the laboratories of M. Margolies and E. Haber. The purified antibodies were injected into A/He mice and rabbits in order to raise antiidiotypic antibodies. To date, the murine responses have been poor. Rabbits which were immunized with three subcutaneous injections of 3 mg antibody given 2 weeks

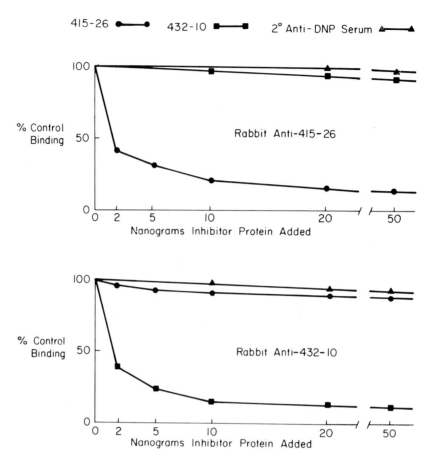

FIGURE 2. Specificity of antiidiotypic antisera. The relative inhibitory patterns of 415-26, 432-10, and a BALB/c secondary anti-DNP antiserum are shown for rabbit anti-415-26 and rabbit anti-432-10.

apart did, however, give a strong response. The serum obtained from these rabbits was adsorbed extensively against ascites fluid containing the nonhomologous IgM hybridoma antibody. The adsorbed sera were then tested for specificity in an inhibition radioimmunoassay against MOPC 104E [IgM(λ)], ABPC 22 [IgM(κ)] and TEPC 15 [IgA(κ)]. No reactivity was seen against these proteins, although the purified homologous hybridoma antibody gave over 90% inhibition (Denis *et al.*, 1979). Preliminary analysis of the anti-DNP antibody present in immunized adult BALB/c mice shows little or no inhibition of this idiotype-specific reaction by the serum antibodies (Fig. 2). In addition, a large array of adult and neonatal monoclonal antibodies were analyzed for the presence of this idiotype. Preliminary evidence indicates that fewer than 5% of adult monoclonal antibodies exhibited even partial reactivity to this antibody (Table II). Since the hybridomas were obtained from neonates at 4–5 days of age, it was anticipated that these hybridomas might express the predominant neonatal clonotypes. Idiotypic analysis with both of these antibodies revealed, however, that only 6% of

TABLE II
Reactivity of Antibodies Derived from Fragment Culture with Antiidiotype Sera

Age of B-cell donor	Rabbit anti-415-26		Rabbit anti-432-10	
	No. positive/ No. tested	Percent positive	No. positive/ No. tested	Percent positive
Day 2–4	16/274	5.8	17/274	6.2
Day 7	1/36	2.7	0/36	0
Adult	1/64	1.6	3/64[a]	4.7

[a]Two of these antibodies were derived from the same adult donor.

early neonatal monoclonal antibodies partially inhibited these antiidiotype antibodies. However, in light of findings using hybridomas containing mixed light chains in better-defined idiotype systems (Claflin, 1980) it is difficult to interpret these results as indicating a paucity of identical or cross-reacting clonotypes in the neonate. Future studies will employ hybridomas derived from nonsecretor myelomas to eliminate the contamination of parental immunoglobulin and thus should clarify the idiotype analysis.

Similar analyses are now being carried out on a large number of monoclonal antibodies derived from neonates of various ages, including those less than 2 days of age. This approach can provide significant numbers of specific probes into the B-cell repertoire at a very early time in ontogeny. Since the use of hybridomas enables analyses at the molecular, amino acid, and nucleic acid levels, it is hoped that continued extensive analyses of this sort will ultimately yield definitive answers to many major questions relevent to the immune mechanism.

ACKNOWLEDGMENT

This work was supported by NIH grants CA-09140, CA-24263, and AI-08778.

References

Cancro, M. P., Sigal, N. H., and Klinman, N. R., 1978a, Differential expression of an equivalent clonotype among BALB/c and C57BL/6, *J. Exp. Med.* **147**:1.

Cancro, M. P., Gerhard, W., and Klinman, N. R., 1978b, The diversity of the influenza-specific primary B-cell repertoire in BALB/c mice, *J. Exp. Med.* **147**:776.

Cancro, M. P., Wylie, D. E., Gerhard, W., and Klinman, N. R., 1979, Patterned acquisition of the antibody repertoire: The diversity of the hemagglutinin-specific B-cell repertoire in neonatal Balb/c mice, *Proc. Natl. Acad. Sci. USA* **76**:6875.

Claflin, J. L., 1980, Analysis of antibodies in the repertoire in pneumococcal phosphocholine using mouse hybridomas, in: *Microbiology—1980* (D. Schlessinger, ed.), American Society for Microbiology, Washington, D.C.

Claflin, J. L., and Williams, K., 1978, Mouse myeloma–spleen cell hybrids: Enhanced hybridization frequencies and rapid screening procedures, *Curr. Top. Microbiol. Immunol.* **81:**107.

Clevinger, B., Hansburg, D., and Davie, J., 1978, Murine anti-a($1 \rightarrow 3$) dextran antibody production by hybrid cells, *Curr. Top. Microbiol. Immunol.* **81:**110.

Cohn, M., Blomberg, B., Geckeler, W., Raschke, W., Riblet, R., and Weigert, M., 1974, First-order considerations in analyzing the generator of diversity, in: *The Immune System: Genes, Receptors, Signals* (E. E. Sercarz, A. R. Williamson, and C. F. Fox, eds.), Academic Press, New York, pp. 89–117.

Cosenza, H., and Köhler, H., 1972, Specific suppression of the antibody response by antibodies to receptors, *Proc. Natl. Acad. Sci. USA* **69:**2701.

Denis, K. A., Kennett, R. H., and Klinman, N. R., 1979, Hybridomas expressing neonatal anti-DNP clonotypes (abstract), *J. Supramol. Struct. [Suppl.]* **3:**312.

D'Eustachio, P., Cohen, J. E., and Edelman, G. M., 1976, Variation and control of specific antigen-binding cell populations in individual fetal mice, *J. Exp. Med.* **144:**259.

Eichmann, K., 1975, Genetic control of antibody specificity in the mouse, *Immunogenetics* **2:**491.

Fernandez, C., and Moller, G., 1978, Immunological unresponsiveness to native dextran B512 in young animals of dextran high responder strains is due to lack of Ig receptor expression, *J. Exp. Med.* **147:**645.

Gearhart, P. J., and Cebra, J. J., 1978, Idiotype sharing by murine strains differing in immunoglobulin allotype, *Nature* **272:**264.

Gearhart, P. J., Sigal, N., and Klinman, N. R., 1975, Heterogeneity of the BALB/c antiphosphorylcholine antibody response at the precursor cell level, *J. Exp. Med.* **141:**56.

Gerhard, W., 1976, The analysis of the monoclonal immune response to influenza virus II. The antigenicity of the viral hemagglutinin, *J. Exp. Med.* **144:**986.

Goidl, E. A., Klass, J., and Siskind, G. W., 1976, Ontogeny of B-lymphocyte function II. Ability of endotoxin to increase the heterogeneity of affinity of the immune response of B lymphocytes from fetal mice, *J. Exp. Med.* **143:**1503.

Imanishi, T., and Makela, O., 1975, Inheritance of antibody specificity II. Anti-(4-hydroxy-5-bromo-3 nitrophenyl)acetyl in the mouse, *J. Exp. Med.* **141:**840.

Ju, S. T., Gray, A., and Nisonoff, A., 1977, Frequency of occurrence of idiotypes associated with anti-p-azophenylarsonate antibodies arising in mice immunologically suppressed with respect to a cross-reactive idiotype, *J. Exp. Med.* **145:**540.

Ju, S. T., Pierres, M., Waltenbaugh, C., Germain, R. N., Benacerraf, B., and Dorf, M. E., 1979, Idiotypic analysis of monoclonal antibodies to poly(Glu^{60}Ala^{30}Tyr^{10}), *Proc. Natl. Acad. Sci. USA* **76:**2942.

Kennett, R. H., Denis, K. A., Tung, A. S., and Klinman, N. R., 1978, Hybrid plasmacytoma production: Fusions with adult spleen cells, monoclonal spleen fragments, neonatal spleen cells and human spleen cells, *Curr. Top. Microbiol. Immunol.* **81:**77.

Klinman, N. R., 1971, Purification and analysis of "monofocal" antibody, *J. Immunol.* **106:**1345.

Klinman, N. R., 1972, The mechanism of antigenic stimulation of primary and secondary clonal precursor cells, *J. Exp. Med.* **136:**241.

Klinman, N. R., and Press, J. L., 1975a, The B-cell specificity repertoire: Its relationship to definable subpopulations, *Transplant. Rev.* **24:**41.

Klinman, N. R., and Press, J. L., 1975b, The characterization of the B-cell repertoire specific for the 2,4-dinitrophenyl and 2,4,6-trinitrophenyl determinants in neonatal BALB/c mice, *J. Exp. Med.* **141:**1133.

Köhler, G., 1976, Frequency of precursor cells against the enzyme β-galactosidase. An estimate of the Balb/c strain antibody repertoire, *Eur. J. Immunol.* **6:**340.

Köhler, G., and Milstein, C., 1975, Continuous cultures of fused cells secreting antibody of predefined specificity, *Nature* **256:**495.

Köhler, G., and Milstein, C., 1976, Derivation of specific antibody-producing tissue culture and tumor lines by cell fusion, *Eur. J. Immunol.* **6:**511.

Kreth, H. W., and Williamson, A. R., 1973, The extent of diversity of antihapten antibodies in inbred mice: Anti-NIP (4-hydroxy-5 iodo-3 nitrophenacetyl) antibodies in CBA/H mice, *Eur. J. Immunol.* **3**:141.

Laskin, J. A., Gray, A., Nisonoff, A., Klinman, N. R., and Gottlieb, P. D., 1977, Segregation at a locus determining an immunoglobulin genetic marker for the light chain variable region affects inheritance of expression of an idiotype, *Proc. Natl. Acd. Sci. USA* **74**:4600.

Laskov, R., and Scharff, M. D., 1970, Synthesis, assembly, and secretion of γ globulin by mouse myeloma cells. I. Adaptation of the MPC11 tumor to culture cloning and characterization of γ globulin subunits, *J. Exp. Med.* **131**:515.

Leon, M., and Young, N. M., 1971, Specificity for phosphorylcholine of six murine myeloma proteins reactive with pneumococcus C polysaccharide and β-lipoprotein, *Biochemistry* **10**:1424.

Lieberman, R., Potter, M., Humphrey, W., and Chien, C. C., 1976, Idiotypes of insulin-binding antibodies and myeloma proteins controlled by genes linked to the allotype locus, *J. Immunol.* **117**:2105.

Makela, O., and Karjalainen, K., 1977, Inherited immunoglobulin idiotypes of the mouse, *Immunol. Rev.* **34**:119.

Marshall-Clarke, S., and Playfair, J. H. L., 1978, Ontogeny of murine B-lymphocytes. Avidity of antigen binding cells in neonatal and adult mice, *Immunology* **34**:1089.

Montgomery, P. C., and Williamson, A. R., 1972, Molecular restriction of antihapten antibody elicited in neonatal rabbits: Antibody production in littermates. *J. Immunol.* **109**:1036.

Nisonoff, A., and Bangasser, S. A., 1975, Immunological supression of idiotypic specificities, *Transplant. Rev.* **27**:100.

Pierce, S. K., and Klinman, N. R., 1977, Antibody-specific immunoregulation, *J. Exp. Med.* **146**:509.

Pierres, M., Ju, S. T., Waltenbaugh, C., Dorf, M. E., Benacerraf, B., and Germain, R. N., 1979, Fine specificity of antibodies to poly(Glu^{60}Ala^{30}Tyr^{10}) produced by hybrid cell lines, *Proc. Natl. Acad. Sci. USA* **76**:2425.

Reth, M., Hammerling, G. J., and Rajewsky, K., 1978, Analysis of the repertoire of anti-NP antibodies in C57BL/6 mice by cell fusion, *Eur. J. Immunol.* **8**:393.

Schulman, M., Wilde, C. D., and Köhler, G., 1978, Introduction and derivation of the Sp2/0-Ag14 cell line for fusion, *Nature* **276**:269.

Sher, A., and Cohn, M., 1972, Inheritance of an idiotype associated with the immune response of inbred mice to phosphorylcholine, *Eur. J. Immunol.* **2**:319.

Sigal, N. H., and Klinman, N. R., 1978, The B-cell clonotype repertoire, *Adv. Immunol.* **28**:255.

Sigal, N. H., Gearhart, P. J., Press, J. L., and Klinman, N. R., 1976, Late acquisition of a germ line antibody specificity, *Nature* **259**:51.

Silverstein, A. M., Uhr, J. W., Kraner, K. L., and Lukes, R. J., 1963, Fetal response to antigenic stimulus II. Antibody production by the fetal lamb, *J. Exp. Med.* **117**:799.

5

The Use of Hybridomas to Localize Mouse Immunoglobulin Genes

Hans Hengartner, Tomaso Meo, and Edith Müller

I. Introduction

The chromosomal assignment of genes for the immunoglobulin (Ig) heavy and light chains has led to very contradictory results over the past few years. Genetic studies clearly demonstrated that the loci for the heavy- and light-chain genes are located on different autosomes (Mage *et al.*, 1973; Weigert and Potter, 1977). By using the V_κ framework peptide marker I_B, Gottlieb mapped the V_κ locus close to the *Ly2,3* region on chromosome 6 (Gottlieb, 1974). This finding was supported by analyzing κ chains of normal antisera (Gibson, 1976) or κ chains of antiphosphorylcholine antibodies (Claflin, 1976; Claflin *et al.*, 1978) and by studies of the inheritance pattern of an idiotype on antibodies to phenylarsonate (Laskin *et al.*, 1977).

More recent results were obtained by somatic cell genetics either by analysis of secreted Ig chains and correlation with the presence of particular human (Smith and Hirschhorn, 1978) or mouse (Hengartner *et al.*, 1978b) chromosomes or by DNA-hybridization analysis with different probes and correlation with the presence of particular mouse chromosomes (Valbuena *et al.*, 1978).

The purpose of this chapter is to describe the approach we used in making chromosomal assignments for the Ig(κ) light-chain and the Ig heavy-chain genes

Hans Hengartner, Tomaso Meo, and Edith Müller • Basel Institute for Immunology, CH-4005 Basel 5, Switzerland.

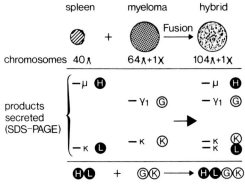

Figure 1. The fusion of a spleen cell with a myeloma cell. Spleen cells of normal mice have 40 acrocentric chromosomes. The cells of two feral mouse populations, CB and CD (Capanna *et al.*, 1976), exhibit karyotypes consisting of 18 metacentric plus 4 acrocentric chromosomes. The Heavy (μ) and the Light (κ) chains are of spleen, the Gamma (γ₁) and Kappa chains of myeloma origin.

in the mouse. Cell hybrids were obtained by fusing spleen cells with the myeloma cell line P3/X63-Ag8, and loss of Ig chain expression was correlated with mitotic loss of individual chromosomes of spleen cell origin.

II. The Experimental System

A. General Concept: Somatic Cell Genetics

Somatic cell hybrids between the mouse myeloma P3/X63-Ag8 and spleen cells usually secrete two sets of Ig heavy and light chains (Fig. 1). One is of myeloma (GK) and the other of spleen cell (HL) origin (Köhler and Milstein, 1976). Chain loss mutants of such hybrids can be obtained by analyzing randomly selected subclones or by screening for subclones which lost a certain antibody activity (Köhler and Milstein, 1976).

The sequence of chain losses follows a pattern (Köhler *et al.*, 1978). The first loss is always either one of the two heavy chains, H or G. After this initial loss, the remaining heavy chain or the two light chains can be lost. While there are no myelomas or hybridomas which secrete only Ig heavy chains, secretors of only light chains are rather frequent. Aside from the above restriction the loss of the ability to secrete an Ig chain is a random event. When hybridomas which secrete the two complete sets of Ig heavy and light chains are selected right after the fusion event, they regularly show much higher chromosome numbers than hybridomas after several subclonings, which secrete only one or two of the original four Ig chains.

Technically it is extremely difficult to correlate chain loss with chromosome loss, since such hybridomas theoretically contain one metacentric plus 104 acro-centric chromosomes: 40 acrocentric chromosomes of the normal mouse cell and one metacentric plus 64 acrocentric chromosomes of the myeloma cell P3/X63-Ag8. In addition, there is no way of determining whether a particular chromosome was derived from the spleen cell or from the myeloma. The cytoge-netic analysis of hybridomas and their variants was greatly facilitated by using lymphocytes from two feral mouse populations, CB and CD (Capanna *et al.*, 1976), instead of normal mice for fusions with the myeloma cell line. As a result of extensive centric fusions (Robertsonian translocations) the karyotypes of both CB and CD consist of nine pairs of metacentric chromosomes. The nine meta-centric chromosomes of CB mouse origin are formed from the following com-binations of normal acrocentrics: 18/1, 17/2, 11/4, 7/6, 13/3, 15/5, 14/8, 12/10, 16/9; for the CD mouse the combinations are: 7/1, 8/3, 13/6, 15/4, 11/10, 18/2, 17/5, 14/12, 16/9. Chromosome 19 and the two sex chromosomes are the only acrocentric chromosomes in both CB and CD mice. With the exception of one chromosome 16/9, the chromosomes of CB and CD mice represent different combinations of the original acrocentric chromosomes. The involvement of the same chromosomes in different translocations allows us in principle to assign genes to all murine chromosomes except 16, 9, and the sex chromosomes. The

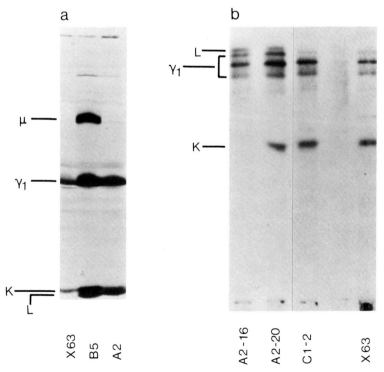

FIGURE 2. Analysis of radioactive cell products by (a) SDS-PAGE and (b) isoelectric focusing pH 5–9. The letters refer to subclones of clone XCD9-C5, X63 to the myeloma X63–Ag8.

metacentric chromosomes of CB and CD mice show no alterations in banding patterns following trypsin G staining (Buckland et al., 1976) when compared to the corresponding acrocentric chromosomes of normal mice. The secreted products can easily be traced by SDS–polyacrylamide gel electrophoresis (SDS–PAGE) or isoelectric focusing (Fig. 2) to the myeloma or lymphocyte.

B. Derivation and Characterization of Hybridomas and Their Variants

Following the protocol of Köhler and Milstein (1975, 1976), a number of hybridomas were prepared by fusing spleen cells of CB and CD mouse origin with the cell line P3/X63-Ag8. Three different hybridomas were selected on the basis of good cell growth and good distinguishability of the secreted products for a detailed biochemical and cytogenetic analysis: XCD9, XCB23, and XCB1, where the prefix XCB and XCD denote strains derived by fusion with CB and CD cells, respectively. These cell hybrids were cloned and subcloned on soft agar (Cowan et al., 1974; Hengartner et al., 1978a), and a large number of clones were analyzed in order to get chain loss variants. The screening was carried out by SDS–PAGE (Cowan et al., 1974) and isoelectric focusing (Köhler et al., 1976) of ^{14}C-labeled intracellular and secreted Ig (Fig. 2). Figure 3 shows the different hybridomas and their chain loss variants.

The cells of the clones listed in Fig. 3 were arrested at mitosis by colchicine treatment, and the chromosomes were prepared using conventional cytogenetic techniques (Hengartner et al., 1978b). The chromosomes were stained by a trypsin G banding technique (Buckland et al., 1976). Karyograms of the different hybrids were made from photographs of randomly selected metaphases. Only the metacentric chromosomes were analyzed. Hybrids were considered to have retained a given pair of the nine metacentric chromosomes when more than 70% of the metaphases analyzed contained both homologous chromosomes, whereas they were considered to have retained one copy of the homologous metacentric chromosomes when more than 90% of metaphases showed the presence of only one copy.

The metacentric chromosome of P3/X63-Ag8 could be distinguished very easily from the metacentric ones of CB or CD mouse origin. Table I shows an example of karyotype analysis of two hybrids: (1) the analysis of a hybrid which secretes HLGK, and (2) the analysis of its LGK chain loss variant. The complete karyotype and biochemical analyses of all the different clones are summarized in Tables II and III.

The 29 karyograms of clone ACD9-C5-C2 (Table I) and the analysis of XCD9-C5 and XCD9-C5-B5 show a consistent loss of one copy of chromosome 8/3 without affecting the secretion of the H or the L chain. The 28 karyograms of the LGK-secreting subclone XCD9-C5-A2 (Table I) is representative for the karyograms for the further subclones A4, B2, C4, D1, and A4-5 of clone XCD9-C5 (Table II). All the subclones which lack the expression of the H chain lost one copy of chromosome 14/12.

The analogous analysis of HLGK and LGK-secreting subclones of XCB23

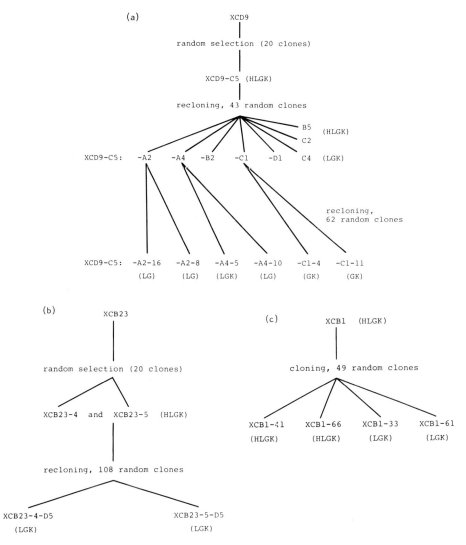

FIGURE 3. Derivation of subclones from hybridomas (a) XCD9, (b) XCB23, and (c) XCB1. [Taken from Hengartner *et al.*, 1978b.]

shows that the loss of one copy of chromosome 12/10 leads to the loss of the expression of the heavy chain *H* (Table III). The common cytogenetic feature of the XCD and XCB LGK-secreting variants was the loss of one copy of chromosome 12. But one copy of chromosome 12 is sufficient to express the same heavy chain as visualized by clones XCB1-41 and XCB1-66 (Table III). Several light-chain (L and K) variants of XCD9 origin were selected. The LG variants, the ones which lost the ability to secrete the myeloma κ light chain, show, as expected, identical karyograms with respect to the metacentric chromosomes as the LGK variants. The two GK variants C1-11 and C1-4 of XCD9-C5 origin, which

Table I
Karyotype Analysis of the Metacentric Chromosomes of an HLGK and of a LGK Secretor[a]

Preparation	7/1	8/3	13/6	15/4	11/10	18/2	17/5	14/12	16/9	Acro-centrics
				Clone: XCD9-C5-C2 (HLGK)						
28/1	X	X	X							67
27/6		X		X		X				69
28/2		X		X					X	60
28/5		XX	X			X			X	64
28/3		X	X							65
28/4		X							X	58
28/7		X							57	
27/10		X		X						64
27/8		X		X						67
27/11		X		X						67
27/1		X			X			X		63
27/2		X							X	62
27/4		X								63
27/5		XX							X	62
27/7		X								63
27/9		X					X			60
29/6		X		X						59
28/8		X								66
29/8		X								67
29/9		X					X	X		64
29/2		XX							X	71
29/3		X					X		X	65
29/4		X							X	63
29/5		X					X			69
29/1		X								62
29/7		XX								59
13/2		X								68
13/7	X	X	XX							68
13/6		X								68
				Clone: XCD9-C5-A2 (LGK)						
30/3		X	X				X	X	X	64
29/10		X				X		X		62
30/8		X				X		X	X	59
30/5		X						X		95
32/6		XX				X		X		55
31/4		X								56
32/4		X		X			X	X	X	61
32/7		X			X			X		62
31/3		X						X		65
32/5		X						X	X	65
31/2		X	X					X		62
32/1		X					X		57	
32/3		X						X		64
31/1		X						X		64
31/7		X		X				X		50
31/6		X					X	X		61

TABLE I
(Continued)

Preparation	7/1	8/3	13/6	15/4	11/10	18/2	17/5	14/12	16/9	Acro-centrics
			Clone: XCD9-C5-A2 (LGK) *(continued)*							
31/5		X						X		60
31/8		X						X		63
30/4		X						X		64
30/7		X					X	X		96
32/2		X						X		59
30/6		X						X		63
30/1		X			X			XX		66
30/9		X						X		56
32/8		XX						X		62
15/7		XX		X			X	X		57
16/5		X						X		66
16/1		XX	X					X		66

[a]X refers to a loss of one copy of the two autosomes.

TABLE II
Distribution of CD Metacentric Chromosomes in XCD9-C5 and Selected Subclones[a]

Hybrid clones (karyotyped metaphases)		Set of Ig chains	Metacentric chromosomes of CD origin								
			7/1	8/3	13/6	15/4	11/10	18/2	17/5	14/12	16/9
XCD9-C5	(6)	HLGK	2	1	2	2	2	2	2	2	2
XCD9-C5-C2	(29)	HLGK	2	1	2	2	2	2	2	2	2
XCD9-C5-B5	(5)	HLGK	2	1	2	2	2	2	2	2	2
XCD9-C5-A2	(28)	LGK	2	1	2	2	2	2	2	1	2
XCD9-C5-A4	(18)	LGK	2	1	2	2	2	2	2	1	2
XCD9-C5-B2	(8)	LGK	2	1	2	2	2	2	2	1	2
XCD9-C5-C4	(7)	LGK	2	1	2	2	2	2	2	1	2
XCD9-C5-D1	(6)	LGK	2	1	2	2	2	2	2	1	2
XCD9-C5-A4-5	(8)	LGK	2	1	2	2	2	2	1	1	2
XCD9-C5-A2-16	(10)	LG	2	1	2	2	2	2	2	1	2
XCD9-C5-A4-10	(5)	LG	2	1	2	2	2	2	2	1	2
XCD9-C5-C1-4	(13)	GK	2	1	1	2	2	2	2	1	2
XCD9-C5-C1-11	(4)	GK	2	1	1	2	2	2	2	1	2

[a]Taken from Hengartner *et al.* (1978b).

TABLE III
Distribution of CB Metacentric Chromosomes in Selected Clones of XCB23 and XCB1

Hybrid clones (karyotyped metaphases)		Set of Ig chains	Metacentric chromosomes of CB origin								
			18/1	17/2	11/4	7/6	13/3	15/5	14/8	12/10	16/9
XCB23-4-B5	(21)	HLGK	2	2	2	2	2	2	2	2	2
XCB23-4-C1	(6)	HLGK	2	1	2	2	1	2	2	2	2
XCB23-5-B1	(7)	HLGK	2	2	2	2	1	2	1	2	2
XCB23-5-B3	(8)	HLGK	2	2	2	2	1	2	2	2	2
XCB23-4-D5	(30)	LGK	2	2	2	2	1	2	2	1	2
XCB23-5-D5	(8)	LGK	2	2	2	2	2	2	1	1	2
XCB1	(6)	HLGK	2	2	2	2	2	2	2	2	2
XCB1-41	(8)	HLGK	2	1	1	1	–	2	1	1	2
XCB1-66	(10)	HLGK	2	1	1	1	–	2	1	1	2
XCB1-33	(7)	LGK	2	1	1	1	1	2	1	1	1
XCB1-61	(10)	LGK	2	1	1	1	–	2	1	1	2

no longer secrete the light chain of CD origin, lost one copy of chromosome 13/6.

The three subclones -41, -66, and -61 of XCB1 still secreting the CB type of light chain L lost both copies of chromosome 13/3, whereas all of them retained one copy of chromosome 7/6. The analogous conclusion can be drawn as for the heavy chain: The presence or absence of one copy of chromosome 6 is responsible for the expression of the light chain (L). The light chain L is of κ-light-chain type.

III. Discussion

The experiments described demonstrate that hybrid cells between myeloma and spleen cells of the two populations of feral mice, CB and CD, provide the means of correlating the presence of a particular chromosome and the expression of a biochemical marker. Using hybridomas of CB or CD and myeloma cells, it is possible to distinguish between chromosomes of myeloma and spleen cells for all but chromosome 19 and the sex chromosomes, and the metacentric chromosomes can be identified with much less ambiguity than acrocentric chromosomes.

The analyzed biochemical markers encoded on the metacentric chromosomes of the hybridomas were the μ and the κ chains. We assigned the genes responsible for the μ heavy chain production to chromosome 12 (Hengartner et al., 1978b). In the mouse there is close linkage of the Ig-1 (γ_{2a}), Ig-2 (α), Ig-3 (γ_{2b}), Ig-4 (γ_1), Ig-5 (δ), and Ig-6 (μ) loci (Herzenberg et al., 1977), as well as linkage between the prealbumin marker *Pre-1* and *Ig-1* (γ_{2a}) (Taylor *et al.*, 1975). Hence, we are able to conclude that all the genetic markers *Ig-1* to *Ig-6* plus *Pre-1* are located on chromosome 12.

Genetic studies also implied that the genes for the heavy and light chain structures are located on different autosomes and that the loci for the κ- and the λ-type light chains are not genetically linked (Weigert and Potter, 1977). Our experiments suggest that the gene for the κ-type light chain is located on chromosome 6 (Hengartner *et al.*, 1978b), a result which is concordant with earlier studies (Gottlieb, 1974; Claflin, 1976; Gibson, 1976; Claflin *et al.*, 1978; Laskin *et al.*, 1977).

In complete disagreement are hybridization studies by Valbuena *et al.* (1978). The authors used cDNA of conventionally purified mRNA for κ-, λ-, γ_{2b}-, and α-Ig chains as probes to hybridize extracted DNA of nine different mouse–man hybrid cell lines. These hybrids showed segregation of the acrocentric mouse chromosomes. The probable and possible locations of the mouse constant region genes C_K and C_H exclude chromosome 6 and 12, respectively. The degree to which the hybridization probes are pure is very critical for such experiments and might be one of the factors related to the discordant results.

A. Regulatory or Structural Genes

The obvious question is, do the identified chromosomes carry structural or regulatory genes for the expression of Ig chains? Our data as well as the findings of others (Köhler *et al.*, 1976; Margulies *et al.*, 1977) are most easily interpreted using the assumption that they are structural genes. The heavy chain H and light chain L can be lost without affecting the G and K chain production and vice versa. A regulatory gene showing these characteristics would have to act within each set of the parental genes of the hybrid cell. Further support comes from fusion experiments between chain loss variants and myelomas or hybridomas which secrete the same Ig chain subclass type as the one which was lost in one of the fusion partners. No reexpression of the lost Ig chain has ever been observed (Köhler *et al.*, 1976; Margulies *et al.*, 1977). Complementation of genes by fusion even within the same subclass of heavy chains does not occur.

B. Allelic Exclusion of Allotypes

The cytogenetic analysis clearly demonstrated that the loss of one copy of chromosome 6 or 12 causes the loss of the expression of the Ig light and heavy chain expression, respectively. The presence of one copy of chromosome 6 or 12 can be sufficient to express the light or the heavy chain, respectively. Hence, we conclude that the Ig gene complexes on the two homologous chromosomes are in different stages of differentiation. One copy may contain the gene(s) that code(s) for an Ig chain in an "active" form, the other in an "inactive" form.

The molecular analysis of DNA suggests that there are at least two possible arrangements of variable and constant region genes. One is an embryonic form, and the other is characteristic for myeloma cells (Brack *et al.*, 1978; Hozumi and Tonegawa, 1976). The phenomenon of allelic exclusion of allotypes could be explained if the variable and constant region genes are rearranged on one copy of the two chromosomes only, the inactive form remaining in the embryonic state. Alternatively, it is possible that the variable and constant region genes are rearranged on both chromosomes but on one copy in an abortive way. Molecular analysis of the light- and heavy-chain DNA from the various chain loss variants should aid in further explaining the presented observations.

ACKNOWLEDGMENTS

We acknowledge the critical reading of the manuscript by Dr. Jack Haar and Professor Charles Steinberg from the Basel Institute for Immunology and Dr. Hansjakob Müller, Kinderspital Basel. We thank Dr. E. Cupanna, University of Rome, for kindly supplying us with CB and CD mice. The excellent technical assistance of Regina Taslimi and the secretarial assistance of Ms. Sharon Buser and Ms. Mariella Imrie are gratefully acknowledged.

References

Brack, C., Hirama, M., Lenhard-Schuller, R., and Tonegawa, S., 1978, A complete immunoglobulin gene is created by somatic recombination, *Cell* **15**:1.

Buckland, R. A., Fletcher, J. M., and Chandley, A. C., 1976, Characterization of the domestic horse karyotype using G- and C-banding techniques, *Experientia* **32**:1146.

Capanna, E., Gropp, A., Winking, H., Noack, G., and Civitelli, M. V., 1976, Robertsonian metacentrics in the mouse, *Chromosoma* **58**:341.

Claflin, J. L., 1976, Uniformity in the clonal repertoire for the immune response to phosphorylcholine in mice, *Eur. J. Immunol.* **6**:669.

Claflin, J. L., Taylor, B. A., Cherry, M., and Cubberley, M., 1978, Linkage in mice of genes controlling an immunoglobulin kappa-chain marker and the surface alloantigen Ly-3 on T lymphocytes, *Immunogenetics* **6**:379.

Cowan, N. J., Secher, D. S., and Milstein, C., 1974, Intracellular immunoglobulin chain synthesis in nonsecreting variants of a mouse myeloma: Detection of inactive light-chain mRNA, *J. Mol. Biol.* **90**:691.

Gibson, D., 1976, Genetic polymorphism of mouse immunoglobulin light chains revealed by isoelectric focusing, *J. Exp. Med.* **144**:298.

Gottlieb, P. D., 1974, Genetic correlations of a mouse light chain variable region marker with a thymocyte surface antigen, *J. Exp. Med.* **140**:1432.

Hengartner, H., Luzzati, A. L., and Schreier, M., 1978a, Fusion of *in vitro* immunized lymphoid cells with X63-Ag8, in: *Current Topics in Microbiology and Immunology*, Vol. 81 (F. Melchers, M. Potter, and N. Warner, eds.), Springer-Verlag, Berlin, Heidelberg, p. 92.

Hengartner, H., Meo, T., and Müller, E., 1978b, Assignment of genes for immunoglobulin kappa and heavy chains to chromosomes 6 and 12, *Proc. Natl. Acad. Sci. USA* **75**:4494.

Herzenberg, L. A., Herzenberg, L. A., Black, S. J., Loken, M. R., Okumura, L. K., van der Loo, W., Osborne, B. A., Hewgill, D., Goding, J. W., Gutman, G., and Warner, N. L., 1977, Surface markers and functional relationships of cells involved in murine B-lymphocyte differentiation, *Cold Spring Harbor Symp. Quant. Biol.* **41**:33.

Hozumi, N., and Tonegawa, S., 1976, Evidence for somatic rearrangement of immunoglobulin genes coding for variable and constant regions, *Proc. Natl. Acad. Sci. USA* **73**:3628.

Köhler, G., and Milstein, C., 1975, Continuous cultures of fused cells secreting antibody of predefined specificity, *Nature* **256**:495.

Köhler, G., and Milstein, C., 1976, Derivation of specific antibody-producing tissue culture and tumor lines by cell fusion, *Eur. J. Immunol.* **6**:511.

Köhler, G., Howe, S. C., and Milstein, C., 1976, Fusion between immunoglobulin secreting and nonsecreting myeloma cell lines, *Eur. J. Immunol.* **6**:292.

Köhler, G., Hengartner, H., and Milstein, C., 1978, The sequence of immunoglobulin chain losses in mouse (myeloma × B-cell) hybrids, in: *Protides of the Biological Fluids* (H. Peeters, ed.), Pergamon Press, Oxford and New York, pp. 545–549.

Laskin, J. A., Gray, N. R., Nisonoff, N. R., Klinman, N. R., and Gottlieb, P., 1977, Segregation at a locus determining an immunoglobulin V$_L$-region genetic marker affects inheritance of expression of an idiotype, *Proc. Natl. Acad. Sci. USA* **74**:4600.

Mage, R., Lieberman, R., Potter, M., and Terry, W. D., 1973, in: *The Antigens* (M. Sela, ed.), Academic Press, New York, pp. 299–376.

Margulies, D. H., Cieplinski, W., Dharmgrongartama, B., Gefter, M. L., Morrison, S. L., Kelly, T., and Scharff, M. D., 1977, Regulation of immunoglobulin expression in mouse myeloma cells, *Cold Spring Harbor Symp. Quant. Biol.* **41**:781.

Smith, M., and Hirshhorn, 1978, Location of the genes for human heavy chain immunoglobulin to chromosome 6, *Proc. Natl. Acad. Sci. USA* **75**:3367.

Taylor, B. A., Bailey, D. W., Cherry, M., Riblet, R., and Weigert, M., 1975, Genes for immunoglobulin heavy chain and serum prealbumin protein are linked in mouse, *Nature* **256**:644.

Valbuena, O., Marcu, K. B., Croce, C. M., Huebner, K., Weigert, M., and Perry, R. P., 1978, Chromosomal locations of mouse immunoglobulin genes, *Proc. Natl. Acad. Sci. USA* **75**:2883.

Weigert, M., and Potter, M., 1977, Antibody variable-region genetics, *Immunogenetics* **4**:401.

PART III
DETECTION AND ANALYSIS OF HUMAN GENE PRODUCTS

6
Monoclonal Antibodies as Tools for Human Genetic Analysis

E. Solomon and E. A. Jones

I. Introduction

Research in human genetics includes areas such as mRNA and gene isolation; structural studies of enzymes and proteins and the interaction of their subunits; structural and population studies of protein polymorphisms; somatic cell genetics, including gene mapping; development and differentiation involving cell- and tissue-specific cell-surface antigens; chromosome structure and function; immunogenetics; and clinical genetics, including inherited metabolic disorders, chromosome abnormalities, and transplantation antigens. It is safe to predict that monoclonal antibodies will be used in all of these areas within a short time. Their advantages over conventional antisera for human genetic analysis, as for other areas, lie in their monospecificity, high titer, and availability in large quantities. Coupled with this is the fact that these extremely pure and specific antibodies may be produced from immunizations with relatively crude material. Of additional advantage to human genetics is their potential in clinical work for diagnostic and possibly therapeutic purposes.

Many workers in human genetics have already utilized the unique properties of monoclonal antibodies, and some of these studies are discussed in other chapters of this book. Rather than concentrate on one area in this chapter, we have chosen to present a number of different studies so as to demonstrate a variety of approaches and possible types of analysis. The antigens we describe are two components of the classical complement pathway, C1q and briefly C3; the membrane-associated enzyme alkaline phosphatase; determinants coded for

E. Solomon and E. A. Jones • Genetics Laboratory, Department of Biochemistry, University of Oxford, Oxford OX1 3QU, England. *Present address for* E. Solomon: Imperial Cancer Research Fund, P. O. Box 123, Lincoln's Inn Fields, London WC2A 3PX, England. *Present address for* E. A. Jones: Division of Immunology, Stanford University Medical School, Stanford, California 94305.

by the *HLA* region, HLA-A, -B, -C and -DRW, and β_2-microglobulin (β_2m); cell-surface antigens detected in somatic cell hybrids; erythrocyte-specific antigens; and a thymocyte-specific antigen. These areas have little in common other than that the antigens are all products of human genes and have been analyzed by monoclonal antibodies. They were chosen because, first, the work is largely unpublished and we thereby avoid repeating already known data, and, second, they represent a number of different methods of immunization, screening, characterization, and a variety of different uses of the antibodies. These are summarized in Table I.

Immunizations have been carried out with purified soluble proteins, purified membrane proteins, the glycoprotein fraction of membrane preparations, membrane preparations, and whole cells. Screening has been carried out principally by indirect trace-binding assays. Binding is measured either to purified antigen coupled to sheep red blood cells, or flexible plastic microtiter plates, or to whole cells. Characterization and definition of the monoclonal antibodies include inhibition of binding by purified antigen, inhibition of catalytic activity of the antigen, immunoprecipitation of enzymatic activity, and complement-mediated cytotoxicity. Studies with these antibodies include analysis of binding of C1q, biosynthesis of C1q and C3, tissue specificity of alkaline phosphatase, chromosomal location of cell-surface antigens in somatic cell hybrids, analysis of HLA-associated determinants and β_2m, and detection of a thymus-specific antigen in thymic leukemias.

It is difficult to bring these together under any general heading. We have therefore presented each antigen or system as a section on its own. In the discussion we have tried to speculate as to possible future uses for monoclonal antibodies in human genetics.

Many of the same cell lines are used in different sections of this chapter. These lines and their origins are given in Table II.

II. Monoclonal Antibodies against a Variety of Human Gene Products

A. C1q

C1q, a serum protein, is the first subcomponent of the first component (C1) of the classical complement pathway. It is an extremely complicated 18-chain molecule, whose structure has been determined from amino acid sequence data, physical and electron microscopy studies (Reid and Porter, 1976; Reid, 1979; Brodsky-Doyle *et al.*, 1976). The molecule consists of three different protein chains (A, B, C) each represented six times. Each of these chains has a globular region of about 105 amino acid residues, and a region of about 78 residues, which is strikingly like collagen, in that the sequence is $(gly-x-y)_n$, and both

Monoclonal Antibodies Described in This Chapter[a]

Antigen	Antibody	Immunogen	Screening	Characterization	Studies
Clq	48.3M	Purified Clq	Binding to sheep red blood cells, or flexible plastic plates, coated with Clq	Inhibition of Cl hemolytic activity	Binding and biosynthesis of Clq produced by human fibroblasts
C3[b]	WM1	Purified C3	Binding to flexible plastic plates coated with C3	Inhibition of binding by purified C3	Biosynthesis of C3
Alkaline phosphatase	AAP1	Cell membrane (D98/AH2)	Binding to whole cells (D98/AH2)	Immunoprecipitation of alkaline phosphatase activity from cell membrane (D98/AH2)	Tissue specifity of alkaline phosphatase produced by D98/AH2
HLA region determinants (A, B, C and DRW) and β_2 m[c]	W6/32 BBM.1 PA2.1 PA2.2 BB7.1 BB7.2 DA2 3.53	Whole cells; cell membrane; glycoprotein fraction of cell membrane; purified papain-solubilized antigen	Binding to whole cells of immunizing specifity	Inhibition of binding by purified antigen; complement-mediated cytotoxicity; cell type-specific binding (DRW)	Detection and definition of polymorphic determinants by binding and complement-mediated cytotoxicity; genetic analysis with human/mouse somatic cell hybrids; structural studies of the antigens; purification of antigen by affinity chromatography
Chromosome-specific cell-surface antigens	W6/34 W6/45 W6/46 Others	Cell membrane (tonsil)	Binding to whole cells (tonsil)	Binding and complement-mediated cytotoxicity to human/mouse somatic cell hybrids	Definition of cell-surface antigens; genetic mapping of cell-surface antigens
Thymocyte-specific antigen	NA1/34	Thymocytes	Binding to whole cells (thymocytes)	Thymocyte-specific binding and immunoperoxidase staining	Definition of cell type; immunoprecipitation of antigen; definition of thymic-ALL
Erythrocyte-specific antigens	W6/1 W6/28	Cell membrane (tonsil; contaminating erythrocytes)	Binding to erythrocytes, measured by autoradiography	Hemagglutinating activity; erythrocyte-specific binding	Blood group specificity

[a]References are given in the text.
[b]These are preliminary experiments not fully described.
[c]These antibodies are described in detail in Table V.

TABLE II
Cell Lines

	Origin	Reference
Human cell lines		
Bristol 8	B-cell lymphoid line	Goodfellow *et al.* (1976b)
LoVo	Colonic adenocarcinoma	Drewinko *et al.* (1976)
JY	B-cell lymphoid line	Terhorst *et al.* (1976)
Molt 4	Thymus leukemia	Minowada *et al.*(1972)
U937	Macrophage line	Sundstrom and Nilsson (1976)
HT 1080	Fibrosarcoma	Croce (1976)
Butler	Primary fibroblast	Gift of S. Povey
IMR 32	Neuroblastoma	Tumilowicz *et al.* (1970)
JAR	Choriocarcinoma	Patillo *et al.* (1971)
Daudi	B-cell lymphoid line	Klein *et al.* (1967)
HSB2	T-cell lymphoid line	Adams *et al.* (1967)
D98/AH2 (HeLa)	Cervical carcinoma	Szybalski *et al.* (1962)
MAR	Primary fibroblast	Genetics Laboratory, Oxford
ME180	Cervical carcinoma	Sykes *et al.* (1970)
LS174T	Colonic carcinoma	Tom *et al.* (1976)
LKT	B-cell lymphoid line	Genetics Laboratory, Oxford
LNSV	SV40 transformed fibroblast	Croce (1976)
Mouse cell lines		
Clone 1D	L cell	Kit *et al.* (1963)
1.1F	Primary fibroblast	D. Buck, Genetics Laboratory, Oxford

hydroxyproline and hydroxylysine are present (Reid, 1979). Within the assembled molecule the three chains associate to give six "tuliplike" structures. The globular regions of these chains form the "heads" and the collagenlike regions the "stems" by forming a rigid triple helical structure similar to that of collagen (Brodsky-Doyle *et al.*, 1976). Disulfide bonds hold the A—B and C—C chains together. A diagram of the molecule is shown in Fig. 1.

C1q is the molecule that binds to antigen/antibody complexes on the cell surface, and which thereby activates the cascade of the classical complement pathway, resulting in cell lysis. It is believed that binding to the antigen/antibody complex occurs through the "heads" of the C1q molecule and that the subsequent two steps in the complement cascade, the activation of C1r and C1s (second and third subcomponents of C1), occur by the binding of these molecules to the collagenlike tails of C1q (Reid *et al.*, 1977; Knobel *et al.*, 1974; Paques *et al.*, 1979).

Somatic cell genetic techniques have been used to assign the chains of two types of collagen to a particular human chromosome. Preliminary evidence indicates that two chains of Type I collagen [α_1(I) and α_2] and one chain of Type III collagen [α_1 (III)] are coded for by genes on chromosome 7 (Sykes and Solomon, 1978; Solomon and Sykes, 1980). The unique nature of C1q, a soluble serum protein with a collagenlike region, makes it a fascinating molecule to include in studies on the genetics of collagen. It is therefore being mapped with the aim of determining whether it is chromosomally linked to any of the collagen genes.

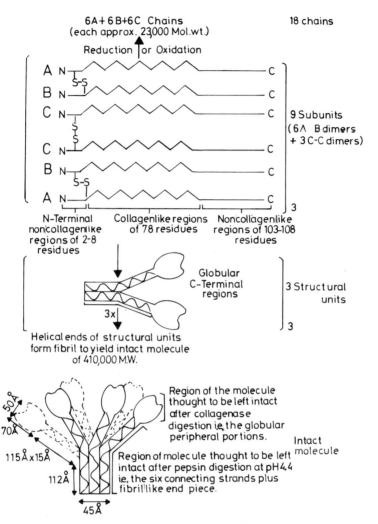

FIGURE 1. Proposed peptide chain structure of human Clq. Dimensions are averages as estimated from electron microscopic studies. $\sim\!\!\!\!\sim\!\!\!\sim$, Proposed triple helix sections, i.e., collagenlike regions of molecule. Length of collagenlike fiber plus fibrillike end piece = 115 Å + 112 Å = 227 Å. Length of triple helix proposed from sequence studies = 80 × 2.9 Å = 232 Å. [Reproduced with permission from Porter and Reid (1978).]

Although several complement components (C2, C4, and Bf) have been shown to be coded for by genes in the *HLA* region (for review see Lachmann and Hobart, 1978) there are currently no data as to the location of Clq. Clq, as well as Clr and Cls, are produced by cultured fibroblasts (Reid and Solomon, 1977). However, it is found that the Clq produced by these cells is of a larger molecular weight form than that found in human serum. The nature of this difference has not so far been determined.

To approach both the structural and genetic questions regarding Clq, monoclonal antibodies are being made to this molecule. First, antibodies specific for different parts of the molecule should be ideal tools for determining the nature of the molecular-weight difference between the serum and fibroblast forms of C1q. Second, the production of a species-specific antibody that will react with human, but not mouse, C1q should enable those genes to be mapped. Rabbit anti-human C1q antiserum cross-reacts with mouse C1q and therefore cannot be used to analyze human/mouse hybrids.

Immunization of mice was carried out with purified C1q (Reid, 1974). Spleen cell/myeloma hybrids were produced by standard methods (see Appendix). Culture medium from possible antibody-producing hybrids was screened for anti-C1q activity by two different methods:

1. Glutaraldehyde-fixed sheep red blood cells were coated with purified C1q (Reid, 1974). A standard trace-binding assay was then performed using [^{125}I]rabbit anti-mouse (RAM) F (ab′)$_2$ as the second antibody. Standard curves and controls were performed with immunized mouse serum, normal mouse serum, culture medium, and uncoated cells. Similar results were obtained with flexible plastic microtiter plates that are passively coated with C1q (Klinman *et al.,* 1976).

2. Serum C1 hemolytic activity was measured by incubation with serum (source of C1) and erythrocytes (E) coated with antibody (A) and C4, giving EAC41 cells. The C1 was activated by heating these cells at 30°C for 60 min. C2 and C3 through C9 are then added, and the degree of lysis of the erythrocytes determined by measuring the $A^{412\text{mm}}_{1\text{cm}}$ of the supernatant (for method see Reid *et al.,* 1977). Inhibition of C1 activity by hybrid-produced anti-C1q antibody was determined by prior incubation of the hybrid medium with the C1 sample and measurement of the degree to which lysis was inhibited.

So far, one monoclonal antibody to C1q has been characterized (Solomon and Reid, unpublished data). Titrations of antibody from cloned hybrid cell medium (48.3) and antibody from mice in which the hybrid was grown as a tumor (48.3M) are shown in Fig. 2. In this assay, performed on flexible plastic microtiter plates, 48.3 typically gives 50% binding at a dilution of about 8×10^{-2} and 48.3M at a dilution of about 2×10^{-5}. The antibody is IgG3.

As shown in Table III, the lysis of antibody-coated sheep red blood cells by human serum C1 is inhibited by 48.3. Lysis by the same number of effective molecules of fibroblast C1q is not inhibited by 48.3. The same results are found with 48.3M. This is consistent with the finding that rabbit anti-human C1q F(ab′)$_2$ has relatively little affinity for fibroblast C1q compared with serum C1q. Both activities are equally inhibited by immune complexes such as ovalbumin/antiovalbumin (Reid and Solomon, 1977).

To determine the position of binding of 48.3 to the serum C1q the antibody is added at different points during the assay. If antibody is added to C1 before binding to the EAC4 cells, inhibition of lysis occurs. If, however, C1 is first incubated with EAC4 cells, and the antibody added subsequently, no inhibition

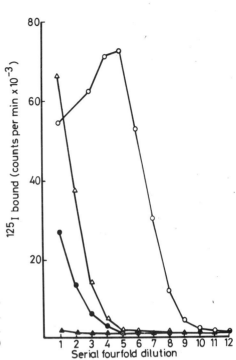

FIGURE 2. Titration of 48.3 and 48.3M in an indirect trace binding assay on plastic microtiter plates. A solution of purified Clq (50 μl, 5 μg) was added to each well. The plates were incubated for 1 hr at room temperature, and then washed four times with phosphate-buffered saline (PBS)/0.11% bovine serum albumin (BSA). The Clq bound is in excess in this assay. Anti-Clq antibody (48.3 and 43.3M) or control solutions (50 μl) were added to each well. The plates were incubated for 1 hr at room temperature and washed three times as above. [^{125}I] RAM F(ab')$_2$ was added to each well (3 $\times$ 10^5 cpm in 50 μl) for 1 hr at room temperature and the plates washed three times. The wells were cut out and counted. (O) 48.3M; (●) normal mouse serum; (Δ) 48.3; (▲) cell culture medium.

TABLE III

Inhibition of Serum and Fibroblast C1 Activity by 48.3[a]

	Percent lysis human serum Cl[b]		Percent lysis fibroblast medium Cl[c]	
Dilution^{-1} of 48.3	+Ab	−Ab	+Ab	−Ab
10	0	100	100	100
20	0		100	
40	0		100	
80	5		100	
100	11		100	
200	23		100	

[a]Cl (human serum or fibroblast medium) was incubated at 30°C for 20 min with EAC4 cells, forming EAC41 cells. These were washed in veronal-buffered saline assay medium at 4°C, resuspended in the same medium, and incubated at 30°C for 60 min. C2 was added; the mixture incubated at 30 °C for 15 min. Ethylenediaminetetraacetic acid (EDTA) was added and then C-EDTA (C3–C9) and incubation continued at 37°C for 1 hr. The degree of lysis of the red blood cells was determined by reading the A$^{412mm}_{1cm}$ (Reid *et al.*, 1977). For inhibition studies dilutions of the antibody were made, and the equivalent amounts (on a hemolytic basis) of either human serum Cl or fibroblast Cl were added to each set of dilutions and the mixtures incubated at 30°C for 20 min, prior to the addition of EAC4 cells. After further incubation at 30°C for 20 min the cells were spun down, resuspended in fresh buffer, and assayed for remaining Cl activity as described above.
  Primary human skin fibroblasts are grown in RPMI 1640 plus 10% inactivated fetal calf serum (FCS). The medium from 5–7-day confluent cultures is the source of fibroblast Cl.
[b]1/10,000 dilution (2 $\times$ 10^9 effective molecules/ml).
[c]2 $\times$ 10^9 effective molecules/ml.

of lysis occurs (see Table IV). These results suggest that 48.3 is specific for the "head" regions of C1q and inhibits the binding of C1q to the antibody/antigen complex. The fact that lysis inhibition does not occur once the C1q is bound to the complex suggests that the antibody does not affect binding of C1r and C1s to the collagenlike tail. Since cultured fibroblast C1q is not inhibited by 48.3, it is possible that this molecule differs from serum C1q in the region that binds to the antibody/antigen complex.

Human serum C1q activity is inhibited by 48.3 at dilutions up to about 1/1500. Mouse serum C1q activity is somewhat inhibited at low dilutions of 48.3, but this inhibition disappears at dilutions of about 1/150. The antibody is therefore species-specific at high dilutions. However, because it is ineffective in inhibiting the fibroblast C1q activity it is not useful for purposes of mapping, using hybrids in which the human parent is a fibroblast. Other antibodies are being prepared for these purposes.

B. C3

Work is also in progress on the production and characterization of monoclonal antibodies to the third (C3) and fourth (C4) components of the classical complement pathway (S. Whitehead, personal communication). As with C1q, one of the purposes is the production of species-specific antibodies for purposes of gene mapping. C3 is a two-chain structure and C4 a three-chain structure. Homology between the A and B chains of C3 and the A and B chains of C 4 has been suggested (see Lachmann and Hobart, 1978). Linkage of C4 to the *HLA* region in man has been shown by family studies, although these do not show which chain is coded for within the region. There is some evidence that the three chains are synthesized as a single-chain precursor, presumably indicating close genetic linkage (Hall and Colten, 1977; Gigli, 1978). Monoclonal antibodies to the individual chains will be of great importance in determining if all three chains are coded for within the *HLA* region and in examining the structure of the precursor molecule. The genetic map location of C3 in man is not known,

TABLE IV

Inhibition of Binding of Serum C1 to EAC4 Cells by 48.3[a]

	First incubation (15 min, 0° C)	Added in second incubation (15 min, 0° C)	Percent lysis
A	C1 + 48.3	EAC4	6
B	C1 + EAC4	48.3	100
C	C1 + EAC4	Buffer	100

[a]Human serum (C1: 2×10^9 effective molecules) was incubated with EAC4 cells at 0° C. At this temperature binding occurs but C1 activation does not. The 48.3 supernatant was used at a dilution of 1/100. After the indicated incubations, the EAC41/antibody complex was spun and the C1 activated by heating to 30° C for 60 min. The assay then continued as described in Table III.

but here, too, chain-specific antibodies will greatly aid in the mapping of the gene for this molecule.

Purified C3 and C4 (Tack and Prahl, 1976; Bolotin *et al.*, 1977) were used for immunizations and monoclonal antibodies to both have been obtained. These are assayed by binding to flexible plastic plates that have been passively coated with C3 or C4. One of the C3 antibodies, WM1, has been used in an inhibition of binding assay to measure C3 production by various cell lines. In an initial screen the following lines do not inhibit the binding of WM1 antibody and are therefore considered negative for C3 production: Bristol 8, LoVo, JY, Molt 4, U937, HT1080, LS174T, 1.1F. Several human fibroblast lines are positive— Butler, FS, MAR, DUV, LNSV—confirming the observation of Senger and Hynes that fibroblastic lines produce C3. The fact that 1.1F, a mouse fibroblast, is negative suggests, as expected, that the antibody is species-specific. This antibody is being used for purposes of gene mapping, using human fibroblast/L-cell hybrids.

C. Alkaline Phosphatase

Immunization of mice with membrane from D98/AH$_2$ and subsequent fusion produced a monoclonal antibody, AAP1, which appears to be against alkaline phosphatase (J. Arklie and J. Trowsdale, personal communication). This tissue-specific enzyme is known to be produced by various lines of HeLa, including D98/AH2 (Benham *et al.*, 1978). Screening by binding on the following lines gives negative results: primary fibroblasts (MAR, Butler), lymphoid lines (Daudi, Bristol 8) and various tumor lines (ME 180, U927, LS174T, LoVo). Positive reactions are seen on D98/AH2, Chang liver, Girardi heart, LV, and FLA (all believed to be derivatives of HeLa).

Butanol extracts of D98 membrane were assayed for alkaline phosphatase activity. Figure 3 shows the results of treating the extracts with AAP1, and

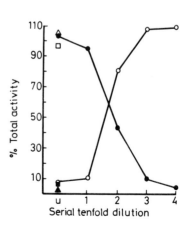

FIGURE 3. Alkaline phosphatase activity in supernatant and pellet, expressed as a percentage of total activity in 20 μl D98/AH2 butanol membrane extract. 10 μl of antibody AAPI was used to precipitate alkaline phosphatase from 20 μl of D98/AH2 extract. This was incubated for 60 min at 4°C, then antigen–antibody complexes precipitated by incubating a further 60 min at 4°C with Staph A cells. The Staph A cells with bound antigen–antibody complex were spun down and washed three times with PBS + 0.1% BSA + 0.5% NP40, then assayed with 0.4 μl p-nitrophenyl phosphate at 37°C for 15 min. The reaction was stopped with 1.2 μl 0.25 N NaOH and read at OD$_{410}$. O, Supernatant from AAPI–Staph A precipitate; ●, AAPI–Staph A precipitate; □, supernatant from X63–NS1–Staph A precipitate; ■, X63–NSI–Staph A precipitate; Δ, supernatant from W6/32–Staph A precipitate; ▲, W6/32–Staph A precipitate. [From J. Arklie and J. Trowsdale, unpublished work.]

precipitation of complex with *Staphylococcus aureus* bearing protein A (Staph A). Alkaline phosphatase activity is measured both in the supernatant and in the precipitate. Increasing amounts of antibody results in increasing amounts of activity in the precipitate and decreasing amounts of the supernatant. Similar results are seen with NP40 extracts. Controls using monoclonal antibody W6/32 (HLA-A, -B, -C) and X63 (mouse myeloma) medium are also shown. In neither case is the alkaline phophatase activity precipitated. Activity of another membrane-associated enzyme, 5'-nucleotidase, is not affected by treatment with antibody AAP1.

Alkaline phosphatases in different lines of HeLa are extremely heterogeneous and include placentalike and liverlike forms, as well as several other forms (Benham *et al.*, 1978). Preliminary results with antibody AAP1, in a screen against various human tissues, including liver, kidney, placenta, lower intestine, and fetal intestine, suggest that the alkaline phosphatase activity recognized is intestinal. Work is in progress to identify more precisely which form(s) of alkaline phosphatase is recognized by this antibody.

D. Antigens of the Major Histocompatibility Complex and Associated Antigens

1. HLA-ABC Antigens and β_2-Microbloblulin

The major human histocompatibility region in man is an extremely complex genetic region coding for at least seven different loci all functionally related within the immune system (Barnstable *et al.*, 1978b). This region, which maps to the short arm of chromosome 6 (Francke and Pellegrino, 1977) codes for the HLA-A, -B, and -C polymorphic determinants, at least one of the two glycoproteins chains that make up the HLA-DRW specificities, some of the complement components of both the classical and alternative pathways, and probably many other determinants involved in cell/cell interactions or the immune system.

The polymorphic HLA-A, -B, and -C antigens consist of two chains. The larger glycoprotein of 43,000 daltons bears the polymorphic determinants and is coded for by a gene within the *HLA* region on chromosome 6 (Crumpton *et al.*, 1978). The smaller is a protein chain of 12,000 daltons coded for by a gene on chromosome 15 (Goodfellow *et al.*, 1975).

The HLA–DRW antigens consist of two noncovalently associated glycoprotein chains of 28,000 and 33,000 daltons (Crumpton *et al.*, 1978). Studies with somatic cell hybrids suggest that possibly only one of these chains is coded for within the *HLA* region (Barnstable *et al.*, 1977). A major aim of those working in this field has been to find a more reliable source of antibodies to HLA-A, -B, -C and DRW determinants for kidney cross-matching, for studies in disease association, and for research on cell/cell interactions. Previous serology has been carried out, using antisera obtained by fetal–maternal stimulation (Bodmer, 1975), by planned immunization of human volunteers (Thorsby and Kissmeyer-Nielsen, 1969) from multiply transfused individuals or, in limited cases, by heteroantisera made either in rabbits or primates, which can in some cases be rendered polymorphic by absorption (Barnstable et al., 1977; Barnstable et al., 1978; Solheim et al., 1978). These antisera all suffer from disadvantages such as limited availability in large quantities, low titer, and multispecificity.

Production of monoclonal antibodies to both polymorphic and nonpolymorphic determinants on these molecules reduces many of these problems and must eventually replace conventional tissue-typing reagents. Furthermore their role in the understanding of in vitro models of cellular interactions such as specific cell-mediated lympholysis (CML) and mixed lymphocyte culture (MLC) must be invaluable. It is for these reasons that many laboratories are devoting considerable effort to the production of monoclonal antibodies against HLA region determinants.

Table V shows the monoclonal antibody-producing cell lines described in this section together with a description of the immunogen and some basic characteristics of the antibodies. The fusion protocol used to produce these hybrids and the method of cloning are essentially those described in the Appendix. Supernatants are assayed by both complement-dependent cytotoxicity, where possible, and by standard indirect binding assays using [^{125}I]RAM immunoglobulin G (IgG) F(ab')$_2$ (see Appendix).

A number of monoclonal antibodies have now been produced to nonpolymorphic HLA-ABC determinants. The first to be well characterized was W6/32 (Barnstable et al., 1978a). This antibody will be used as an example of such reagents; further examples can be found in Brodsky et al. (1979b). This antibody, produced after immunization with human tonsil leukocyte membrane, is of the IgG2a subclass and is active in complement-mediated cytotoxicity. It was initially screened on a wide range of human cell types, including peripheral blood lymphocytes separated by Ficol/Triosil density centrifugation, B-lymphoid lines, T-lymphoid lines, HeLa, IMR 32, JAR, cells grown from a testicular teratoma, and LoVo. It has also been tested on preparations of human sperm.

All the cells tested, except Daudi, JAR, LoVo, the testicular teratoma, and sperm, gave positive results. Daudi is a B-cell line which lacks β$_2$m and therefore does not express HLA-A, -B, or -C determinants at the cell membrane (Arce-Gomez et al., 1978), although heavy-chain precursors probably exist in the cytosol (Ploegh et al., 1979). This suggests that W6/32 might be directed against these determinants or β$_2$m. Lack of the HLA-ABC or β$_2$m antigens on cells of trophoblastic origin also explains the lack of reaction on JAR (Goodfellow et al., 1976a; Faulk and Temple, 1976). Similarly it has been shown that mouse embryonic teratomas lack H.2K and D determinants (Artzt and Jacob, 1974). Thus from tissue distribution alone it seems likely that W6/32 recognizes an nonpolymorphic determinant on the HLA-ABC molecule or β$_2$m.

Figure 4 shows the complete inhibition of W6/32 with papain-solubilized HLA-A2 antigen. These data suggest that the antigenic determinant is on the glycoprotein chain rather than on the β$_2$m molecule. This is supported by similar results on immunoabsorbent columns, which suggest that the determinant is present on all HLA-A, -B, and -C molecules (Parham et al., 1979).

TABLE V

Origin and Nature of Antibodies Directed against Major Histocompatibility Region Determinants

	Specificity	Ig class	Complement fixing	Protein A binding	Immunogen	Reference
W6/32	anti-HLA-ABC glycoprotein	IgG2a	+	+	Human tonsil leukocyte membrane	Barnstable et al. (1978)
BBM.1	anti-β_2m	IgG2a	+	+	Molt 4 cells	Brodsky et al. (1979a)
PA2.1	anti-HLA-A2	IgG1	–	–	Papain-purified HLA-A2	Parham and Bodmer (1978)
PA2.2	anti-HLA-A, -B polymorphic	IgG	–	+	Papain-purified HLA-A2	Parham and Bodmer (1978)
BB7.1	anti-HLA-B7	IgG1	–	–	Papain-purified	Brodsky et al. (1979b)
BB7.2	anti-HLA-A2	IgG2b	+	+	Papain-purified	Brodsky et al. (1979b)
DA.2	anti-HLA-DRW nonpolymorphic	IgG1	–	–	LKT cell membrane	Brodsky et al. (1980)
3.53	anti-HLA-DRW 1,2,6	IgG1	–	–	Glycoprotein fraction from BRI 8 cell membrane	Brodsky et al. (1980)

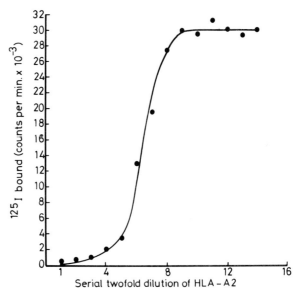

FIGURE 4. Inhibition of binding of W6/32 to Bri8 cells by pure papain-solubilized HLA-A2 antigens. 50 μl of serial dilutions of papain-solubilized HLA-A2 (5 μg/ml) were incubated with 50 μl of a 1 in 500-fold dilution of concentrated W6/32 cell-culture supernatant for 1 hr at room temperature. The inhibited antibody was then tested for indirect trace binding to 10^6 Bri8 cells (Parham *et al.*, 1979).

W6/32 was also tested against a panel of somatic cell hybrids containing limited numbers of human chromosomes. This antibody reacted only with those hybrids containing chromosome 6 or chromosomes 6 and 15, but not those carrying 15 alone. W6/32 does not bind to Horl 9.8R 3.3 (Jones, 1976), which retains only one human chromosome 15 and expresses β_2m.

Data have also been obtained for monoclonal antibodies to β_2m. The first of these antibodies to be characterized is BBM.1, a cytotoxic antibody of the IgG2b subclass (Brodsky *et al.*, 1979a). This was produced by immunization with Molt 4, a T-cell line. This antibody shows identical tissue distribution to W6/32, again showing no reactivity with the Daudi cell line.

Its activity is completely inhibited by papain-solubilized HLA-A, -B, -C antigens and free β_2m (Fig. 5) showing that this antigen is present on both free β_2m and β_2m associated with the polymorphic glycoprotein chain. The reaction of

FIGURE 5. Inhibition of BBM.1 antibody by either free β_2m (■) or papain-solubilized HLA-A, -B antigens (●). Separate preparations of free β_2m (16 μg/ml) and HLA-A, -B antigens (22 μg/ml) were serially diluted and 50-μl aliquots of each dilution preincubated with 50 μl BBM.1 supernatant (diluted 1/100) for 1 hr at 4°C. Residual activity in 50 μl preincubated supernatant was measured by trace binding against 2 × 10^5 Bristol 8 cells. Protein concentrations were estimated by the method of Lowry, using BSA as a standard. [Reproduced with permission from Brodsky *et al.* (1979a).]

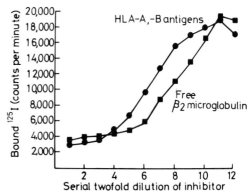

this antibody with somatic cell hybrids is shown in Table VI. This shows a reaction with the hybrid Horl 9.8R 3.3, which contains only human chromosome 15, and which expresses human β_2m. BBM.1 does not react with hybrids containing human chromosome 6 but lacking chromosome 15. Other monoclonal anti-β_2m antibodies have also been characterized (Brodsky *et al.*, 1979b).

Immunization to produce monoclonal antibodies has essentially followed the same patterns as more conventional immunizations in that those antibodies detecting polymorphic determinants are outnumbered by those detecting nonpolymorphic determinants. So far three antibodies to specific polymorphic determinants have been identified: PA2.1, BB7.1, and BB7.2 (Parham and Bodmer, 1978, Brodsky *et al.*, 1979b). A fourth antibody which identifies a somewhat broader polymorphic specificity has also been isolated, PA2.2 (Parham and Bodmer, 1978). PA 2.1 was produced by immunization with papain-solubilized A2, and BB7.2 was produced by immunization with papain-solubilized A2 and B7. Both react in indirect binding assays with lymphoid line cells of HLA-A2 specificity. When tested against four cell lines expressing HLA-A28, the HLA-A2 cross-reacting determinant, only one cell type, IDF, reacts. All other HLA-A28 lines do not react, suggesting that these monoclonal antibodies may be splitting the A28 specificity as previously defined. The reactions of PA2.1 with a panel of lymphoid lines is shown in Fig. 6. BB7.2 is a cytotoxic antibody, the pattern of reactions being identical to those in indirect binding. Both BB7.2 and PA2.1 can be specifically inhibited in trace binding by pure papain-solubilized A2 antigen, but not by A28 antigen prepared from BB7.2 and PA2.1 (Parham and Bodmer, 1978).

BB7.1 was produced in the same fusion as BB7.2. This antibody is noncytotoxic and reacts in trace binding with only those cells expressing HLA-B7. In contrast to many conventional sera against HLA-B7 this serum shows no cross-reaction with cells of the HLA-B40 type.

The antibody PA2.2 derived from the same fusion as PA2.1 shows considerably less specificity than the other polymorphic antibodies defined. This antibody was tested against cells of many different specificities. Only one cell, WT 46 *(HLA-A32, B13)*, does not react, although this line types normally with alloanti-

TABLE VI

Reactions of W6/32 and BBM.1 with Human/Mouse Somatic Cell Hybrids

Hybrid	Mouse parent	Human parent	W6/32	BBM.1	CHRM 6	CHRM 15
DUR4	1R	DUV[a]	−	+	−	+
DUR 5R.1	1R	DUV	−	−	−	−
Horp 27R	1R	Lymphocyte	−	+	−	+
Horl 9.8R	1R	Lymphocyte	−	+	−	+
Horl 9.8R 3.3[b]	1R	Lymphocyte	−	+	−	+
CTP 41	PG19	T lymphocyte	+	+	+	+
CTP 21	PG19	T lymphocyte	+	+	+	+

[a]Contains an X/15 translocation (Solomon *et al.*, 1976).
[b]Contains chromosome 15 as its only karyotypically visible human material.

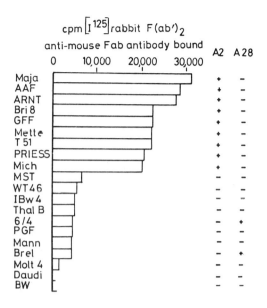

FIGURE 6. Specificity of PA2.1 antibody for cell lines expressing HLA-A2 as measured by indirect trace binding assay. Cells (10⁶) were incubated with 50 μl of PA2.1 culture supernatant for 1 hr at 4°C, washed three times, and then incubated with 300,000 cpm of [¹²⁵I]rabbit F(ab′)₂ anti-mouse Fab antibody for 1 hr at 4°C. The cells were washed four times and then counted for radioactivity. BW is a mouse thymoma cell line, Molt 4 a human T-cell line, and all others are human B-cell lines. [Reproduced with permission from Parham and Bodmer (1978).]

sera. The activity of this antibody can be inhibited by all HLA-A and -B specificities tested, though inhibition with *B* locus antigens is less efficient. Inhibition has not so far been tested with purified HLA-A32 and B13.

2. HLA-DRW

Another class of determinants to which monoclonal antibodies have been raised are the HLA-DRW or Ia antigens. These, in contrast to antibodies directed to the HLA-A, -B, -C or $\beta_2 m$ determinants, have a characteristic restricted tissue distribution (Jones *et al.*, 1975). The noncytotoxic antibody DA2 produced by immunization with membrane derived from the B lymphoid line LKT, reacts strongly with all B-cell lines tested, chronic lymphocytic leukemia (CLL) cells, and purified B lymphocytes from which T lymphocytes have been removed by E rosetting (Wilson *et al.*, 1975). The antibody reacts only weakly with unseparated peripheral blood lymphocytes and not with separated T lymphocytes and the T-cell lines Molt 4 and HSB-2. This restricted tissue distribution parallels that found with pregnancy HLA-DRW sera.

The indirect binding activity of this antibody can be inhibited by detergent solubilized glycoprotein (Brodsky *et al.*, 1980). Furthermore an F(ab′)₂ fragment of a previously defined rabbit anti-human Ia serum (Barnstable *et al.*, 1977) can also inhibit the reaction of this antibody when preincubated with target cells (Fig. 6). Immunoprecipitation from [³⁵S]methionine labeled lymphoid line cells with a whole-serum RAM IgG precipitates two chains with molecular weights of approximately 28,000 and 33,000.

These results strongly suggest that this antibody is directed against a nonpolymorphic determinant on the Ia molecule.

This possibility is further supported by preliminary results with tissue homogenate absorptions which suggest that the activity of PA.2 can be absorbed out with spleen, kidney, and liver homogenates but not with brain or heart. It has been suggested that Ia is present on the liver and kidney of both rat and guinea pig (Hart and Fabre, 1979; Wiman *et al.*, 1978).

Monoclonal antibodies to polymorphic HLA-DRW specificities have also been obtained. One of them, Genox 3.53, obtained by immunization with the glycoprotein fraction from Bristol 8 cell membrane, has been cloned. This antibody recognizes HLA-DRW specificities of the cross-reacting group DRW 1, 2, and 6 clearly defined by conventional alloantisera. This antibody is noncomplement-fixing and reacts with cells which type as DRW-1, -2, or -6. It does not react with cells of other specificities. Its binding to target cells can be inhibited by purified DRW antigens derived from a DRW-4, 6- positive cell line, and it can also be blocked by the F(ab')$_2$ rabbit anti-human Ia antibody (Fig. 7).

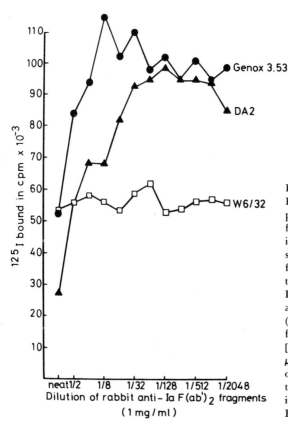

FIGURE 7. Inhibition of Genox 3.53, DA2, and W6/32 antibody binding by preincubation with rabbit anti-Ia F(ab')$_2$ fragments. 5×10^5 fixed PGF cells were incubated for 1 hr at 9°C with 30 μl of serial dilutions of rabbit anti-Ia F(ab')$_2$ fragments (1 μg/ml). After washing three times in 0.5% BSA-PBS, 30 μl of either DA2 antibody (1.2 μg/ml), Genox 3.53 antibody (1.2 μg/ml), or W6/32 antibody (1 μg/ml) was added. Cells were washed four times as before after 1 hr at 4°C and [^{125}I]RAM F(ab')$_2$ fragments added in 25 μl (0.125 μg/ml, 3×10^5 cpm). After another hour at 4°C, cells were washed five times and counted for bound radioactivity. [Reproduced with permission from Brodsky *et al.* (1980).]

III. Somatic Cell Hybrids

Man/mouse somatic cell hybrids undergo a random loss of human chromosomes and then become relatively karyotypically stable (Weiss and Green, 1967). These hybrids are of fundamental importance in human genetic analysis in that they contain and express only part of the human genome. Monoclonal antibodies produced against human material may be characterized by their reactions with such hybrids, and the antigenic determinants that they recognize can be assigned to particular human chromosomes. These antigens may then be used as chromosomal markers, and the monoclonal antibodies as a means of rapidly identifying which chromosomes are present in other hybrids. They can also be used as a means of selecting for or against hybrids carrying particular chromosomes either by the use of the fluorescence-activated cell sorter (Loken and Herzenberg, 1975) or by complement-mediated cytotoxicity (Jones et al., 1976).

Table VII shows some of the characteristics of the monoclonal-antibody-producing cell lines described in this section.

A. SA.1

Antibodies W6/34, 45, and 46 were produced from the same tonsil membrane fusion as W6/32 (Barnstable et al., 1978a). These supernatants were tested by autoradiography, using standard procedures with either whole peripheral blood or tonsil cells. The results are shown in Table VIII. W6/34 and 46 label all morphological cell types, although not all lymphocytes and monocytes. W6/45 labels only a subpopulation of lymphocytes and all eosinophils, but not other cell types tested. When tested on a variety of other tissue culture cells by indirect binding W6/34 and 46 react with all human cells tested, including B-cell lines, T-

TABLE VII
Monoclonal Antibody-Producing Cell Lines

Monoclonal antibody	Chromosome specificity	C' fixing	Immunization	Reference
W6/34	11	+	Human tonsil leukocyte membrane	Barnstable et al. (1978a)
W6/45	11	+	Human tonsil leukocyte membrane	Barnstable et al. (1978a)
W6/46	11	+	Human tonsil leukocyte membrane	Barnstable et al. (1978a)
Genox 4/1	14	ND	AML membrane	Barnstable (1978)
Genox 4/7	22	ND	AML membrame	Barnstable (1978)
Genox 4/21	11	ND	AML membrane	Barnstable (1978)
Genox 4/24	22	ND	AML membrane	Barnstable (1978)

TABLE VIII

Labeling by Chromosome 11-Specific Monoclonal Antibodies of Various Cell Types among
Peripheral Blood or Tonsil Cell Preparations[a]

Monoclonal antibody	Erythrocytes	Polymorphs	Monocytes	Lymphocytes	Eosinophils
W6/34	+	+	−[b]	±	+
W6/45	−	−	−	±	+
W6/46	+	+	−[b]	±	+

[a]+, All cells of one type labeled; −, none labeled; ±, some labeled, others not.
[b]Some very weakly labeled cells were observed.

cell lines, diploid fibroblasts, neuroblastoma cells and HeLa. W6/45 also reacts with a wide range of cell types, suggesting that it is less specific than the autoradiography indicates.

These antibodies were then tested on a panel of somatic cell hybrids by complement-dependent cytotoxicity (Table IX). The only chromosome in common among all the hybrids that react positively is chromosome 11. Identical results are obtained by indirect binding. Assignment is further confirmed using a series of chromosome 11 negative subclones of 4W10. These clones were produced by immunoselection with an antiserum to SA-1, an antiserum defining a chromosome 11 marker (Buck and Bodmer, 1974) and complement. Six independent subclones lost the chromosome 11 markers lactate dehydrogenase-A (LDH-A) and SA-1 and so had presumably lost chromosome 11. These subclones are also negative for W6/34, 45, and 46.

TABLE IX

Segregation of W6/34, 45, and 46 Activity with Chromosome 11 in Human/Mouse
Somatic Cell Hybrids

Hybrid	Mouse parent	Human parent	Chromosome 11	W6/34	W6/45	W6/46
3M4	1R	Lymphocyte	+	+	+	+
3W7	1R	Lymphocyte	+	+	+	+
4W10[a]	1R	Lymphocyte	+	+	+	+
LBT-2-HAT[b]	3T3 (BALB/c)	Fibroblast	+	+	+	+
LBT2-BudR[c]	3T3 (BALB/c)	Fibroblast	−	−	−	−
CTP 41	PG19	Peripheral T lymphocyte	−	−	−	−
DTP 7.5	PG19	Peripheral T	−	−	−	−

[a]Six subclones of 4W10 that had been immunoselected for loss of chromosome 11 with anti-SA-1 and complement no longer reacted with W6/34, 45, and 46.
[b]Hybrid containing one human translocation chromosome (11/17 breakpoints p15 and q21, respectively).
[c]BudR-resistant subclone of LBT2-HAT that has lost the 11/17 chromosome; three other subclones gave similar results.

Regional localization of these antigens on chromosome 11 was obtained using the hybrid LBT2-HAT (Francke and Busby, 1974). This cell contains only one human chromosome that involves a translocation between the short arm of chromosome 11 and the long arm of chromosome 17 (breakpoints p15 and q21, respectively). This hybrid is clearly positive with all three monoclonal antibodies. Since the mouse parent of the hybrid is thymidine kinase-negative, selection of LBT2-HAT in BudR results in the loss of the 11/17 chromosome. Subclones selected in this way (LBT2-BudR) no longer react with W6/34, 45, and 46. This confirms the localization of the three target determinants to chromosome 11 and also places the relevant genes on the short arm of the chromosome. The antigenic determinants recognized by W6/34, 45, and 46 have yet to be defined. It is possible that they recognize the same, or similar, determinants as those of SA-1. Preliminary evidence indicates that the anti-SA-1 serum is inhibited by ceramides, suggesting that the antigenic determinant is a carbohydrate moiety (D. Marcus, personal communication). This raises the intriguing possibility that the SA-1 gene could be coding for a glycosyl transferase. The pattern of inhibition of the monoclonal antibodies is being investigated with this possibility in mind. Puck *et al.* (1971) have defined two cell-surface antigens also on the short arm of chromosome 11. Whether or not these are related to SA-1 or to the antigens recognized by the monoclonal antibodies is also not yet clear.

B. Other Antigens

A second series of hybrids made in Oxford to map antigenic determinants in somatic-cell hybrids were derived from a fusion after immunization with plasma membrane from acute myeloblastic leukemia cells (Barnstable, 1978). Four supernatants give patterns of segregation consistent with the presence or absence of particular chromosomes, namely, 11, 14, and 22. Table X shows these results. These antibodies are as yet uncloned and the nature of their target antigens are unknown.

TABLE X

Segregation of Binding of Genox 4 Antibodies with Individual Human Chromosomes in Human/Mouse Hybrids

Monoclonal antibody	Chromosomal location of gene for antigen	Number of hybrid clones binding/chromosome		Total number of hybrid clones tested
		+/+	−/−	
Genox 4/1	14	8	4	12
Genox 4/7	22	7	5	12
Genox 4/12	11	11	1	12
Genox 4/24	22	7	5	12

IV. Erythrocyte-Specific Antigens

Two antibodies, W6/1 and W6/28, which bind specifically to erythrocytes, were derived from the same fusion that gave rise to W6/32 (Barnstable *et al.*, 1978a). Neither antibody binds to other blood cells tested, including polymorphs, monocytes, lymphocytes, or eosinophils (although W6/28 binds very weakly to some lymphocytes). Presumably both of these antibodies were raised in response to contaminating erythrocyte membrane in the tonsil preparation.

One of these antibodies, W6/28, binds to erythrocytes from all donors tested, and thus appears to be specific for this cell type. The nature of this antigen is not known, but this antibody and others like it may be extremely useful in studies on erythroid cell differentiation.

The second erythrocyte-specific antibody, W6/1, binds only to erythrocytes of blood group types A1 or A2, under conditions of limiting second antibody, as described in Barnstable *et al.* (1978a). When saturating amounts of second antibody are used, however, binding is five times as great on erythrocytes of type A1 than A2. This antibody appears therefore to behave like conventional anti-A1 sera in its specificity (A. Williams, personal communication). The antibody is an IgM antibody and effectively causes hemagglutination of type A1 erythrocytes (C. Milstein, personal communication). This system provides another clear example of the possibility of producing monoclonal antibodies to polymorphic determinants in a xenogeneic immunization.

V. Thymocyte-Specific Antigen

McMichael and others have isolated a monoclonal antibody that identifies another human cell-surface antigen with extremely narrow tissue distribution (McMichael *et al.*, 1979). By immunizing mice with human thymocytes an antibody, NA1/34, has been isolated, which reacts by binding and immunoperoxidase labeling with only thymocytes and the thymus leukemia cell line, Molt 4. The antigen defined by NA1/34 has been called human thymus antigen 1 or HTA-1. The antibody reacts specifically with cortical thymocytes and will therefore be extremely useful in defining and identifying this subclass of T cells.

Figure 8 shows the binding of NA1/34 to a variety of human cells. Molt 4 and thymocytes are the only positive cells. No reaction is seen with red blood cells, platelets, peripheral blood lymphocytes or lymph node cells, among others. The reaction is species-specific in that there is no reaction with rat or dog thymus.

Another feature of this antibody is the fact that it reacts reciprocally with W6/32, the monoclonal antibody against HLA-A, -B, -C determinants. That is,

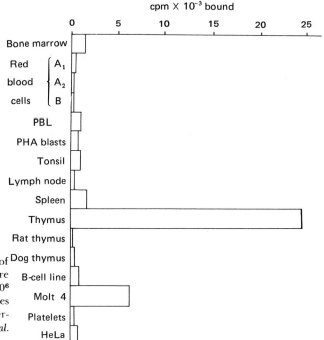

FIGURE 8. Tissue distribution of NA1/34 binding, 25 μl of culture supernatant assayed on 2.5×10^6 cells from each of the sources shown. [Reproduced with permission from McMichael et al. (1979).]

using immunoperoxidase labeling, it can be demonstrated that 85% of thymocytes from the cortex react with NA1/34 and weakly or not at all with W6/32. The remaining 15% of cells react with W6/32 and not NA1/34. When both antibodies are used simultaneously, 99% of cells are labeled. Those cells that react with W6/32 appear larger than those reacting with NA1/34. Interestingly, Molt 4 reacts with both W6/32 and NA1/34. HTA-1 therefore appears to be present on a subclass of thymocytes, and the antibody NA1/34 may be extremely useful in following the differentiation of this cell type and of T cells in general.

Conventional antisera have recently been used to classify leukemias in a large number of patients (Janossy et al., 1980). Monoclonal antibodies have now also been used in further studies of this type (Bradstock et al., 1980). Significant binding of NA1/34 antibody is observed only in Thy-ALL (thymic-ALL) cases and in no other leukemias, including non-T, non-B ALL, acute and chronic myeloid leukemias, B-type CLL, and lymphomas. Immunofluorescence studies show, however, that in patients with Thy-ALL only a proportion of the leukemic blasts develop typical characteristics of cortical thymocytes, including staining with NA1/34. These studies demonstrate the extreme specificity of the monoclonal antibodies in analyzing subclasses of hemopoietic lymphoid cells, and demonstrate their potential for diagnostic purposes.

VI. Discussion

A. Chemistry

For certain types of structural studies, where immunization is carried out with purified protein and conventional multispecific sera can easily be obtained, the principle advantage of monoclonal antibodies lies in their monospecificity. Purification of specific antibodies from conventional sera by multiple absorptions or affinity chromatography is often limited by availability of antigenic protein, or the essential fragment of protein. With monoclonal antibodies it is possible to obtain large amounts of high-titer pure antibody reactive with specific parts of a molecule. These antibodies may then be used as reagents for identifying, purifying, or studying particular functional sites. Our studies on C1q are an example of the way in which a monoclonal antibody may specifically inhibit a binding site. Monoclonal antibodies to other portions of the C1q molecule, particularly to the "collagenlike" region which binds C1r and C1s, will, we hope, clarify whether this portion of the molecule is also altered in fibroblast C1q, or whether in this region it is the same as serum C1q. Similar approaches could be taken in identifying precursor and variant forms of molecules in other systems.

Monoclonal antibodies with defined chemical specificity can also be used in simple, single-step purification procedures, using affinity chromatography to purify molecules present in very low quantities. For example, W6/32 has been used (Parham *et al.*, 1979) to purify HLA-A, -B, -C molecules present in very small amounts from normal human serum.

B. mRNA Isolation

When minority species mRNAs are translated *in vitro* these can be recognized by specific immunoprecipitation of the translated products. In this sort of study a monoclonal antibody of defined specificity that recognizes the translated product is clearly an advantage over conventional sera in that it is more likely to identify the correct protein rather than a contaminating or cross-reacting one. If, however, the antibody is made to a protein in its native form, such as a membrane-bound protein, or multimeric protein, it may not recognize the nascent form of a translation product *in vitro*. Care must therefore be taken in the selection of the monoclonal antibodies used for this purpose. This system is being applied to the HLA-A, -B, -C chains and $\beta_2 m$ (Pleogh *et al.*, 1979; J. Trowsdale, personal communication) with the eventual aim of cloning the *HLA* region. In addition, isolation of mRNA from polysomes (Palacious *et al.*, 1972) should also be possible with monoclonal antibodies, which again have the advantage of high titers and defined specificities. Obviously, the same precautions mentioned above apply here.

C. Protein Polymorphisms

In the HLA system the production of monoclonal antibodies to the polymorphic determinants has been more successful using purified or partially purified material rather than whole cells (Brodsky et al., 1979b). While this is not a substantial difficulty, it does mean that more time will be needed until conventional typing sera can be replaced by monoclonal antibodies. One possible means of avoiding the purification step is immunization with whole cells that have been coated with antibody to the nonpolymorphic determinants (Jones, 1976).

Not surprisingly, immunization with whole cells tends to result in the production of antibodies such as W6/32, which react with the nonpolymorphic sites in the HLA-A, -B, -C chains. This type of antibody has not been found before in this system and may only be produced by immunizing across widely separated species such as man and mouse. Monoclonal antibodies therefore are also proving of great interest in revealing the portion of the molecule that these allogeneic chains have in common. Some of these antibodies have been used in the analysis of various primate species and the evolutionary significance of these findings are discussed by Brodsky et al. (1979b).

Presumably this sort of analysis will be possible in other systems as well. Antibodies that are specific to the variant and nonvariant regions of allelic proteins or proteins from duplicated genes should provide interesting evolutionary insight into a large number of both structural and enzymatic proteins.

D. Somatic Cell Genetics

The development of somatic cell genetics provides an experimental system for human genetics. Because breeding experiments are obviously not feasible, the discovery of a method of inducing chromosome segregation in cultured cells has enormously increased the potential of human genetic analysis. Monoclonal antibodies will increase the scope of this field even further. These antibodies should provide easily identifiable markers for each human chromosome, or each arm of each chromosome, and a means of positive and negative selection for these chromosomes. Several such antibodies have already been discovered for antigens on chromosomes 11, 14, and 22. Several approaches may be taken to the production of these antibodies. Whole human cells may be used for immunization and antibodies screened on a panel of somatic cell hybrids to determine which chromosome codes for the gene for a particular antigen. There is some evidence (Brodsky et al., 1979b) that immunizing with whole cells rather than purified soluble-membrane antigen is more likely to result in cytotoxic antibodies, so that it seems likely that this approach might yield antibodies useful for chromosome selection.

Another approach is immunization with human/mouse hybrids that contain a single human chromosome, a broken human chromosome, or a small fragment of human material translocated to a mouse chromosome. These may be used to produce antibodies to an antigen coded for by the small piece of human chromosome. In this way antibodies may be produced to known gene products without further purification. Another possible use of such an antibody would be to identify and isolate a gene on a small fragment of chromosome. This could then be used to isolate adjacent genes on that fragment by isolation of sequential overlapping fragments.

E. Cell- and Tissue-Specific Antibodies

The advantages of monoclonal antibodies for studying development and differentiation are that they may provide very specific markers for particular cell types and particular stages of development or embryogenesis. Immunization with relatively crude material, which would produce conventional multispecific sera of extreme complexity, can be used for the production of monoclonal antibodies specific for cell or tissue markers. These antibodies can be used to follow differentiation of teratocarcinomas *in vitro,* both as fluorescent and cytotoxic markers for particular cell types, and also as a means of blocking and thereby identifying particular steps in development. Antibodies to specific cell types such as NA1/34, the thymocyte-specific antigen, will also be of great importance in following cellular differentiation, and in particular, hemopoietic stem-cell differentiation.

F. Chromosome Structure

Another area of human genetics likely to benefit from monoclonal antibodies is that of chromosome structure. For example, there will almost certainly be monoclonal antibodies produced to the nonhistone proteins. While conventional sera could not be specific enough to pick out particular proteins *in situ* without extensive purification, it is possible that monoclonal antibodies can be used as fluorescent probes to examine the position of these proteins in metaphase chromosomes. Similar approaches with spindle protein may provide information about the mitotic apparatus.

G. Clinical Applications

Just as monoclonal antibodies are likely to replace tissue-typing reagents, it also seems probable that they will be used as diagnostic reagents. Many diseases are currently identified by radioimmunoassay and immunoelectrophoresis, and monoclonal antibodies could provide standardized pure reagents for these assays. In addition, as with the thymocyte-specific antibody, they may be useful in diagnosing particular forms of diseases such as leukemia. Clear distinction of these forms may greatly help in choice of treatment and hence prognosis. Monoclonal antibodies may eventually also replace antilymphocyte serum as immuno-suppressive agents and in the treatment of aplastic anemia.

Many inborn errors of metabolism exist in both CRM-negative and CRM-positive forms. Monoclonal antibodies to the enzymes that are deficient in these diseases may help in diagnosing them and also in determining the extent and nature of their heterogeneity.

It has been found that amniotic fluid cultures contain cells of different morphological types and certain of these may be related to the presence of neural tube defects (Gosden and Brock, 1978; Bobrow *et al.*, 1978). Immunization with these cells and production of cell-specific monoclonal antibodies could also be of tremendous diagnostic value.

VII. Conclusion

The list of possible uses of monoclonal antibodies in human genetics is long, and this discussion is very far from exhaustive. We have tried to present some of the concrete results obtained with them and to mention some possible future directions for their use. It is clear that within the next few years their use will become quite routine in some areas and that they will provide valuable information in areas which would be otherwise very difficult to approach.

ACKNOWLEDGMENTS

We would like to thank S. Whitehead, J. Arklie, J. Trowsdale, A. McMichael, and K. Reid for allowing us to use their unpublished data. We are grateful to W. F. Bodmer, P. N. Goodfellow, and M. Bobrow for helpful discussions. We would also like to thank Mrs. P. Allen for her help in the preparation and typing of this manuscript.

References

Adams, R. A., Foley, E. E., Uzman, B. G., Farber, S., Lazarus, H., and Kleinman, L., 1967, Leukemia: Serial transplantation of human leukemic lymphoblasts in newborn Syrian hamsters, *Cancer Res.* **27**:772.

Arce-Gomez, B., Jones E. A., Barnstable, C. J., Solomon, E., and Bodmer, W. F, 1978, The genetic control of HLA-A and B antigens in somatic cell hybrids: Requirements for β_2 microglobulin, *Tissue Antigens* **11**:96.

Artzt, K., and Jacob, F., 1974, Absence of serologically dectectable H.2 on primitive teratocarcinoma cells in culture, *Transplantation* **17**:632.

Barnstable, C. J., 1978, Genetic and biochemical analysis of human cell surface antigens, D. Phil. thesis, Oxford University.

Barnstable, C. J., Jones, E. A., Bodmer, W. F., Bodmer, J. G., Arce-Gomez, B., Snary, D., and Crumpton, M. J., 1977, Genetics and serology of HLA-linked human Ia antigens, *Cold Spring Harb or Symp. Quant. Biol.* **41**:443.

Barnstable C. J., Bodmer, W. F., Brown, G., Galfre, G., Milstein, C., Williams, A. F., and Ziegler, A., 1978a, Production of monoclonal antibodies of Group A erythrocytes, HLA and other human cell surface antigens, *Cell* **14**:9.

Barnstable, C. J., Jones, E. A., and Crumpton, C., 1978b, Chemistry and genetics of HLA antigens, *Br. Med. Bull.* **34**(3):241.

Barnstable, C. J., Snary, D., Crumpton, M. J., Balner, H., and Bodmer, W. F., 1980, Antisera recognising HLA.A,B & DRW antigens raised in rhesus monkeys, *Tissue Antigens* (in press).

Benham, F. J., Povey, S. M., and Harris, H., 1978, Heterogeneity of alkaline phosphatases in different HeLa lines, *Somat. Cell Genet.* **4**:13.

Bobrow, M., Evans, C. J., Noble, J., and Patel, C., 1978, Cellular content of amniotic fluid as a predictor of central nervous system malformations, *J. Med. Genet.* **15**:97.

Bodmer, J. G., 1975, The A.B.C. of HLA, in: *Histocompatibility Testing 1975* (F. Kissmeyer-Nielsen, ed.), Munksgaard, Copenhagen, pp. 21–99.

Bolotin, C., Morris, S., Tack, B., and Prahl, J., 1977, Purification and structural analysis of the fourth component of human complement, *Biochemistry* **16**(9):2008.

Bradstock, K. F., Janossy, G., Pizzolo, G., Hoffbrand, A. V., McMichael, A., Pilch, J. R., Milstein, C., Beverly, P., Bollum, F. J., 1980, Subpopulations of normal and leukemic human thymocytes: An analysis using monoclonal antibodies, *J. Natl. Cancer Inst.* (in press).

Brodsky, F. M., Bodmer, W. F., and Parham, P., 1979a, Characterization of a monoclonal anti β_2-microglobulin and its use in genetic and biochemical analysis of major histocompatibility antigens, *Eur. J. Immunol.* **9**:536.

Brodsky, F. M., Parham, P., Barnstable, C. J., Crumpton, M. J., and Bodmer, W. F., 1979b, Monoclonal antibodies for analysis of the HLA system, *Immunol. Rev.* **47**:3.

Brodsky, F. M., Parham, P., and Bodmer, W. F., 1980, Monoclonal antibodies to HLA-DRW determinants, *Tissue Antigens* (in press).

Brodsky-Doyle, B., Leonard, K. R., and Reid, K. B. M., 1976, Circular-dichroism and electron-microscopy studies of human subcomponent Clq before and after limited proteolysis, by pepsin, *Biochem. J.* **159**:279.

Buck, D., and Bodmer, W. F., 1974, The human species antigen on chromosome 11, *Cytogenet. Cell Genet.* **14**:257.

Croce, C. M., 1976, Loss of mouse chromosomes in somatic cell hybrids between HT-1080 human fibrosarcoma cells and mouse peritoneal macrophages, *Proc. Natl. Acad. Sci. USA* **73**:3248.

Croce, C. M., Girardi, A. J., and Koprowski, H., 1973, Assignment of the T-antigen gene of simian virus 40 to human chromosome C7, *Proc. Natl. Acad. Sci. USA* **70**:3617.

Crumpton, M. J., Snary, D., Walsh, F. S., Barnstable, C. J., Goodfellow, P. N., Jones, E. A., and Bodmer, W. F., 1978, Molecular structure of the gene products of the human HLA system: Isolation and characterization of HLA-A,B,C and Ia antigens, *Proc. R. Soc. Lond. [Biol.]* **202**:159.

Drewinko, B., Romsdahl, M. M., Yang, L. Y., Ahearn, M. J., Trujillo, J. M., 1976, Establishment of a human carcinoembryonic antigen-producing colon adenocarcinoma cell line, *Cancer Res.* **36**:467.

Faulk, W. P., and Temple, A., 1976, Distribution of β_2-microglobulin and HLA in chorionic villi of human placentae, *Nature* **262**:799.

Francke, U., and Busby, N., 1975, Assignments of the human genes for lactate dehydrogenase A and thymidine kinase to specific chromosomal regions, in: Rotterdam Conference 1974: 2nd International Workshop on Human Gene Mapping, *Birth Defects* **2**(3):143.

Francke, U., and Pellegrino, M. A., 1977, Assignment of the major histocompatibility complex to a region of the short arm of human chromosome 6, *Proc. Natl. Acad. Sci. USA* **74**:1147.

Gigli, I, 1978, A single chain precursor of C4 in human serum, *Nature* **272**:836.

Goodfellow, P. N., Jones, E. A., van Heyningen, V., Solomon, E., Bobrow, M., Miggiano, V., and Bodmer, W. F., 1975, The β_2-microglobulin gene is on chromosome 15 and not in the HLA region, *Nature* **254**:267.

Goodfellow, P. N., Barnstable C. J., Bodmer, W. F., Snary, D., and Crumpton, M. J., 1976a, Expression of HLA system antigens on placenta, *Transplantation* **22**(6):595.

Goodfellow, P., Barnstable, C., Jones, E. A., Bodmer, W. F., Crumpton, M. J., and Snary, D., 1976b, Production of specific antisera to human B lymphocytes, *Tissue Antigens* **7**:105.

Gosden, C., and Brock, D. J. H., 1978, Combined use of α foetoprotein and amniotic fluid cell morphology in early prenatal diagnosis of foetal abnormalities, *J. Med. Genet.* **15**:262.

Hall, R. E., and Colten, H. R., 1977, Cell-free synthesis of the fourth component of guinea pig complement (C4): Identification of a precursor of serum C4 (pro-C4), *Proc. Natl. Acad. Sci. USA* **74**:1707.

Hart, D., and Fabre, J., 1979, Quantitative studies on the tissue distribution of Ia and SD antigens in the DA and Lewis rat stains, *Transplantation* **27**:110.

Janossy, G, Hoffbrand, A. V., Greaves, M. F., Ganeshaguru, K., Pain, C., Bradstock, K., Prentice, H. G., Kay, H. E. M., 1980, *Br. J. Haematol.* **44**:221.

Jones, E. A., 1976, A genetic and serological study of the major human histocompatibility complex, D. Phil. thesis, Oxford University.

Jones, E. A., Goodfellow, P. N., Kennett, R. H., and Bodmer, W. F., 1975, Serological identification of HLA linked human "Ia-type" antigens, *Nature* **256**:250.

Jones, E. A., Goodfellow, P. N., Kennett, R. H., and Bodmer, W. F., 1976, The independent expression of HLA and β_2-microglobulin in human–mouse hybrids, *Somat. Cell Genet.* **2**(6):483.

Kit, S., Dobbs, D. R., Piekarsk, L. J., Hsu, T. C., 1963, Deletion of thymidine kinase activity from L cells resistant to bromodeoxyuridine, *Exp. Cell Res.* **31**:297.

Klein, E., Klein, G., Nadkarni, J. S., Nadkarni, S., Wigzell, H., and Clifford, P., 1967, Surface IgM specificity on cells derived from a Burkitt's lymphoma, *Lancet* **2**:1068.

Klinman, N. R., Pickard, A. R., Sigal, N. H., Gearhart, P. J., Metcalf, E. S., and Pierce, S. K. 1976, Assessing B cell diversification by antigen receptor and precursor cell analysis, *Ann. Immunol.* **127C**:489.

Knobel, H. R., Heuser, C., Rodnick, M. L., and Isliker, H., 1974, Enzymatic digestion of the first component of human complement C1q, *J. Immunol.* **112**:2094.

Lachmann, P. J., and Hobart, M. J. 1978, Complement genetics in relation to HLA, *Br. Med. Bull.* **34**(3):247.

Loken, M. R., and Herzenberg, L. A., 1975, Analysis of cell populations with a fluorescence activated cell sorter, *Ann. NY Acad. Sci.* **254**:163.

McMichael, A. J., Pilch, J. R., Galfré, G., Mason, D. Y., Fabre, J. N., and Milstein, C., 1979, A human thymocyte antigen defined by a hybrid myeloma monoclonal antibody, *Eur. J. Immunol.* **9**:205.

Minowada, J., Ohnuma, T., and Moore, G. E., 1972, Rosette-forming human lymphoid cell lines. 1. Establishment and evidence for origin of thymus-derived lymphocytes, *J. Natl. Cancer Inst.* **49**:891.

Palacious, R., Palmiter, R. D., Schimke, R. T., 1972, Identification and isolation of ovalbumin-synthesizing polysomes, *J. Biol. Chem.* **247**:2316.

Paques, E. P., Huber, R., and Priess, H., 1979, Isolation of the globular region of the subcomponent q of the C1 component of complement, *Hoppe-Seylers Z. Physiol. Chem.* **360**:177.

Parham, P., and Bodmer, W. F., 1978, Monoclonal antibody to a human histocompatibility alloantigen, HLA-A2, *Nature* **276**:397.

Parham, P., Barnstable, C. J., and Bodmer, W. F., 1979, Use of a monoclonal antibody W6/32 in structural studies, *J. Immunol.* **123**:342.

Patillo, R. A., Ruckert, A., Hussa, R., Bernstein, R., and Delss, E., 1971, The Jar cell line—continuous human multihormone productions and controls, *In Vitro* **6**:389.

Ploegh, H. L., Canon, L. E., Strominger, J. L., 1979, Cell-free translation of the mRNA's for the heavy and light chains of HLA-A and HLA-B antigens, *Proc. Natl. Acad. Sci. USA* **76**:2273.

Porter, R. R., and Reid, K. B. M., 1978, The biochemistry of complement, *Nature* **275**:699.

Puck, T. T., Wuthier, P., Jones, C., and Kao, F., 1971, Genetics of somatic mammalian cells: Lethal antigens as genetic markers for study of human linkage groups, *Proc. Natl. Acad. Sci. USA* **68**:3102.

Reid, K. B. M., 1974, A collagen-like amino acid sequence in a polypeptide chain of Human Clq (a subcomponent of the first component of complement), *Biochem. J.* **141**:189.

Reid, K. B. M., 1979, Complete amino acid sequences of the three collagen-like regions present in subcomponent Clq of the first component of human complement, *Biochem. J.* **179**:367.

Reid, K. B. M., and Porter, R. R., 1976, Subunit composition and structure of subcomponent Clq of the first component of human complement, *Biochem. J.* **155**:19.

Reid, K. B. M., and Solomon, E., 1977, Biosynthesis of the first component of complement by human fibroblasts, *Biochem. J.* **167**:647.

Reid, K. B. M., Sim, R. B., and Faiers, A. P., 1977, Inhibition of the reconstitution of the haemolytic activity of the first component of human complement by a pepsin-derived fragment of subcomponent Clq, *Biochem. J.* **161**:239.

Senger, D. R., and Hynes, R. O., 1978, C3 component of complement secreted by established cell lines, *Cell* **15**:375.

Solheim, B. G., Fuks, A., Smith, L., Strominger, J. L., and Thorsby, E., 1978, Possible detection of HLA-DR alloantigenic specificities in man with unabsorbed rabbit antisera, *Scand. J. Immunol.* **8**:15.

Solomon, E., and Sykes, B., 1980, Assignment of $a_1(I), a_2$ and possibly $a_1(III)$ chains of human collagen to chromosome 7, Edinburgh Conference 1979: Fifth International Workshop on Human Gene Mapping, *Cytogenet. Cell Genet.* (in press).

Solomon, E., Bobrow, M., Goodfellow, P., Bodmer, W. F., Swallow, D. M., Povey, S., and Noel, B., 1976, Human gene mapping using an X/autosome translocation, *Somat. Cell Genet.* **2**:125.

Sundstrom, C., and Nilsson, K., 1976, Establishment and characterization of a human histiocytic lymphoma cell line (U937), *Int. J. Cancer* **17**:565.

Sykes, B., and Solomon, E., 1978, Assignment of a type I collagen structural gene to human chromosome 7, *Nature* **272**:548.

Sykes, J. A., Whitescarver, J., Jernstrom, P., Nolan, J. F., and Byatt, P., 1970, Some properties of a new epithelial cell line of human origin, *J. Natl. Cancer Inst.* **45**:107.

Szybalski, W., Hunter, E., Szybalski, E. H., and Ragni, G., 1962, Genetic studies with human cell lines, *Natl. Cancer Inst. Monogr.* **7**:75.

Tack, B. F., and Prahl, J. W., 1976, Third component of human complement: Purification from plasma and physicochemical characterization, *Biochemistry* **15**(20):4513.

Terhorst, C. T., Parham, P. R., Mann, D. L., and Strominger, J. L., 1976, Structure of HLA antigens: Amino acid and carbohydrate compositions and NH_2-terminal sequences of four antigen preparations, *Proc. Natl. Acad. Sci. USA* **73**:910.

Throsby, E., and Kissmeyer-Nielsen, F., 1969, Production of HLA typing antisera of desired specificity, *Vox. Sang.* **17**:102.

Tom, B. H., Rutzky, L. P., Jakstys, M. M., Oyasu, R., Kaye, C. E., Kahan, B. D., 1976, Human colonic adenocarcinoma lines. I. Establishment and description of a new line, *In Vitro* **12**:180.

Tumilowicz, J., Nichols, W., Cholon, J., Green, A., 1970, Definition of a continuous human cell line derived from neuroblastoma, *Cancer Res* **30**:2110.

Weiss, M. C., and Green, H., 1967, Human–mouse hybrid cell lines containing partial complements of human chromosomes and functioning human genes, *Proc. Natl. Acad. Sci, USA* **58**:1104.

Wilson, A. B., Haegert, D. G., and Coombs, R. R. A., 1975, Increased sensitivity of the rosette forming reaction of human T lymphocytes with sheep erythrocytes afforded by papain treatment of sheep cells, *Clin. Exp. Immunol.* **22**:179.

Wiman, K., Curman, B., Forsum, U., Klareskog, L., Malmvias-Tjeinlund, U., Rask, L., Trägardh, L., and Peterson, P. A., 1978, Occurrence of Ia antigens on tissue of non-lymphoid origin, *Nature* **276**:711.

7

The Use of Hybridomas in Enzyme Genetics

C. A. SLAUGHTER, M. C. COSEO, C. ABRAMS,
M. P. CANCRO, AND H. HARRIS

I. Introduction

A. The Field of Enzyme Genetics

The genome of every individual contains a large number of "structural" genes which determine the amino acid sequences of polypeptide chains of enzymes. Mutations at such loci involve some change in the nucleotide sequence of the DNA and will often result in a change in the amino acid sequence of the encoded polypeptide, and hence in the structure and properties of the enzyme. During the last two decades a considerable effort has gone into studying the nature of such enzyme variants and their distribution among individual members of various human and animal populations. Much of this work has relied on the use of relatively simple physicochemical techniques for the discrimination of variants, chief among which has been electrophoresis. From this work, two important generalizations have emerged.

First, it has become clear that polymorphism due to the existence of multiple alleles at enzyme loci is a very widespread phenomenon. In a survey of the incidence of electrophoretic enzyme variation, for example, Harris and Hopkinson (1972, 1976) showed that polymorphism, defined as occurring when the frequency of heterozygotes in the population is 2% or greater, occurs in human populations at some 25–30% of loci coding for enzyme structure. The average

C. A. SLAUGHTER, M. C. COSEO, C. ABRAMS, AND H. HARRIS • Department of Human Genetics, University of Pennsylvania, School of Medicine, Philadelphia, Pennsylvania 19104. M. P. CANCRO • Department of Pathology, University of Pennsylvania, School of Medicine, Philadelphia, Pennsylvania 19104.

heterozygosity per locus for such alleles, taken over both polymorphic and non-polymorphic loci, was found to be around 6%. It was further shown (Harris *et al.*, 1974) that multiple rare alleles (those with gene frequencies of less than 0.005) occur at both polymorphic and nonpolymorphic loci and probably exist at virtually all loci. The physiological significance of high levels of allelic variation in the structure of enzymes is largely unknown, and the nature of the evolutionary pressures which have given rise to them is still a hotly contested issue (see, for example, Lewontin, 1974).

The second generalization to have emerged from the study of enzyme variants is that, although many enzymes appear to be determined by single gene loci, there are frequent examples in which two or more different loci determine the structures of a set of enzyme proteins which have the same or very similar catalytic properties but which are structurally distinct from one another. In a recent review of 83 different enzymes, selected only in that all had been studied by electrophoresis, Harris (1979) found evidence that as many as 35% of the enzymes are encoded by two or more loci, and about 56% of the loci determining the 83 enzymes are involved in coding for such multilocus enzyme systems. In evolutionary terms the most plausible general explanation of the existence of such "multilocus enzyme systems" is that in each case the two or more genes involved are descended from a common ancestral gene which has undergone duplication during the course of evolution. That the protein products of the different loci, although very similar, now differ in some degree in their structures and enzymic and physical properties, can be explained in terms of subsequent mutational divergence of the original duplicate genes. In many cases there is a marked degree of tissue differentiation in the expression of the different loci of the set, implying that there has been an evolution of specific genetic regulatory elements along with the evolution of the structural genes themselves. In other cases, differences in the subcellular localization of the enzymes are found.

Enzyme genetics is concerned in large measure with developing an understanding of the role of multiple alleles and multiple gene loci in determining enzyme protein structure and function. These questions, which of course also apply to nonenzymic proteins, have an important bearing on theories of the organization of structural genes in the genome as a whole and are of direct relevance to the problem of enzyme evolution and molecular evolution in general. They are also relevant to an understanding of enzyme regulation with respect to both subcellular localization and tissue differentiation, and are pertinent in determining the relationship of genotype to phenotype in a variety of genetically determined diseases.

B. *Immunology and Enzyme Genetics*

The application of immunology in enzyme genetics is based upon the expectation that enzymes which differ by one or a few amino acid substitutions will differ only slightly in immunological properties, whereas large sequence differences will result in more extensive differences in immunochemical characteristics. Detailed studies of cytochrome c (Margoliash et al., 1970) and lysozyme (Prager and Wilson, 1971a,b) have supported the existence of a correlation between the number of amino acid differences between genetically homologous proteins in different species and the cross-reactivities of the corresponding antisera raised against them. Subsequent work has shown that this correlation is general, at least for globular monomeric proteins which differ in sequence by less than 30% of their amino acid residues. Indeed, essentially the same calibration line relating the percentage of amino acid sequence differences and the immunological distance estimated by microcomplement fixation has been found to hold for several proteins, including bird lysozymes (Prager and Wilson, 1971a, Jollès et al., 1976), bacterial azurins (Champion et al., 1975), plant plastocyanins (Wallace and Boulter, 1976), and mammalian ribonucleases (Welling et al., 1976).

This relationship has been exploited in many studies involving the structural comparison of enzymes and proteins, and the results continue to demonstrate that a considerable amount of information can be obtained by the application of standard immunochemical methods. General reviews of this work have appeared (e.g., Arnon, 1973; Crumpton, 1974), and other publications dealing with particular aspects of the research are also available. For example, Wilson and his colleagues have engaged in an extensive program of taxonomic investigations into the structural diversification of genetically homologous proteins between different animal species. Most of the work has involved the technique of microcomplement fixation and has been described by Champion et al. (1974) and Wilson et al. (1977). Other groups have focused attention on various examples of multilocus enzyme systems. For example, Taylor and colleagues have used inhibition of enzyme activity by antisera to measure immunological cross-reactivities in a study of the structural relationships of the tissue-specific enolases, a system of enzymes encoded by three separate gene loci (Rider and Taylor, 1974, 1975; Fletcher et al., 1976). In another case, Christen and his colleagues have used microcomplement fixation to study the structural relationships between the mammalian cytoplasmic and mitochondrial aspartate aminotransferases, which are encoded by separate gene loci (Sonderegger et al., 1977; Sonderegger and Christen, 1978).

All such studies involving standard immunochemical methods, however, are subject in some degree to problems which arise inevitably from certain characteristics of the immune system and its response to complex protein antigens. Whole antisera contain a very wide range of specific antibodies, which possess different antigen-combining sites capable of interacting with the immunogen. Although antibodies with the same antigen-combining sites share specificity for the same immunological determinant, whole antisera containing a heterogeneous mixture of antibodies are capable of interacting with many different determinants on the immunogen. The overall reactivity of an antiserum is determined by the relative and the absolute abundances and affinities of the different determinant-specific antibodies which comprise it. Unfortunately, these are ill-defined and highly variable quantities. This state of affairs leads to various difficulties.

1. Different antigens which bear distinct but overlapping subsets of antigenic determinants may not be resolved by heterogeneous antisera. It is generally impossible to assess the effect that variation in the immunogenicity of different determinants on a protein antigen may have on the immunological cross-reactivities of an antiserum raised against it. However, such variation is almost certainly important in determining whether or not amino acid substitutions which occur within different determinants are discriminated by an antiserum (Margoliash et al., 1970).

2. Changes in both the abundances and affinities of specific antibodies take place during immune responses and these may result in changes in the cross-reactivities of successive antiserum samples collected from a given animal (Prager and Wilson, 1971a). Moreover, the repertoire of antibodies an individual can make varies from one animal to another, and cross-reactivities measured with antisera collected from different individuals may vary accordingly (Prager and Wilson, 1971a). In some cases, reciprocal measurements of immunological distance made between pairs of antigens may also show poor agreement (Margoliash et al., 1970; Prager and Wilson, 1971a). Compensation for these difficulties can only be made by comparing and combining results obtained with antisera from several different animals at various stages during the course of an immune response and by averaging data from all possible reciprocal measurements.

The cross-reactivities displayed by whole antisera are thus influenced by a number of variables, which are only indirectly related to sequence dissimilarity. They can therefore provide only a general indication of relative degrees of structural relatedness of protein antigens at the level of amino acid sequence.

The technique of fusing B lymphocytes from the spleens of immunized mice with appropriate plasmacytoma cells and subsequently isolating clonal hybrid plasmacytoma lines (hybridomas) which secrete antibodies specific for the immunogen has rendered practical the use of elicited monoclonal antibodies as immunochemical reagents (Köhler and Milstein, 1975). The use of these reagents may overcome many of the difficulties involved with whole-serum antibodies in the structural comparison of proteins.

With possible rare exceptions, hybridomas secreting antigen-specific immunoglobulins carry just one clonotype out of the repertoire of antigen-specific immunoglobulins produced by the mouse. Unlike whole antisera, which are heterogeneous mixtures of different immunoglobulins, hybridoma antibodies are therefore homogeneous antibodies with definite chemical structure. The antibodies produced by hybridomas are available in potentially unlimited quantity and can therefore be universally employed as standard serological reagents with essentially invariant properties. Moreover, they open the way for immunological comparison of proteins on a determinant-by-determinant basis (Laver et al., 1979; Yewdell et al., 1979). At the level of antigenic determinants small changes in protein structure may be expected to produce relatively large changes in immunological reactivity, a circumstance which suggests that monoclonal antibodies may provide exquisitely sensitive probes for discriminating between structurally related proteins.

With these potential advantages in view, preliminary experiments with monoclonal antibodies produced by hybridomas have been carried out, using a model system of enzymes as antigens. The results suggest that hybridomas will provide effective and versatile tools in enzyme genetics and related fields.

C. The Human Alkaline Phosphatases as an Experimental System

The human alkaline phosphatases (E.C. 3.1.3.1) have been selected as a model multilocus enzyme system for study by monoclonal antibodies. The system is especially interesting for two reasons. The first is that one of the gene loci encoding these enzymes is extraordinarily polymorphic in human populations, yet no polymorphism has been identified at the other alkaline phosphatase loci. The second is that in certain malignant tumors and cultured cell lines derived from malignancies one may find aberrant expression of an alkaline phosphatase not normally expressed in the tissue of origin.

The alkaline phosphatases (ALPs) catalyze the hydrolysis of a wide range of monophosphate esters to give inorganic phosphate and the corresponding alcohol, phenol, or sugar, etc. They are distinguished from a separate group of enzymes, the acid phosphatases, by their pH optima in the alkaline range.

The ALPs exist in a number of different forms which show striking organ specificity and are usually referred to as liver, bone, kidney, intestinal, placental ALPs, etc. (Fishman, 1974). All these forms share in common a variety of distinctive properties, which suggest that they are evolutionarily related to one another by common ancestry (for review, see Fernley, 1971). They are membrane-associated glycoproteins with subunit sizes in the range 64,000–86,000. The subunits are associated in enzymatically active dimers, but enzymatically active aggregates with higher molecular weights can usually also be demonstrated. The isoelectric points are in the acidic range of 4.0–4.7, although after treatment with neuraminidase the pIs of some forms rise considerably. At room temperature the ALPs are generally stable and some forms (e.g., human placental ALP) are spectacularly stable to heat denaturation. The enzymes are also very similar in their catalytic properties, including substrate specificities and pH optima.

The present genetic evidence suggests that at least three gene loci are concerned with coding for the different ALPs in man; one locus for placental ALP, at least one locus for intestinal ALP, and at least one locus for liver, bone, and kidney ALPs. The evidence falls into two parts:

1. It has been shown that a considerable number of electrophoretically distinct variants of placental ALP determined by a series of alleles at a single autosomal locus can be demonstrated (Robson and Harris, 1965, 1967; Donald and Robson, 1973). Three common alleles giving six common phenotypes occur in most human populations, and an extensive

series of rare alleles, most of which are found in heterozygous combination with one or other of the common alleles, have also been identified. Thus the locus coding for placental ALP is highly polymorphic. In contrast, electrophoretic surveys of intestinal, liver, bone, and kidney ALPs have not as yet revealed any such variants (Harris *et al.*, 1974). This indicates that these other ALPs must be determined by loci different from that which codes for placental ALP.

2. In the rare bone disease hypophosphatasia, which is inherited as an autosomal recessive, there is a gross deficiency of the bone and also the liver and kidney ALPs (Rathbun, 1948; Frazer, 1957). The clinical abnormalities appear to be due to a defect in ossification, apparently the consequence of the deficiency of bone ALP. The severest form of the disease becomes manifest *in utero,* the infants being stillborn or dying shortly after birth. Several studies have indicated that intestinal ALP and also placental ALP, which is determined by the genome of the fetus and not that of the mother (Robson and Harris, 1965), are not affected in this condition (e.g., Mulivor *et al.*, 1978a). Thus the mutation in hypophosphatasia does not affect the placental or intestinal ALP loci.

The enzyme products of the three ALP loci, although very similar to one another in many respects, differ in a variety of biochemical properties. Thermostability studies, inhibition studies, and electrophoretic studies before and after treatment of the enzymes with neuraminidase have all shown that it is possible to discriminate sharply between the three categories of ALP: placental, intestinal, and liver/bone/kidney ALPs (Fishman, 1974; Harris and Hopkinson, 1976; Mulivor *et al.*, 1978b). Purified liver and placental ALPs have further been shown to differ in their peptide fingerprint maps, their overall amino acid composition and the N-terminal amino acid sequences (Badger and Sussman, 1976). Peptide fingerprint maps of liver, kidney, and bone ALPs have been found to be very similar, if not identical, but different from those for intestinal or placental ALP (Seargent and Stinson, 1979). Placental and intestinal ALPs have been shown to differ in amino acid composition (Hirano *et al.*, 1977). These results provide further evidence that the three categories of human ALP are encoded by different gene loci.

Antisera raised in various species against preparations of ALP from different human organs have also been used to characterize the several ALPs. It has generally been found that antisera to placental ALP do not cross-react with liver or bone ALP but usually cross-react with intestinal ALP (Sussman *et al.*, 1968; Lehmann, 1975; Doellgast *et al.*, 1976). Similarly, antisera against intestinal ALP do not cross-react with liver or bone ALP but cross-react with placental ALP (Khattab and Pfleiderer, 1976). Antisera raised against liver ALP (Sussman *et al.*, 1968) and against bone ALP (Singh and Tsang, 1975), fail to cross-react with both placental and intestinal ALP. The immunochemical relationship between placental and intestinal ALP has been studied qualitatively by Ouchterlony double diffusion (Lehmann, 1975; Khattab and Pfleiderer, 1976; Doellgast *et al.*, 1976) and quantitatively by immunoprecipitation of enzyme activity (Lehmann,

1975). The qualitative studies indicate that a relationship of partial identity exists between the two enzymes, and the quantitative data show that a greater quantity of antiplacental ALP antiserum is needed to precipitate intestinal ALP than placental ALP when the amounts of these antigens are standardized by enzyme activity. Different allelic forms of placental ALP could not be discriminated by immunoprecipitation using whole-serum antibodies (Lehmann, 1975), but Doellgast (1979) has demonstrated the existence of allotype-specific antibodies to the rare "D variant" of placental ALP in homologous antisera after extensive absorption with other allelic forms of placental ALP.

In our study of the human ALPs we have undertaken to use monoclonal antibodies produced by hybridomas for determinant-by-determinant comparisons of the following:

1. Different allelic forms of placental ALP
2. Organ-specific products of the different ALP gene loci
3. Various organ-specific ALPs in nonhuman animals
4. Aberrantly expressed ALPs in some cancers and cell lines derived from malignancies

Most of the work so far has been concerned with the allelic variants of placental ALP, and the remainder of this chapter deals principally with this aspect of the research.

II. Methodology for Production and Detection of Antibodies against Human Placental Alkaline Phosphatase

A. Immunizations

The purpose of an immunization scheme for producing hybridomas is to generate within the animal which is to be used as a spleen cell donor an expanded population of B lymphocytes bearing high-affinity, antigen-specific immunoglobulins at a stage when the cells are capable of undergoing fusion with plasmacytoma cells.

Mice of the BALB/c strain are most commonly used as spleen cell donors, providing an appropriate immune response can be mounted by these animals. The mice are first immunized with a preparation of the enzyme or protein of interest in order to generate expanded populations of specific cells. Normally this is done by one or more subcutaneous or intraperitoneal injections of the immunogen in Freund's adjuvant. Following this, and just prior to fusion, the animal is challenged with immunogen in such a way as to capture the maximum number of specific activated B cells in a state that is optimal for cell fusion. This is achieved with an intravenous injection of the immunogen in saline 3 days prior to fusion.

The present report describes hybridomas produced in two fusions, each employing spleen cells from a single immune BALB/c mouse. In both experiments the immunogen consisted of pure ALP isolated from pooled extracts of two human placentas, each of which showed the heterozygous ALPp2-1 electrophoretic phenotype. The ALP was purified in a four-stage procedure involving butanol extraction of the tissue followed by affinity chromatography with concanavalin A–Sepharose (Pharmacia), diethylaminoethyl (DEAE) ion exchange chromatography on Whatman DE52, and gel filtration on Sephacryl S-200 (Pharmacia). The resulting protein was homogeneous to sodium dodecyl sulfate (SDS)-polyacrylamide gel electrophoresis and showed enzymatically active components as the only bands resolved by conventional gel electrophoresis.

Two different immunization procedures were employed. In the first procedure the mouse was primed (Day 0) by intraperitoneal injection of 80 μg of ALP together with 4 mg of alum as adjuvant and was challenged on Day 22 with an intravenous injection of 50 μg of ALP in saline for fusion on the third day following. In the second procedure the mouse was primed (Day 0) by subcutaneous injection of 70 μg of ALP in Freund's complete adjuvant and reinjected on Day 22 with a further 70 μg of ALP in Freund's incomplete adjuvant by the same route. Subsequent challenge was on Day 88 with an intravenous injection of 70 μg of ALP in saline for fusion on the third day following.

B. Fusion and Culture Methods

The methods for fusion of mouse spleen cells with plasmacytoma cells and the subsequent selection and culturing of the hybrids have become relatively standard and are detailed in the Appendix of this volume. The hybridomas described in the present report were produced in fusions with 8-azaguanine-resistant cells of the lines P3/X63-Ag8 (Köhler and Milstein, 1975) and Sp2/0-Ag14 (Shulman *et al.*, 1978).

The procedures used were identical to those described by Kennett *et al.* (1978). Briefly, on the third day after intravenous challenge with the immunogen the spleen was removed and a cell suspension was made by perfusion. After lysing red blood cells, the remaining cells were counted for viability and approximately 10^8 cells were used to make a mixture with 10^7 plasmacytoma cells from a culture in log phase. Following a single wash with serum-free medium the cell mixture was centrifuged in the presence of 0.2 ml of 30% polyethylene glycol 1000 in serum-free medium. The cells were then resuspended in 30 ml of "hybridoma" (HY) medium (Kennett *et al.*, 1978) lacking aminopterin and were distributed, one drop per well, into 96-well culture plates. The following day hypoxanthine–aminopterin–thymidine (HAT) selective medium was completed by adding one further drop of double-strength aminopterin in HY medium to each well. Hybrid clones began to appear macroscopically 10–20 days after fusion.

Culture fluids from hybridomas which arose were tested for antiplacental ALP binding activity (see Section II.C) and positive hybrids were cloned as early as possible in soft agarose over a fibroblast feeder layer (Coffino *et al.*, 1970; Kennett *et al.*, 1978). Individual foci of cell growth were removed and retested for specific antibody production. Then 4–5 positive clones were expanded for collection of large volumes of culture fluids and for injection into pristane-primed BALB/c mice (Potter *et al.*, 1972; Cancro and Potter, 1976) for collection of ascites fluids. Both sources of specific monoclonal antibody were retested periodically for continued antigen-binding activity. Several vials of each separate clone were also frozen for storage in liquid nitrogen.

C. Methods for Assay and Cross-Reactivity Testing

Various methods which are employed for the assay of serum antibodies can be adapted for use with monoclonal antibodies. However, binding assays are particularly suitable for monoclonal antibody work because they are simple and sensitive while being applicable, in principle, to all classes of antibody and most protein antigens.

Binding assay methods usually make use of artificially labeled antigen or antibody, or employ a labeled second antibody. The most commonly used labels are radioisotopes, which have given rise to various types of radioimmunassay (Skelley *et al.*, 1973), and enzymes, which provide the basis for the enzyme-linked immunosorbent assays (Wisdom, 1976). In either case some system is required for separating bound and free labeled molecules. Various procedures have been described (Ratcliffe, 1974), but those in which antigen or antibody is first bound to a solid support have become increasingly popular. The component to be immobilized is either physically adsorbed to plastic tubes; microtiter plates; or glass, cellulose ester (Millipore), or nylon filter discs, or covalently coupled to cellulose fibers or to polyacrylamide, dextran, or agarose beads (Wisdom, 1976).

In preliminary experiments with solid-phase radioimmunoassays for antibodies to human placental ALP, three different methods for immobilizing the pure antigen were compared, namely, covalent coupling to cyanogen bromide-activated filter paper discs prepared by the method of Manson *et al.* (1978), covalent coupling to cyanogen bromide-activated Sepharose 4B (Pharmacia) and noncovalent adsorption to the wells of polyvinyl microtiter plates (Dynatech). All three methods were found to provide the basis for successful binding assays, but the plate assay was the most convenient to perform, as it avoided manipulative problems associated with the other two methods. Despite its convenience, however, the plate assay suffered from the disadvantage that relatively small quantities of placental ALP were adsorbed to the plastic under conditions in which other proteins, such as immunoglobulins, were readily taken up. Sufficient antigen for a working assay could be immobilized only by using extravagantly high concentrations of antigen solution. However, this problem was circumvented by employing an indirect absorption method in which placental ALP was allowed to bind to plastic which had been precoated with a specific antiplacental ALP antiserum raised in rabbits. The plastic shows superior adsorption properties for immunoglobulins, although variation in adsorptive capacity between different batches of plates does occur. This high adsorptive capacity could thus be used to increase the quantities of placental ALP bound to the plate, and much lower concentrations of the antigen were therefore required. High sensitivity of detection of mouse antiplacental ALP serum antibodies in this system indicated that potential masking of determinants on the placental ALP by the rabbit antiserum used to immobilize it was not a serious problem. Also in this method the specificity of the rabbit antiserum could in principle be exploited to produce purification of placental ALP *in situ* from crude tissue and cell extracts, providing nonspecific adsorption of other tissue proteins was first blocked by treating the plastic with a protein such as bovine serum albumin (BSA). The potential use of unpurified antigen samples would in turn make rapid testing of placental ALP from large numbers of different individuals in a genetic screening program feasible.

The detailed protocol for a solid-phase binding assay for monoclonal antiplacental ALP antibodies based upon indirect antigen immobilization and the use of a labeled second antibody is given in the Appendix. This assay is convenient and applicable in principle to the analysis of antigenic determinants on a wide variety of enzyme and protein antigens.

III. Results and Discussion

A. Production and Specificity of Monoclonal Antibodies

Preliminary results obtained with hybridomas from two fusions are reported here. In the first, P3/X63-Ag8 cells were fused with spleen cells from a mouse which had been immunized with two injections of pure human placental ALP of the heterozygous electrophoretic phenotype 2-1 (Section II.A). In the second, Sp2/0-Ag14 cells were fused with spleen cells from a mouse immunized by three injections with the same antigen (Section II.A).

From the first fusion culture fluids from 20 wells showing cell growth were tested for antibodies to pure human placental ALP in the solid-phase binding radioimmunoassay described in the Appendix. For the purposes of screening for specific antibody, binding in excess of twice the background level in "no antigen" controls was regarded as positive, and one hybridoma was found to satisfy this criterion. From the second fusion, culture fluids from 30 wells were tested, and 4 showed positive binding. However, the cells from one of these wells subsequently ceased production of specific antibody during the initial passages. The remaining hybridomas were cloned in soft agarose, and supernatants from six or more clones from each line were collected for testing in the radioimmunoassay. All these showed positive binding to pure placental ALP. Representative clones from each line were also passaged in pristane-primed BALB/c mice and all ascites fluids collected were shown to give positive binding.

In recognition of their status as stable hybridomas the four lines have been given the generic names $ALP_p/P3/1$, $ALP_p/Sp2/2$, $ALP_p/Sp2/3$ and $ALP_p/Sp2/4$. The first part of these designations refers to human placental ALP, which was used to immunize the spleen cell donor. The second part represents the plasmacytoma line with which the spleen cells were fused, and the last part is a number specifying the particular hybridoma line.

Establishing the relative effectiveness of the two immunization procedures used here, as well as other possible regimes for this and other enzymes, must await further experiments. However, it is to be expected that the best protocol to follow in any particular case will depend on the special immunogenic characteristics of the antigen being used. The optimum number and frequency of injections, the doses of immunogen required, and the nature of the adjuvant employed will probably have to be determined empirically for each new system studied.

The solid-phase assay propounded in this chapter relies for its specificity on the specificity of the antiserum used for selective immobilization of the ALP and on efficient blocking of unwanted protein adsorption to the plastic. A convenient preliminary test for the assay's specificity was performed, using a murine antiserum raised against pure placental ALP in A/He strain mice. Binding by this antiserum was shown to be the same whether purified placental ALP or the corresponding crude placental extracts containing the same quantity of ALP enzyme activity were supplied for testing. Subsequent binding assays could therefore be performed with unpurified enzyme as the source of antigen, since all binding in excess of the level observed in "no-antigen" controls could be attributed specifically to ALP protein alone. However, it was felt that it was unwise to extrapolate from the specificity of the assay with respect to binding by whole antisera to specificity with respect to binding by individual monoclonal antibodies. Therefore, each separate monoclonal antibody was also tested using the procedure with purified and unpurified placental ALP as an extra precaution.

B. Characteristics of Binding in Radioimmunoassay

Binding curves given by supernatants from representative cultures that grew to more than 10^6 cells per ml were obtained. All gave positive binding at dilutions of 1/1000 or greater. The solid-phase assay system thus showed adequate sensitivity for our purposes and allowed saturation analysis to be conducted with economical use of monoclonal antibody.

Levels of background binding in "no-antigen" controls were low for three of the antibodies but relatively higher for $ALP_p/P3/1$. In the fusions carried out with P3 and the Sp2 plasmacytoma lines, unusually high levels of background binding were also observed for supernatants from several wells not showing the presence of antiplacental ALP antibodies. The same high background binding was observed in the absence of precoating antiserum and was also unaffected by changing the conditions under which the blocking protein, BSA, was allowed to adsorb to the plastic. Replacing BSA by gelatin, fetal calf serum, or agamma horse serum, also had no effect. Apparently, therefore, some monoclonal antibodies have higher affinity for polyvinyl chloride than any blocking agent so far tested. This reinforces the necessity of performing "no antigen" controls for each culture supernatant during screening for specific antibody production and in cross-reactivity testing.

Binding curves given by representative ascites fluids containing the four monoclonal antibodies all displayed positive binding to higher dilutions than the corresponding *in vitro* cell culture fluids. Three of the hybridomas (ALP_p/P3/1, ALP_p/Sp2/2, and ALP_p/Sp2/3) showed positive binding to dilutions of 1/64,000 or greater, and the fourth (ALP_p/Sp2/4) was positive to a dilution of 1/10,000.

C. Antibody Classes

The class of antibodies produced by the hybridomas was determined in Ouchterlony double-diffusion tests using commercial antisera monospecific for different classes of murine immunoglobulins (Research Products International Corp.). ALP_p/P3/1 and ALP_p/Sp2/3 were both found to produce IgG (γ1 heavy chain only) and ALP_p/Sp2/2 produced IgG (γ2b heavy chain). ALP_p/Sp2/4 also made IgG but the specific subclass of γ chains has not yet been determined with certainty. All four hybridomas produced κ light chains.

ALP_p/P3/1 produced the MOPC21 myeloma protein which bears the IgG1 isotype, as well as the antigen-specific immunoglobulin. Since the latter may carry a different class specificity, unrecognized in the Ouchterlony test owing to its possible low relative abundance in the total immunoglobulin secreted by the hybridoma, a separate test was carried out. ALP_p/P3/1 culture fluid was incubated with immobilized placental ALP in the solid-phase radioimmunoassay system and specifically bound mouse antibodies were then tagged with ^{125}I-labeled rabbit antibodies against different murine immunoglobulin classes. In this way labeling would be restricted to immunoglobulin molecules with at least one antigen-specific combining site. Again, however, antibodies with the γ1 heavy chain were the only ones detected.

D. Cross-Reactivities with ALP from Different Human Placentas

Electrophoretic screening of placental ALP in human populations has revealed the existence of a large number of structural variants of the enzyme, which are determined by different alleles at a single autosomal gene locus (Section I.C). Three common alleles, ALP_p^1, ALP_p^2, and ALP_p^3, giving rise to six phenotypes, occur in most human populations. In addition, an extensive series of rarer alleles, most of which are found in heterozygous combination with one or other of the common alleles has also been identified (Section I.C). Quantitative studies of the level of enzyme activity in individuals of the six different common electrophoretic phenotypes have also been made (Beckman, 1970) and from the data it appears that the level of enzyme activity associated with the

$ALP_p{}^3$ allele is close to one half that associated with either the $ALP_p{}^1$ or the $ALP_p{}^2$ alleles. Since the specific activity of pure ALP isolated from placentas with the ALP_p3 phenotype is similar to the specific activity of ALP isolated from ALP_p1 and ALP_p2 placentas (Holmgren *et al.*, 1977), it is probable that the reduced levels of enzyme activity associated with the $ALP_p{}^3$ allele are a consequence of reduced quantities of the corresponding enzyme protein.

Prior to the studies reported here, ALP from a series of nearly 300 unselected placentas had been phenotyped by electrophoresis and were available for screening with the four hybridomas shown to produce specific antibody against placental ALP. Only a proportion of these different ALP samples have been examined so far. However, some interesting results have been obtained, which indicate that the general method is indeed capable of detecting enzyme polymorphism.

Antigen was supplied for assay using dialyzed butanol extracts of single placentas, diluted to provide a uniform level of enzyme activity for selective immobilization. Saturation binding of monoclonal antibodies from the hybridoma culture fluids to the ALPs from different individuals was then measured.

1. Hybridoma $ALP_p/P3/1$

$ALP_p/P3/1$ was the first positive hybridoma to be found and has so far been studied in somewhat more detail than the others. It has been tested against 61 placental ALP specimens selected to include representatives of each of the six "common" electrophoretic phenotypes and all the "rare" phenotypes in the original series. Of these specimens 57 showed high levels of binding with the antibody, but in 4, no significant binding could be detected at all. These 4 samples each had the electrophoretic phenotype 3 (genotype $ALP_p{}^3ALP_p{}^3$) and were in fact the only 4 ALPs of this phenotype in the original series of nearly 300. When whole antiserum from A/He strain mice immunized with placental ALP was used in place of the monoclonal antibody, the level of binding with the four phenotype 3 samples was essentially the same as with the other samples. Thus it appeared that $ALP_p/P3/1$ was detecting a determinant present on the enzyme protein products of the $ALP_p{}^1$ and $ALP_p{}^2$ alleles, but absent from the ALP coded by $ALP_p{}^3$.

If this conclusion is correct, then one would expect the ALPs of phenotypes 3-1 and 3-2 to show, on average, lower levels of binding with the hybridoma culture fluids than phenotypes 1, 2-1, and 2. To examine this question, and also to test whether different clones of $ALP_p/P3/1$ were giving the same results, the following experiment was carried out. Placental extracts of each of the six electrophoretic phenotypes (1, 2, 3, 2-1, 3-1, 3-2) were assayed against seven of the different $ALP_p/P3/1$ clones. The findings are summarized in Table I. Because the absolute counts obtained varied from day to day, the results for the different clones were standardized by expressing the mean level of binding (cpm minus background) of the various ALP phenotypes relative to the mean level of binding of ALP type 1 in each experiment. Culture fluid from the original uncloned hybridoma was also tested in the same way.

The relative antibody binding values for the various ALP phenotypes obtained with the different clones and uncloned hybridoma are consistent with each other. The values for types 1, 2-1, and 2 are not significantly different from each other, nor are values for types 3-1 and 3-2. However, the average for types 3-1 and 3-2 is only 66% of the average value for types 1, 2-1, and 2, and this difference is statistically highly significant ($t = 8.17$, $p < 0.001$). As expected the value for ALP type 3 is not significantly different from zero.

It has already been pointed out that there is evidence based on total activity and specific activity determinations, which suggests that the alleles ALP_p^1, ALP_p^2, and ALP_p^3 produce enzyme protein in the ratio 2:2:1. If this is so, and if this particular antibody detects a specific determinant on ALP phenotype 1 and ALP phenotype 2 which is not present on ALP phenotype 3, then one would expect that the average level of binding with 3-1 and 3-2 placentas would only be about two thirds of the average level of binding with types 1, 2-1, and 2 placentas, since the same amount of ALP is present in each well. Thus there is good agreement between the observed values (Table I) and those expected. The findings therefore support the conclusion that $ALP_p/P3/1$ antibody recognizes a determinant which is present on the enzyme protein product of ALP_p^1 and ALP_p^2 but absent from the enzyme protein product of ALP_p^3.

2. Hybridomas $ALP_p/Sp2/2$, $ALP_p/Sp2/3$, and $ALP_p/Sp2/4$

The antibodies from each of these hybridomas have been tested against about 100 different placental ALPs selected to include representatives of each of the six common electrophoretic phenotypes and also the rare phenotypes. All the ALPs give significant positive binding with each of the antibodies. In the case of $ALP_p/Sp2/3$ the level of binding appeared to be consistently lower with ALPs of phenotype 2 than with the other phenotypes and ALPs of phenotype 2-1 and 3-2 gave intermediate values, though there was much overlap of the distributions. The situation requires further study and more detailed analysis, but the preliminary results suggest that $ALP_p/Sp2/3$ may be discriminating quantita-

TABLE I

Relative Binding of the Six "Common" ALP Types to Antibodies in Culture Fluids of Seven Different Clones and Uncloned Cells of Hybridoma $ALP_p/P3/1$[a]

Alkaline phosphatase phenotype	Clones							Uncloned hybridoma	m	SD	SEM
	1	2	3	4	5	6	7				
1	1.000	1.000	1.000	1.000	1.000	1.000	1.000	1.000	1.000	—	—
2-1	0.819	0.805	1.350	0.945	0.890	0.880	1.056	0.959	0.963	0.176	0.062
2	0.798	0.916	1.203	0.932	0.852	0.871	0.930	0.998	0.938	0.123	0.043
3-1	0.528	0.637	0.831	0.536	0.545	0.644	0.779	0.664	0.646	0.113	0.040
3-2	0.647	0.751	0.876	0.358	0.511	0.629	0.670	0.628	0.633	0.154	0.054
3	0.103	0.072	0.081	−0.0002	−0.040	0.043	−0.057	−0.137	0.008	0.082	0.029

[a]The values given were obtained by dividing the mean c.p.m. minus background for the particular phenotype with a specific clone by the corresponding cpm minus background for ALP type 1.

tively between the enzyme protein products of $ALP_p{}^1$ and $ALP_p{}^3$ on the one hand, and $ALP_p{}^2$ on the other. A possible explanation is that it recognizes a determinant in the ALP proteins determined by $ALP_p{}^1$ and $ALP_p{}^3$ which is present in a structurally modified form in the ALP protein determined by $ALP_p{}^2$, the structural change involved being sufficient to reduce the level of antibody binding, but insufficient to destroy binding entirely. In the cases of $ALP_p/Sp2/2$ and $ALP_p/Sp2/4$, no gross differences between the various electrophoretic phenotypes were noted, but further studies will be required to exclude the existence of polymorphic differences among the placentas in their behavior with these antibodies.

In summary then, one may conclude that the general method is capable of detecting polymorphic differences between enzyme proteins determined by alleles at a particular locus and that it is also capable of differentiating quantitatively between heterozygotes and homozygotes. Further, $ALP_p/P3/1$ is evidently recognizing a different determinant from the determinants recognized by the other three antibodies. $ALP_p/Sp2/3$ may also be recognizing a different determinant from those recognized by other antibodies.

IV. Concluding Remarks

We have described a solid-phase radioimmunoassay which permits screening of particular enzymes and proteins from large numbers of individuals for structural variation with monoclonal antibodies produced by hybridomas. Four hybridomas have been produced which specifically recognize antigenic determinants on human placental ALP. Polymorphic variation, certainly at one and possibly at two of the determinant sites has been identified, and the value of quantitative studies as opposed to a simple all-or-none classification of the reactions has been exemplified. We propose to extend these genetic surveys both by screening more individuals and by producing further hybridomas for the study of additional determinants. In each case any variation discovered will be correlated with the presence of electrophoretically defined allelic forms in order to (1) assess the incidence of multiple allelism not revealed electrophoretically, and (2) estimate the extent of structural differences between the allelic variants. The hybridomas should also prove extremely valuable in characterizing the aberrant placentallike ALPs which occur in certain malignancies and cell lines originally derived from malignancies.

We also propose to use the hybridomas to investigate the antigenic relationships between placental ALP and ALPs determined by other loci. Intestinal ALP is of particular interest here because it has been shown to cross-react with whole antiserum raised against placental ALP and so presumably has some common antigenic determinants, yet it differs quite markedly in various physicochemical characteristics from placental ALP and is evidently coded at a separate locus. Solomon and Jones (this volume) report the production of a monoclonal antibody after immunization of mice with membrane of D98/AH2 cells, which appears to react with human intestinal ALP, an enzyme known to be produced by this cell line (Benham and Harris, 1979). We will also extend the investigations to ALPs derived from tissues of other animal species in order to examine the power of the method for studies in molecular evolution.

Finally, the hybridomas will be used to investigate the surface topology of the glycoprotein. Whether, for example, the particular determinants detected by the various antibodies are in the protein or carbohydrate moiety of the molecule; whether particular monoclonal antibodies extinguish the enzyme's catalytic activity or block the binding of specific inhibitors; and whether and to what degree binding by one monoclonal antibody reduces binding by another. The sensitivity of hybridomas against denatured as opposed to native enzyme will also be tested to determine the relative incidence of "conformation-dependent" as opposed to "sequence-dependent" monoclonal antibodies.

ACKNOWLEDGMENTS

We wish to thank Drs. N. R. Klinman and R. H. Kennett for valuable discussions during the work.

The research was supported by Grant CA-20296 from the National Cancer Institute DHEW, and Grant VC-231A from the American Cancer Society.

References

Arnon, R., 1973, Immunochemistry of enzymes in: *The Antigens*, Vol. 1 (M. Sela, ed.), Academic Press, New York, Chapter 2, pp. 88–159.

Badger, K. S., and Sussman, H., 1976, Structural evidence that human liver and placental alkaline phosphatase isoenzymes are coded by different genes, *Proc. Natl. Acad. Sci. USA* **73**:2201–2205

Beckman G., 1970, Placental alkaline phosphatase, relation between phenotype and enzyme activity, *Hum. Hered.* **20**:74.

Benham, F., and Harris, H., 1979, Human cell lines expressing intestinal alkaline phosphatase, *Proc. Natl. Acad. Sci. USA* **76**:4016–4019.

Cancro, M. P., and Potter, M., 1976, The requirement of an adherent cell substratum for the growth of developing plasmacytoma cells *in vivo*, *J. Exp. Med.* **144**:1554–1567.

Champion, A. B., Prager, E. M., Wachter, D., and Wilson, A. C., 1974, Microcomplement fixation, in: *Biomedical and Immunological Taxonomy of Animals* (C. A. Wright, ed.), Academic Press, New York, pp. 397–416.

Champion, A. B., Soderberg, K. L., Wilson, A. C., and Ambler, R. P., 1975, Immunological comparison of azurins of known amino acid sequence, *J. Mol. Evol.* **5**:291–305.

Coffino, P., Laskov, R., and Scharff, M. D., 1970, Immunoglobulin production: Method for detecting and quantitating variant myeloma cells, *Science* **167**:186–188.

Crumpton, M. J., 1974, Protein antigens: The molecular bases of antigenicity and immunogenicity, in: *The Antigens*, Vol. 2 (M. Sela, ed.), Academic Press, New York, Chapter 1, pp. 1–78.

Doellgast, G. J., 1979, Preparation of variant-specific anti-human placental phosphatase antisera by immunoabsorption, *Biochem. Biophys. Res. Commun.* **86**:661–666.

Doellgast, G. J., Silver, M. D., Fishman, L., and Guenther, R. A., 1976, Homogeneous human placental alkaline phosphatase shares antigenic determinants with human intestinal alkaline phosphates, in: *Onco-Developmental Gene Expression* (W. M. Fishman and W. Soll, eds.), Academic Press, New York, pp. 737–741.

Donald, L. J., and Robson, E. B., 1973, Rare variants of placental alkaline phosphatase, *Ann. Hum. Genet.* **37:**303–313.

Fernley, H. N., 1971, Mammalian alkaline phosphatase, in: *The Enzymes*, 3rd ed., Vol. 4 (P. D. Boyer, ed.), Academic Press, New York, pp. 417–447.

Fishman, W. H., 1974, Perspectives on alkaline phosphatase isoenzymes, *Am. J. Med.* **56:**617–650.

Fletcher, L., Rider, C. C., and Taylor, C. B., 1976, Enolase isoenzymes III. Chromatographic and immunological characteristics of rat brain enolase, *Biochem. Biophys. Acta* **452:**245–252.

Frazer, D., 1957, Hypophosphatasia, *Am. J. Med.* **22:**730–746.

Harris, H., 1979, Multilocus enzymes in man, in: *Human Genetics: Possibilities and Realities, Ciba Found. Symp. 66 [N. S],* Excerpta Medica, Amsterdam, pp. 187–199.

Harris, H., and Hopkinson, D. A., 1972, Average heterozygosity per locus in man: An estimate based on the incidence of enzyme polymorphisms, *Ann. Hum. Genet.* **36:**9–20.

Harris, H., and Hopkinson, D. A., 1976, *Handbook of Enzyme Electrophoresis in Human Genetics*, North-Holland, Amsterdam.

Harris, H., Hopkinson, D. A., and Robson, E. B., 1974, The incidence of rare alleles determining electrophoretic variants: Data on 43 enzyme loci in man, *Ann. Hum. Genet.* **37:**237–253.

Hirano, K., Sugiura, M., Miki, K., Iino, S., Suzuki, H., and Oda, T., 1977, Characterization of tissue-specific isozyme of alkaline phosphatase from human placenta and intestine, *Chem. Pharm. Bull. (Tokyo)* **25:**2524–2529.

Holmgren, P. K., Stigbrand, T., and Beckman, G., 1977, Purification and partial characterization of the I variant of placental alkaline phosphatase, *Biochem. Genet.* **15:**521–530.

Jollès, J., Schoentgen, F., Jollès, P., Prager, E. M., and Wilson A. C., 1976, Amino acid sequence and immunological properties of Chachalaca egg white lysozyme, *J. Mol. Evol.* **8:**59–78.

Kennett, R. H., Denis, K. A., Tung, A. S., and Klinman, N. R., 1978, Hybrid plasmacytoma production: Fusions with adult spleen cells, monoclonal spleen fragments, neonatal spleen cells and human spleen cells, *Curr. Top. Microbiol. Immunol.* **81:**77–91.

Khattab, M., and Pfleiderer, G., 1976, Alkaline phosphatase of human and calf small intestine. Purification and immunochemical characterization, *Hoppe-Seylers Z. Physiol. Chem.* **357:**377–391.

Köhler, G., and Milstein, C., 1975, Continuous cultures of fused cells secreting antibody of predefined specificity, *Nature* **256:**495–497.

Laver, W. G., Gerhard, W., Webster, R. G., Frankel, M. E., and Air, G. M., 1979, Antigenic drift in type A influenza virus: Peptide mapping and antigenic analysis of APR8 34 (HON 1) variants selected with monoclonal antibodies, *Proc. Natl. Acad. Sci. USA* **76:**1425–1429.

Lehmann, F.-G., 1975, Immunological relationship between human placental and intestinal alkaline phosphatase, *Clin. Chim. Acta* **65:**257–269.

Lewontin, R. C., 1974, *The Genetic Basis of Evolutionary Change,* Columbia University Press, New York. (Columbia Biological Series, no. 25.)

Manson, L. A., Verastegui-Cerdan, E., and Sporer, R., 1978, A quantitative disc radioimmunassay for antibodies directed against membrane-associated antigens, *Curr. Top. Microbiol. Immunol.* **81:**232–234.

Margoliash, E., Nisonoff, A., and Reichlin, M., 1970, Immunological activity of cytochrome c. 1. Precipitating antibodies to monomeric vertebrate cytochome c, *J. Biol. Chem.* **254:**931–939.

Mulivor, R. A., Mennuti, M., Zackai, E. H., and Harris, H., 1978a, Prenatal diagnosis of hypophosphatasia: Genetic, biochemical and clinical studies, *Am. J. Hum. Genet.* **30:**271–282.

Mulivor, R. A., Plotkin, L. I., and Harris, H., 1978b, Differential inhibition of the products of the human alkaline phosphatase loci, *Ann. Hum. Genet.* **42:**1–13.

Potter, M., Pumphrey, J., and Walters, J., 1972, Growth of primary plasmacytomas in the mineral oil conditioned peritoneal environment, *J. Natl. Cancer Inst.* **49:**305–308.

Prager, E. M., and Wilson, A. C., 1971a, The dependence of immunochemical cross-reactivity upon sequence resemblance among lysozymes. 1. Micro-complement fixation studies, *J. Biol. Chem.* **246:**5978–5989.

Prager, E. M., and Wilson, A. C., 1971b, The dependence of immunological cross-reactivity upon sequence resemblance among lysozymes. II. Comparison of precipitin and micro-complement fixation results, *J. Biol. Chem.* **246:**7010–7017.

Ratcliffe, J. G., 1974, Separation methods in saturation analysis, *Br. Med. Bull.* **30:**32–37.

Rathbun, J. C., 1948, "Hypophosphatasia." A new developmental anomaly, *Am. J. Dis. Child.* **75:**822–831.

Rider, C. C., and Taylor, C. B., 1974, Enolase isoenzymes in rat tissues. Electrophoretic, chromatographic, immunological and kinetic properties, *Biochim. Biophys. Acta* **365:**285–300.

Rider, C. C., and Taylor, C. B., 1975, Enolase isoenzyme II. Hybridization studies, developmental and phylogenetic aspects, *Biochim. Biophys. Acta* **405:**175–187.

Robson, E. B., and Harris, H., 1965, Genetics of the alkaline phosphatase polymorphism of human placenta, *Nature* **207:**1257–1259.

Robson, E. B., and Harris, H., 1967, Further studies on the genetics of placental alkaline phosphatase, *Ann. Hum. Genet.* **30:**219–232.

Seargeant, L. E., and Stinson, R. A., 1979, Evidence that three structural genes code for human placental alkaline phosphatases, *Nature* **281:**152–154.

Shulman, M., Wilde, C. D., and Köhler, G., 1978, A better cell line for making hybridomas secreting specific antibodies, *Nature* **276:**269–270.

Singh, I., and Tsang, K. Y., 1975, An *in vitro* production of bone specific alkaline phosphatase, *Exp. Cell Res.* **95:**347–358.

Skelley, D. S., Brown, L. P., and Besch, P. K., 1973, Radioimmunassay, *Clin. Chem.* **19:**146–186.

Sonderegger, P., and Christen, P., 1978, Comparison of the evolution rates of cytosolic and mitochondrial aspartate aminotransferase, *Nature* **275:**157–159.

Sonderegger, P., Gehring, H., and Christen, P., 1977, Interspecies comparsion of cytosolic and mitochondrial aspartate aminotransferases. Evidence for a more conservative evolution of the mitochondrial isoenzyme, *J. Biol. Chem.* **252:**609–612.

Sussman, H. H., Small, P. A., and Cotlove, E., 1968, Human alkaline phosphatase. Immunochemical identification of organ-specific isoenzymes, *J. Biol. Chem.* **243:**160–166.

Wallace, D. G., and Boulter, D., 1976, Immunological comparisons of higher plant plastocyanins, *Phytochemistry* **15:**137–141.

Welling, G. W., Groen, G., Beintema, J. J., Emers, M., and Schröder, F. P., 1976, Immunologic comparison of pancreatic ribonucleases, *Immunochemistry* **13:**653–658.

Wilson, A. C., Carlson, S. S., and White, T. H., 1977, Biochemical evolution, *Ann. Rev. Biochem.* **46:**573–639.

Wisdom, G. B., 1976, Enzyme-immunoassay, *Clin. Chem.* **22:**1243–1255.

Yewdell, J. W., Webster, R. G., and Gerhard, W. U., 1979, Antigenic variants in three distinct determinants of an influenza type A hemagglutinin molecule, *Nature* **279:**246–248.

8
Characterization of a Human T-Cell Population Identified and Isolated by a Monoclonal Antibody

RICHARD A. GOLDSBY, BARBARA A. OSBORNE, AND EDGAR G. ENGLEMAN

I. Introduction

The surface properties of human lymphocytes are of great interest because they identify populations of lymphocytes which conduct different functions of the immune system. Thus B lymphocytes carry an array of immunoglobulin (Ig) molecules on their surface (Froland and Natvig, 1972; Fu et al., 1974). Human peripheral T cells and thymocytes bear receptors for sheep erythrocytes and are thus capable of forming rosettes when mixed with sheep red blood cells (Brain et al., 1970; Coombs et al., 1970; Jondal et al., 1972). With the application of appropriate rosetting techniques, complement receptors can be demonstrated on the surface of human B cells and null cells (Perlman et al., 1975). Additionally, immune-response-associated (Ia) alloantigens are expressed in human B cells (Jones et al., 1975; Winchester et al., 1975). Antisera to these determinants have been shown to block stimulation in mixed lymphocyte cultures (Winchester et al., 1975) and to inhibit antibody-dependent cellular cytotoxicity (Chess et al., 1976). These considerations make it apparent that highly specific, high-titer antibody preparations to particular human lymphocyte-surface antigens would

RICHARD A. GOLDSBY • Department of Chemistry, University of Maryland, College Park, Maryland 20742. BARBARA A. OSBORNE • Department of Genetics, Stanford University Medical Center, Stanford, California 94305. EDGAR G. ENGLEMAN • Department of Pathology, Stanford University Medical Center, Stanford, California 94305.

assist greatly in extending our ability to detect changes in lymphocyte subpopulations.

Until the advent of successful approaches to the construction of monoclonal antibody-producing hybrid cell lines one of two standard methods of obtaining antibodies to cell-surface antigens were employed. One of these, immunization with cells bearing the target antigens across xenogeneic or allogeneic barriers, requires an absorption protocol deemed sufficient to remove unwanted activities and render the antisera specific. The other approach involves simplification of the immunogen by isolation and purification of the cell-surface antigen(s) of interest and subsequent use of the purified antigen(s) in a program of immunization.

In this report we describe the derivation of a monoclonal antibody which reacts with a subpopulation of human peripheral T cells. In addition, by immunoprecipitation and two-dimensional gel analysis we have demonstrated that the antigen, which we have called Ta, recognized by the subpopulation-specific, monoclonal anti-Ta antibody is part of, or firmly associated with, a protein of the plasma membrane. We also note that Ta^+ peripheral T cells respond to the mitogens phytohemagglutinin (PHA), pokeweed mitogen (PWM), and concanavalin A (Con A) while Ta^- peripheral T cells respond poorly to PHA and PWM and give no detectable response to Con A.

II. Production and Selection of Antibodies to Human T Cells

A. Production of Antibody-Secreting Hybrids

Hybrids were derived by fusing spleen cells from three 12- to 16-week-old female BALB/c mice which had been immunized as follows: mice were primed by i.p. injection of 1×10^7 peripheral blood mononuclear leukocytes (PBMLs) obtained from fresh peripheral blood by centrifugation over Ficoll–Hypaque gradients (Boyum, 1968) and 10 days later boosted with a second i.p. injection of 5×10^6 PBMLs. Four days after boosting, spleens were removed from the immunized animals and spleen cells harvested by grinding between glass slides and washed in serum-free Dulbecco's Modified Eagle's Medium (DMEM). Pooled spleen cells (2×10^8) were fused to 2×10^7 cells of the line P3/NS1-AG4-1 (Köhler et al., 1976), a nonsecreting variant of MOPC 21, as detailed in Goldsby et al. (1977). Following fusion, the cells were resuspended in DMEM which contained the following additives at the indicated concentrations: 2 mM glutamine, 100 units/ml penicillin, 100µg/ml streptomycin 10% fetal calf serum (FCS), and the hypoxanthine–aminopterin–thymidine (HAT) (Littlefield, 1964) selective system. Then 0.2-ml aliquots of this suspension containing 2×10^6 spleen cells were dispensed to 96 wells of Falcon multiwell plates. At 1 and 2 weeks posthybridization, two thirds of the medium was removed from each well and replaced with fresh HAT medium. After 16 days each well contained two or more clones which were visible to the naked eye. At this point samples of culture fluid from each well were assayed for cell-binding activity by a cell-binding assay conducted as outlined by Levy and Dilley (1977), except we employed an iodinated rabbit anti-mouse Ig as a second step.

B. Binding of Mouse Anti-Human Ig to Human Cell-Surface Antigens

Initial screening assays of hybrid culture fluids were conducted using a cell-binding radioimmunoassay performed as follows: 50 μl of a putative antibody preparation or an appropriate control is added to the wells of a 96-place, flexible U-bottom microtiter plate. Each well then receives 2–5 × 10⁵ PBL target cells in a volume of 50 μl of phosphate-buffered saline (PBS) containing 0.1% bovine serum albumin (BSA) and 0.1% NaN_3 (PBS–BSA–N_3). Following a 1-hr incubation at 25°C the assay plates are centrifuged at 800 × g for 10 min, after which the supernatant is removed by inverting the plate with a single abrupt flick. Cell pellets are resuspended by the rapid simultaneous addition of 200 μl of PBS–BSA–N_3 to all 96 wells of the assay plate with the syringe replicator (Fig. 1) and again centrifuged at 800 × g for 10 min, after which the wash liquor is flicked from the plate. After three washes, 20 μl of [¹²⁵I]rabbit anti-mouse Ig (1000 cpm/μl) is added to each well and the system is incubated for an additional hour. Following the incubation with tracer, the pellets are washed three times as previously described. The plates are then dried, cut with a hot-wire device and the individual wells counted in a gamma counter. Samples were judged to be positive when they exceeded the mean of the growth medium control by more than 3 standard deviations.

When mouse serum samples were assayed the procedure described above was followed with this exception: the activity in the binding assay of a series of dilutions of a sample suspected of containing an anti-human cell antibody is compared with the activity of a comparable series of dilutions of normal serum. Positive sera have significantly (nonoverlapping standard deviations) higher titration curves than control sera.

C. Isolation of Human T and Non-T Cells of Peripheral Blood

Human peripheral blood mononuclear leukocytes were isolated from normal volunteers by Ficoll–Hypaque density gradient centrifugation. The PBMLs were resuspended in 40% FCS in PBS and mixed with an equal volume of 3% sheep erythrocytes previously washed and resuspended in 40% FCS–PBS. This mixture was immediately sedimented over a second Ficoll–Hypaque gradient in order to separate the rosetted T cells from the nonrosetted (non-T) cells. Cells recovered from the rosetted pellet by treatment with 0.155 M NH_4Cl were 96–100% E-rosette-positive and contained fewer than 3% surface-Ig-positive cells on the basis of a direct fluoresceinated antibody-binding assay. In addition, fewer than 1% of this T-enriched fraction were monocytes based on staining with α-naphthyl acetate. Nonrosetting (non-T) cells consisted of 85–93% surface-Ig-positive cells, including 33–45% monocytes.

D. Analysis and Cell Separation on the Fluorescence-Activated Cell Sorter (FACS)

The binding specificity of monoclonal anti-Ta was studied by indirect immunofluorescence with fluorescein-labeled rabbit anti-mouse Ig which had been adsorbed on a column of Sepharose-conjugated human Ig. Cells were stained by resuspending 1×10^6 cells in 0.1 ml of the indicated dilution of serum from normal BALB/c mice or a mouse bearing the anti-Ta-secreting hybrid. All dilutions were made with PBS to which sodium azide had been added to a level of 0.1% to prevent capping. The cells were incubated for 20 min at 25°C, washed twice with PBS-azide and indirectly stained by incubation for an additional 20 min with the fluoresceinated rabbit anti-mouse Ig. After washing, the labeled cells were analyzed in an FACS III (Becton Dickinson Electronic Laboratories, Mountain View, Calif.). For separation experiments T cells were labeled as described and then sorted in populations falling into the upper and lower 30th percentiles of fluorescence intensity.

E. Proliferative Responses of T Cells to Mitogens

Stimulation of the indicated populations was conducted in RPMI 1640 supplemented with 25 mM HEPES buffer, 2 mM glutamine, 100 μ/ml each of penicillin and streptomycin and 10% heat-inactivated FCS under an atmosphere of 5% CO_2/95% air for 3–6 days at 37°C. Round-bottom microtiter wells were seeded with 10^5 cells in 0.2 ml of the supplemented RPMI 1640 containing either no added mitogens or one of the following mitogens at the indicated concentration: Con A (Pharmacia Fine Chemicals, Sweden), 50 μg/ml; PHA (Burroughs Welcome, Beckingham Kent, England), 1 μg/ml; and PWM (Grand Island Biological Company, Grand Island, N.Y.) at a final dilution of 1:100. Assays were performed in triplicate and 1μ Ci/well of [³H]thymidine was added 18 hr before harvesting.

F. Labeling, Immunoprecipitation, and Two-Dimensional Gel Electrophoresis

1. [³⁵S]Methionine Labeling of Human T Cells

Purified peripheral T cells were labeled by adding 500 Ci/mM [³⁵S]methionine (New England Nuclear Corp., Boston, Mass.) to a final activity of 250μ Ci/

ml to 5×10^7 T cells in 1 ml of methionine-free DMEM containing 2 mM glutamine and 5% heat-inactivated FCS. The cells were incubated at 37°C for 4 hr with occasional agitation under a humidified atmosphere of 10% CO_2/90% air. Incorporation of label was terminated by the addition of 5 ml of cold Dulbecco's PBS containing 2 mM methionine and the cells were harvested by centrifugation and washed twice in this medium.

2. Immunoprecipitation

The cell pellet was resuspended at 1×10^7 cells/0.1 ml in 0.5% NP-40 (Particle Data Inc., Elmhurst, Ill.) in Tris-buffered saline (150 mM NaCl, 50 mM tris, 0.2% NaN_3, pH 7.0) and incubated 15 min at 4°C. Insoluble material was removed by centrifugation at 45,000 $\times$ g for 1 hr. Immunoprecipitation was conducted by a procedure in which antigen–antibody complexes are harvested by binding to *Staphylococcus aureus*, Cowan I strain (SaC). Specifically, 100-μl aliquots of the NP-40 extract were treated with 5 μl of serum from a mouse bearing the anti-Ta secreting hybrid as a tumor or with 5 μl of normal BALB/c mouse serum and incubated at 4°C for 15 min. Subsequently, each sample received 200 μl of SaC (a 10% w/v suspension) in PBS (0.2 M NaCl, 0.0125 M $K_3 PO_4$, 0.2% NaN_3, pH 7.6) containing 1 mg/ml BSA and was incubated 10 min at 4°C. The samples were then diluted in the PBS–BSA buffer, centrifuged 10 min at 2000 $\times$ g and subsequently washed 3$\times$ in PBS–BSA. After each wash, the pelleted bacteria were resuspended and transferred to a clean tube. The bound antigen–antibody complexes were eluted from the SaC by addition of 50 μl of isoelectric focusing buffer [9.5 M urea, 2% (w/v) NP-40, 2% pH range 3.5–10 ampholines and 5% β-mercaptoethanol] followed by centrifugation for 10 min at 2000 $\times$ g at 25°C. Samples (1 l) were removed from each eluate for determination of trichloroacetic acid (TCA) precipitable radioactivity.

3. 2D Gel Electrophoresis and Autoradiography

First-dimension isoelectric focusing was performed, using the nonequilibrium pH gradient electrophoresis (NEPHGE) technique of O'Farrell *et al.* (1977). For the second dimension, the NEPHGE gels were embedded in a 4.5% stacking gel and electrophoresed into a 10% acrylamide slab gel as described by Jones (1977). Following electrophoresis the gels were dried *in vacuo* and autoradiographed by permitting them to expose Kodak No-screen X-ray film for 28 days.

G. A Mechanical System for Cloning, Feeding, and the Performance of Washing Operations during Cell-Binding Assays

Figure 1 is a picture of the syringe replicator, a rigid matrix of 96 disposable tuberculin syringes outfitted with dropping tips and concentric with the 96 wells of a microtiter dish. This apparatus is used for the mechanical performance of

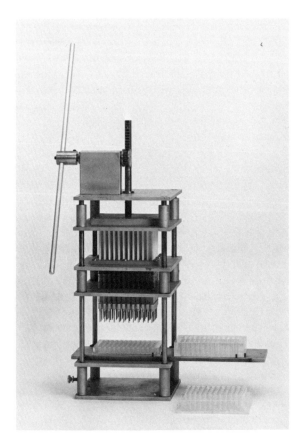

FIGURE 1. Syringe replicator with a chambered trough and 96-well microtiter dish on ways.

such tasks as the seeding of cells, for cloning at limiting dilution, feeding, replica plating, and the precise collection and transfer of measured aliquots of culture fluid during screening procedures.

1. Seeding for the Isolation of Single Clones

Generally it is desirable to seed the wells of microtiter dishes at an average density of 1 cloning unit per well. In practice one usually does not have knowledge of cloning efficiencies of the hybrid lines one wishes to clone. This difficulty is overcome by adding suspensions containing different numbers of cells to the several chambers of a trough such as that pictured in Fig. 1 and using the replicator to transfer samples of each suspension to a group of wells on a microtiter dish. This is accomplished by immersing the syringe replicator's matrix of transfer elements into the cell suspensions and drawing an appropriate volume of the suspension into the syringes by rotation of the handle (see Fig. 1) which drives the rack-and-pinion assembly. The microtiter dish to be loaded is then placed on the ways and moved into position under the transfer elements of the syringe replicator in such a fashion as to place its 96 wells directly beneath the 96 transfer elements. The adjustable platform of the replicator is then raised so as to place the transfer elements of the replicator in the wells of the matrix. The syringe replicator is then made to deliver the desired volume of suspension (±7%) to the wells of the incubation matrix by appropriate rotation of the handle driving the rack-and-pinion assembly.

2. Replica Plating

When the syringe replicator is used in the production of replica plates, the master plate from which cloned patterns are to be transferred is placed on the ways and the needles of the replicator are inserted into the wells of the microtiter dish. The hybrid clones are suspended by rotating the handle back and forth and after dispersion, a measured volume of each cell suspension, usually 0.05 ml, is pulled into the syringe replicator and expelled into a second plate containing 0.2 ml of the desired incubation medium. While clone transfer and feeding can be accomplished with Pasteur pipettes outfitted with dropping bulbs, a considerable saving in time and effort, as well as a more uniform pattern of addition, is obtained when one uses the syringe replicator. Using this procedure 3 or 4 replicas of a master plate may be obtained within 5–10 min. When more than one master plate is to be replica plated, the replicator is freed of contaminating cells by first filling the 96 syringes with sterile 0.85% saline, and subsequently filling the syringes with 70% ETOH to kill any cells which may have been trapped in the apparatus, and finally by filling the syringes with 0.85% saline to remove the alcohol.

III. Characterization of a Human T-Cell Antigen Defined by a Monoclonal Antibody

A. Production of Anti-Human Mononuclear Leukocyte-Secreting Hybrids

Out of 93 initial hybrid populations, 60 produced antibodies which demonstrated reactivity to glutaraldehyde-fixed human MLs when tested in the cell-binding radioimmunoassay as described. After three or more passages in culture some of the hybrids which retained activity were successfully cloned by limiting dilution in microtiter dishes (Goldsby and Zipser, 1967), grown to mass cultures, and inoculated into BALB/c mice where they gave rise to antibody-producing tumors. The sera obtained from mice bearing these tumors yielded the results shown in Table I. Three of the hybrids, Tumor I, # 28, and α-Ta reacted with fixed or unfixed human MLs but failed to react with human or mouse erythrocytes. Another group of hybrids 23-6, 7e, and 21b reacted with fixed human MLs, human red blood cells (RBCs), and mouse RBCs but failed to react with unfixed preparations of these cells. The results summarized in Table II show

TABLE I

Reactivity toward Different Cell Populations[a]

Hybrid	Mixed HMLs[b]		Mixed HRBCs[c]		Fixed HRBCs				BALB/c RBCs[d]		Fixed BALB/c thymocytes
	Fixed	Unfixed	Fixed	Unfixed	A+	O+	A-	O-	Fixed	Unfixed	
Tumor I	+	+	-	-	-	-	-	-	-	-	-
28	+	+	-	-	-	-	-	-	-	-	-
α-Ta	+	+	-	-	-	-	-	-	n.d.	n.d.	-
23-6	+	-	+	-	+	+	+	+	n.d.	n.d.	-
7e	+	-	+	-	+	+	+	+	+	-	+/-
21b	+	-	+	-	+	+	+	+	+	-	+/-
7S2[e] (anti-DNP)	-	-	-	-	-	-	-	-	-	-	-

[a] The pattern of reactivity of several monoclonal antibodies to fixed and unfixed cells of a variety of types.

[b] Human mononuclear leukocytes from 3 to 5 unrelated donors.

[c] Human red blood cells from 3 to 6 unrelated donors.

[d] n.d.: Not determined.

[e] 7S2 is a hybrid which resulted from the hybridization of the myeloma P3/X63-Ag8 with spleen cells from BALB/c mice immunized with DNP–KLH. This hybrid, which produces an anti-DNP molecule devoid of specific reactivity to human cell-surface antigens, provides a negative control.

TABLE II

Reactivity of Various Monoclonal Antibodies to
Human Serum or Human Hemoglobin A[a]

Hybrid	Human serum	Human hemoglobin A
Tumor I	−	−
28	−	−
αTa	−	−
23-6	−	+
7e	−	+
21b	−	+
7S2	−	−

[a]The reactivity of several monoclonal antibodies to polystyrene plates coated with the indicated antigen is shown.

that these hybrids are reacting with hemoglobin, which is bound as an artifact of fixation during the glutaraldehyde treatment. The binding of mouse cells reflects cross-reaction between mouse and human hemoglobin. We feel that these data provide an example of the pitfalls inherent in the use of fixed cells for any purpose other than initial screening.

B. α-Ta Recognizes a Subpopulation of Human T Cells

When the ML-specific hybrids Tumor I, # 28, and α-Ta were screened to determine their suitability for use in immunofluorescence analysis, one of them, α-Ta, which secreted an IgG that focused at pH 6.5 ± 0.2 in the microcolumn technique of Press and Klinman (1973), stained a subpopulation of peripheral T cells but failed to stain peripheral B cells (see Fig. 2). In a survey of 8 healthy adults 30–35% of the T cells stained in 7 individuals and 50% were stained in the eighth member of this population.

Although anti-Ta discriminates between T and B lymphocytes, and even between peripheral T-lymphocyte subpopulations, this specificity does not extend to cultured lymphoid cell lines. As shown in Table III, the antibody binds with similar efficiency to the T-cell-derived lines Molt 4, HUT 78, and HUT 333 and to the B-cell-derived lines RPMI 1788 and HUT 91. The issue of antigenic differences between dividing or transformed cell lines and the nondividing and untransformed normal somatic cells from which they were derived is addressed in Section IV.

C. Immunoprecipitation of the Antigen Ta from Peripheral T Cells by α-Ta

When NP-40 extracts of [35S]methionine-labeled T cells are immunoprecipitated and analyzed by two-dimensional polyacrylamide gel electrophoresis, an

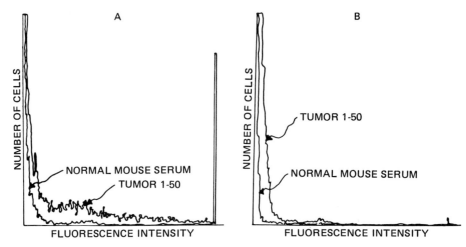

FIGURE 2. FACS analysis of the reactivity of serum from BALB/c mice in which a-Ta (Tumor 1-50) grew as an antibody-secreting tumor. Panel A: Pattern of staining obtained on human peripheral T cells purified by rosetting with sheep erythrocytes. Serum harvested from the tumor-bearing animals, which gave detectable staining at a dilution of 1/160, was used at a dilution of 1/20 to stain 1 × 10^6 human T cells. Normal serum from BALB/c mice at a dilution of 1/20 was used as a control. Panel B: The lack of reactivity of a-Ta against the B-cell-containing, nonrosetting peripheral leukocyte population. The indicated sera were used at a dilution of 1/20.

TABLE III

Reactivity of a Ta with Various Cell Types[a]

	Treatment	
Cell	a-Ta[b]	Normal BALB serum[c]
BW 5147	142 ± 7 cpm	85 ± 17 cpm
Unfixed human MLs	2354 ± 89	143 ± 4
Molt 4	1059 ± 28	73 ± 20
HUT 78	1866 ± 353	91 ± 8
HUT 333	957 ± 53	146 ± 46
RPMI 1788	1816 ± 13	125 ± 4
HUT 91	2114 ± 193	102 ± 4

[a]Binding of hybrid anti-Ta produced antibody by a variety of cell types. MLs were obtained from fresh blood; Molt 4, a human T-cell line, and RPMI 1788, a human B-cell line, were obtained from the American type culture collection; HUT 78, a human T-cell line, HUT 333, a human T-cell line,and HUT 91, a human B-cell line all were donated by Dr. Adi Gazedar of the National Cancer Institute. BW 5147, an AKR T lymphoma, was a gift of Dr. Robert Hyman of the Salk Institute. All determinations were performed in duplicate using 2 × 10^5 target cell of the indicated type and 13,000 cpm of an ^{125}I-labeled rabbit anti-mouse Ig per determination.

[b]Serum from tumor-bearing BALB/c mice at a dilution of 1/800.

[c]Serum from normal BALB/c mice at a dilution of 1/800.

antigen is specifically precipitated from cultures treated with α-Ta (see Fig. 3). Since the ^{35}S label was incorporated into protein, it may be concluded that the antigenic determinant recognized by this monoclonal antibody is a part of, or in firm association with, a polypeptide chain. It is also clear that the polypeptide backbone to which the determinant recognized by α-Ta is attached is of high molecular weight (95,000–115,000) and has a basic pI.

D. Response of Ta$^+$ and Ta$^-$ Cells to Mitogens

To determine if Ta$^+$ and Ta$^-$ cells were functionally distinct, sorted populations of each cell type were tested for their capacity to proliferate when exposed to appropriate concentrations of mitogens. The data in Table IV demonstrate that, although Ta$^+$ and Ta$^-$ cell populations responded equally well to alloantigens in the mixed lymphocyte reaction, the response of Ta$^+$ cells to PHA, PWM, and Con A was significantly greater than that of Ta$^-$ cells. In fact, the Ta$^-$ cell populations failed to give a detectable response to Con A. Also note that the response of Ta$^+$ cells to Con A is significantly greater than that given by the same number of unsorted cells.

IV. Discussion

We have established that the monoclonal antibody, α-Ta, distinguishes and allows isolation of a subpopulation of human T cells. The Ta$^+$ population, which appears to represent 30–35% of peripheral T cells in most individuals, responds well to the mitogens Con A, PHA, and PWM. By contrast, the Ta$^-$ population, while fully responsive to allogeneic stimulation in an MLR, is refractory to mitogenic stimulation by PHA and PWM and fails to respond detectably to incubation with Con A. These observations provide a demonstration of one of the ways in which monoclonal antibodies may be used to identify and isolate particular, functional subpopulations of human T cells from the several such populations present in peripheral blood.

Using the techniques of immunoprecipitation and 2D gel electrophoresis, it was possible to employ the monoclonal antibody we have described to effect biochemical resolution of the α-Ta reactive antigen, Ta, from the mixture of antigens present in peripheral T cells. Whether the Ta of peripheral T cells is the same as the α-Ta-reactive antigen found on some transformed B- and T-cell lines, or whether it is a cross-reacting antigen of different pI or molecular weight, awaits further analysis by 2D gel electrophoresis. If the α-Ta reactive antigen of these transformed cell lines is identical to Ta, such lines will be useful as starting materials for the isolation of this antigen. In this regard it should be emphasized that the reaction of α-Ta with both B- and T-cell lines does not (as demonstrated by the FACS and functional data above) in any way argue against

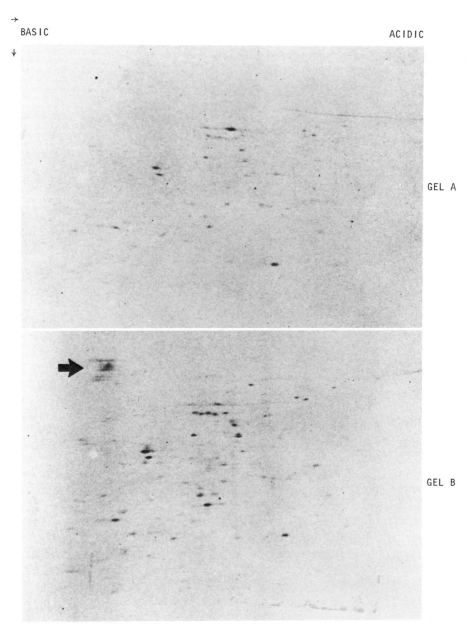

Figure 3. Autoradiograms of 2D gels of immunoprecipitated extracts of [³⁵S]methionine-labeled human peripheral T cells. The gels were run in the first dimension using nonequilibrium pH gradient electrophoresis (NEPHGE). For the second dimension NEPHGE gels were embedded in a 4.5% stacking gel and electrophoresed into a 10% acrylamide slab gel. The direction of electrophoresis is indicated by arrows at the extreme left. The basic end of the gels is on the left. A: Autoradiogram of 2D gel of an extract of human T cells immunoprecipitated with normal mouse serum. 6900 cpm of the extract was applied in a volume of 20 μl. B: Autoradiogram of a 2D gel of an extract of human T cells immunoprecipitated with the monoclonal anti-T cell subpopulation antibody α-Ta. 20 μl of the extract containing 4040 cpm was applied to the gel. The autoradiograms shown in A and B were produced by exposure of the gels to Kodak No-screen X-ray film for 28 days.

TABLE IV
Response of Ta+ and Ta− Cells to Mitogens[a]

Responder population	No mitogen	Con A	PHA	PWM	Allogenic cells
Unsorted T cells	230	3,527	20,688	5,031	52,773
Unsorted T cells +a-Ta + Rabbit a-MIG[b]	−	3,810	22,890	7,114	44,668
Ta+	71	18,947	27,435	4,702	37,612
Ta−	172	845	3,610	880	46,833

[a]Functional characteristics of Ta+ and Ta− cells. The indicated T-cell population from a normal donor were stimulated by PHA (1 μg/ml), Con A (50 μg/ml); and PWM (diluted 1 : 100). Values in cpm. The standard errors of the means never exceeded 15%.
[b]MIG, mouse immunoglobulin.

the ability of this antibody to discriminate between the *untransformed* B and T lymphocytes of peripheral blood. The appearance of new surface markers on lymphoid cells as a consequence of activation by mitogens such as Con A or by viral transformation (Person *et al.*, 1970) has been well documented. As an example of the appearance of nonviral markers as a consequence of activation, recall that surface-insulin receptors are induced in human-lymphocyte cultures by Con A activation (Krug *et al.*, 1972). These considerations make it apparent that differences in the surface-antigen profiles of a peripheral blood lymphocyte and its transformed, *in vitro* counterpart are not surprising but rather to be expected. Therefore, the appearance of an antigen on a transformed B-cell line that is identical to or cross-reactive with a subpopulation-specific antigen of peripheral T cells does not gainsay the usefulness of such an antigenic moiety for differentiating between the B and T lymphocytes of peripheral blood.

It is appropriate that a great deal of effort has been invested in the development of methods which permit the recognition and isolation of human-lymphocyte subsets. The importance of the problem lies in the realization that specific T-cell subsets perform such effector and regulatory functions as help, suppression, proliferation in response to allogeneic stimulation, cytotoxic activities, and the elaboration of certain lymphokines. The detailed analysis of the mechanisms underlying the conduct of these T-cell-mediated processes depends heavily on the ability to identify and isolate the involved T-cell subsets. Steps to resolve T-lymphocyte subpopulations have been taken, and some useful heteroantisera capable of identifying different human T-cell populations have been prepared by immunizing rabbits with T-cell leukemias or purified peripheral T cells and removing unwanted activities from the resultant antisera by programs of absorption (Chess and Schlossman, 1977). Additionally, it has been demonstrated that subpopulations of T cells that help or suppress the response of B cells to PWM bear surface Fc receptors with specificity for different immunoglobulin isotypes (Moretta *et al.*, 1977). To these existing approaches one can now add a monoclonal antibody which allows the identification and isolation of a specific functional subpopulation of peripheral T cells. Undoubtedly, the construction of antibody-producing hybrids for the production of highly specific, high-titer antibody preparations to cell-surface antigens will provide a number of such subset-specific reagents. These will assist greatly in extending our ability to detect and quantitate changes in human T-cell populations and, by so doing, will contribute, decisively, to the analysis of the roles played in the immune response by various human T-cell subpopulations.

ACKNOWLEDGMENTS

We thank Ms. Claudia Benike for excellent technical assistance in cell preparation and assays of T-cell function. We also thank Mr. Frances Assisi for expert assistance in the operation of the FACS. We are grateful to Mrs. Clare Wendal for her careful and patient typing of this manuscript. This work was supported by Grant CA 24607 from the National Institutes of Health, by Grant SBGH from the National Aeronautics and Space Administration, and, in part, by a grant from the Veterans Administration.

References

Boyum, A., 1968, Isolation of mononuclear cells and granulocytes from human blood, *Scand. J. Clin. Lab. Invest.* **21** [suppl. 97]:77.

Brain, P., Gordon, J., and Willetts, W. A., 1970, Rosette formation by peripheral lymphocytes, *Clin. Exp. Immunol.* **6**:681.

Chess, L., and Schlossman, S. F., 1977, Human lymphocyte subpopulations, in: *Advances in Immunology*, Vol. 25 (H. G. Kunkel and F. J. Dixon, eds.) Academic Press, New York, pp. 213–241.

Chess, L., Evans, R., Hymphreys, R. E., Strominger, J. L., and Schlossman, S. F., 1976, Inhibition of antibody-dependent cellular cytotoxicity and immunoglobulin synthesis by an antiserum prepared against a human B-cell Ia-like molecule, *J. Exp. Med.* **144**:113.

Coombs, R. R. A., Gurner, B. W., Wilson, A. B., Holm, G., and Lindgren, B., 1970, Rosette formation between human lymphocytes and sheep red cells not involving immunoglobulin receptors, *Int. Arch. Allergy Appl. Immunol.* **39**:658.

Froland, S. S., and Natvig, J. B., 1972, Class, subclass, and allelic exclusion of membrane-bound Ig of human B-lymphocytes, *J. Exp. Med.* **136**:409.

Fu, S. M., Winchester, R. J., and Kunkel, H. G., 1974, Occurrence of surface IgM, IgD and free light chains on human lymphocytes, *J. Exp. Med.* **139**:451.

Goldsby, R. A., and Zipser, E., 1967, The isolation and replica plating of mammalian cell clones, *Exp. Cell Res.* **54**:271.

Goldsby, R. A., Osborne, B. A., Simpson, E., and Herzenberg, L. A., 1977, Hybrid cell lines with T cell characteristics, *Nature* **256**:707.

Jondal, M., Holm, G., and Wigzell, H., 1972, Surface markers on human B and T lymphocytes—Large population of lymphocytes forming nonimmune rosettes with sheep red blood cells, *J. Exp. Med.* **136**:207.

Jones, E. A., Goodfellow, P. N., Bodmer, J. G., and Bodmer, W. F., 1975, Serological identification of HLA-linked human "Ia-type" antigens, *Nature* **256**:650.

Jones, P. P., 1977, Analysis of H-2 and Ia molecules by 2-dimensional gel electrophoresis, *J. Exp. Med.* **146**:1261.

Köhler, G., Howe, S. C., and Milstein, C., 1976, Fusion between immunoglobulin secreting and nonsecreting lines, *Eur. J. Immunol.* **6:**292.

Krug, U., Krug, F., and Cuatrecasas, P., 1972, Emergence of insulin receptors on human lymphocytes during *in vitro* transformation, *Proc. Natl. Acad. Sci. USA* **69:**2604.

Levy, R., and Dilley, J., 1977, *In vitro* antibody response to cell surface antigens: I. The xenogeneic response to human leukemia cells, *J. Immunol.* **119:**387.

Littlefield, J. W., 1964, Selection of hybrids from matings of fibroblasts *in vitro* and their presumed recombinants, *Science* **145:**709.

Moretta, L. O., Webb, S. R., Grossi, C. E., Lydard, P. M., and Cooper, M. D., 1977, Functional analysis of two human T-cell subpopulations: Help and suppression of B-cell responses by T cells bearing receptors for IgM or IgG, *J. Exp. Med.* **146:**184.

O'Farrell, P. Z., Goodman, H. M., and O'Farrell, P. H., 1977, High resolution two-dimensional electrophoresis of basic as well as acidic proteins, *Cell* **12:**1133.

Pearson, C., Dewey, F., Klein, G., Henle, G., and Henle, W., 1970, Relation between neutralization of Epstein-Barr virus and antibodies to cell membrane antigens induced by the virus, *J. Natl. Cancer Inst.* **45:**989.

Perlman, P., Perlman, H., and Müller-Eberhard, H. J., 1975, Cytolytic lymphocytic cells with complement receptor in human blood: Induction of cytolysis by IgG antibody but not by target cell bound C_3, *J. Exp. Med.* **141:**287.

Press, J. L., and Klinman, N. R., 1973, Isoelectric analysis of neonatal monofocal antibody, *Immunochemistry* **10:**621.

Winchester, R. S., Fu, M., Wernet, P., Kunkel, H. G., DuPont, B., and Jerslid, G., 1975, Recognition by pregnancy serums of non-HLA alloantigens selectively expressed on B-lymphocytes, *J. Exp. Med.* **141:**924.

9
Mouse × Human Hybridomas

Ronald Levy, Jeanette Dilley, Sherri Brown, and Yehudit Bergman

I. Introduction

Much of the original success of Köhler and Milstein in obtaining antibody-secreting hybridomas can be attributed to their development of suitable myeloma cell lines to be used as hybridization partners. It is clear that earlier failures to obtain antibody-secreting cell hybrids resulted from the use of cell lines that were themselves at an inappropriate state of differentiation to support antibody synthesis and secretion. A series of mouse myeloma cell lines, most of them derivatives of the original MOPC-21 or MPC-11 tumors, are now available. They fuse efficiently and support high-level synthesis and secretion by their hybridized partners. Thus, mouse monoclonal antibodies are now available in great variety and abundance. It would be of obvious interest to obtain human monoclonal antibodies for various diagnostic and therapeutic applications in clinical medicine. However, no suitable human cell line is currently available for the production of antibody-secreting human × human hybridomas. A high priority should be placed on the development of such human myeloma cell lines. In the meantime, it has become clear that interspecies hybrids between mouse cells and human cells can serve as a stable source of human immunoglobulin (Ig) production (Schwaber, 1975; Levy and Dilley, 1978), indicating that specific human antibodies will be obtainable from such mouse × human hybridomas.

In the present chapter, we will review a series of experiments with mouse × human hybridomas with an emphasis primarily on the characterization of the hybrid cells and their secreted products. The original impetus for these experiments was not the production of human antibodies, but rather the study of human B-cell malignancies and their cell-surface Ig. Specifically, the goal was to

Ronald Levy, Jeanette Dilley, Sherri Brown, and Yehudit Bergman • Howard Hughes Medical Institute Laboratories and Department of Medicine, Stanford University Medical Center, Stanford, California 94305.

develop an approach to human B-cell tumors that would take advantage of their Ig idiotype as a tumor-specific marker.

II. Mouse Myeloma Cells Hybridized with Human B-Cell Tumors

A. Cell Types

Approximately 80% of adults with lymphoproliferative malignancies have Ig-containing or Ig-producing tumors (Table I) (Levy and Kaplan, 1978; Filippa *et al.*, 1978). These tumor cell populations can be regarded as relatively homogeneous prototypes of various stages of normal B-cell maturation (Salmon and Seligmann, 1974). The Ig produced by these maligant populations is monoclonal, i.e., restricted to a single V_L, V_H, and light-chain type, either κ or λ.

The Ig is in some cases secreted in large amounts (i.e., multiple myeloma or Waldenström's macroglobulinemia) and in other cases found only intracytoplasmically or on the cell membrane (i.e., chronic lymphocytic leukemia, nodular lymphoma, etc.). We have focused our studies on the latter group, in which there is no significant secretion of Ig. The first question was: Could Ig secretion be rescued from these nonsecreting tumor cells by hybridization with mouse myeloma cells? Initially, the Ig-secreting mouse myeloma cell line P3/X63-Ag8 was fused to human chronic lymphocytic leukemia (CLL) or lymphosarcoma cells. In each case hybrids were obtained, and over 50% of them secreted human Ig as well as mouse Ig (Table II) (Levy and Dilley, 1978). In subsequent work, the nonsecreting myeloma line NS-1/Ag4 was used as the mouse hybridization part-

TABLE I
Human B-Cell Tumors

	Endogenous Ig secretion	Hybridized with mouse myeloma[a]	Human Ig secretion by hybrids[a,b]
Chronic lymphocytic leukemia	−	+	+
Lymphosarcoma-cell leukemia	−	+	+
Nodular lymphoma	−	+	+
Large-cell lymphoma	−	+	+
Burkitt's lymphoma	−	NT	NT
Hairy-cell leukemia	−	NT	NT
"Undifferentiated" lymphoma	−	NT	NT
Acute lymphocytic leukemia of pre-B-cell type	−	NT	NT
Multiple myeloma	+	NT	NT
Waldenström's macroglobulinemia	+	NT	NT

[a]NT, Not tested.
[b]Ig secretion was detected by radioimmunoassay.

ner and it gave a similar frequency of human Ig-secreting cell hybrids (Table II, Fig. 1). In each case the human light-chain type of all of the secreting hybridomas was identical to that on the cell surface of the human tumor cell parent. In addition, the light-chain mobility of the rescued human Ig was identical for all the hybrids from a given patient and different for each patient (Fig. 1). Thus, the secreting hybridomas were derived from the tumor cell population and not from contaminating nontumor cells (see also discussion of the production of antiidiotype reagents in Section VI). Listed in Table I are the various types of human B-cell tumors that have been successfully hybridized to produce human Ig-secreting hybridomas. We have succeeded in rescuing secretion from all of the types of human B-cell tumors that we have tested so far, although there is variability in the secretion success rate among hybridomas made from individual patients. For example, the cells from some patients consistently failed to yield human Ig-secreting hybrids, even though they did rescue secretion of mouse light chain of the nonsecreting NS-1 parent.

Is preexisting Ig secretion and/or cell division necessary before a B cell can successfully fuse with a myeloma cell and continuously secrete antibody? The results of these human × mouse hybridomas would suggest that neither cell division nor prior Ig secretion are necessary, since CLL cells will work. However, the fusion frequency in these experiments is only on the order of $1/10^5$. It is possible that the tumor populations contain dividing or secreting cells at low levels and that it is these cells which preferentially form hybrids. Recent results of Eshhar *et al.* (1979), who rescued Ig secretion from nonsecreting mouse B lymphoma cells, would tend to make this explanation unlikely, since no Ig-secreting cells could be detected in their input population by a technique that could detect secreting cells at a level of $1/10^6$. Furthermore, our own results on the molecular form of the "rescued" μ chain (see Section IV) would suggest that the true parent was indeed a nonsecreting cell. Table III lists other successful attempts to rescue Ig secretion from nonsecreting cells by hybridization to myelomas.

TABLE II

Rescue of Human Ig Secretion

Patient	Disease[a]	Cell-surface Ig light chain type	Mouse myeloma cell partner	Hybrids isolated	Secreted human Ig light chain type	
					κ	λ
M	CLL	κ	P3/X63-Ag8	27	19	0
S	CLL	κ	P3/X63-Ag8	21	14	0
H	LSCL	κ	P3/X63-Ag8	200	200	0
E	LSCL	λ	P3/X63-Ag8	11	0	4
W	LSCL	λ	NS1-Ag4	8	0	5
K	NL	λ	NS1-Ag4	98	0	74

[a]CLL, chronic lymphocytic leukemia; LSCL, lymphosarcoma cell leukemia; NL, nodular lymphoma.

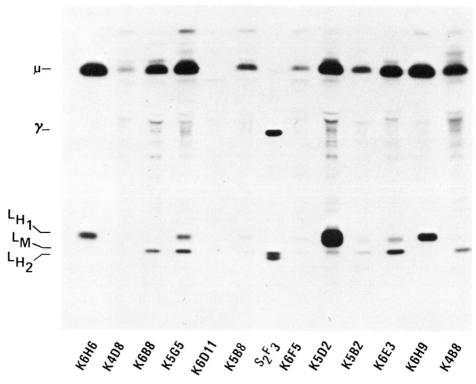

FIGURE 1. Secreted products of mouse × human hybridomas. Hybrids were cultured for 16 hr in leucine-free medium containing [^{14}C]leucine. Unpurified supernatants were analyzed by SDS-PAGE under reducing conditions in 10% acrylamides. S$_2$F$_3$ was a hybrid between mouse P3/X63-Ag8 and a human CLL patient. A prominent mouse γ and light (L$_M$) chain can be seen as well as a human μ and a human light chain (L$_{H_2}$). All other lanes represent independent hybrids between mouse NS-1/Ag4 and human lymphoma cells from patient Ka. All of these hybrids except K6D11 show a prominent human μ chain and at least one light chain—either mouse (L$_M$) or human (L$_{H_1}$). Note the similar mobility of the human light chain from all Ka hybrids (L$_{H_1}$) and their distinction from the light chain of patient S (L$_{H_2}$).

B. Stability of Human Ig Production

With continued growth in culture, many of the human × mouse hybridomas that initially secrete human Ig fail to continue secreting. The failure rate for these human × mouse hybridomas has shown variation with the particular input parental cell, some cases resulting in extremely rapid loss of production and other cases yielding persistent secretors at high frequencies. Overall, the failure rate is greater than that for mouse × mouse hybridomas. The most obvious explanation for loss of Ig production, both in mouse × mouse and in mouse × human hybridomas, is chromosome segregation, although a number of other mechanisms involving control of Ig gene expression are possible. Remarkably, by subcloning and sib-selection, it has been possible to establish mouse × human hybridoma lines that have continued human Ig production for more than 6

TABLE III

Fusion of Myeloma Cells and B Cells

Parental cells	Hybridization products	Reference
Mouse myeloma RPC 5.4 × human PBL from normal and immunodeficient patients	Myeloma protein, human Ig and chain-shuffled products	Schwaber (1975); Schwaber and Rosen (1978)
Mouse myeloma P3/X63-Ag8 or NS1-Ag/4 × human B cell leukemia (nonsecreting)	Myeloma protein, human monoclonal Ig, and chain-shuffled products (no γ– μ molecules). Membrane μ chain secreted	Levy and Dilley (1978)
Mouse myeloma P3/X63-Ag8 or NS1-Ag/4 × mouse B-cell leukemia (nonsecreting)	Myeloma protein, Ig from B-cell tumor, no membrane μ chain secreted	Eshhar *et al.* (1979)
Mouse myeloma MPC-11 × mouse B-cell leukemia (nonsecreting)	Myeloma protein, Ig from B-cell tumor	Laskov *et al.* (1979)

months of continuous culture. An extensive analysis of the human chromosomes of these stable producers is underway, but no assignment of the requisite human chromosomes is possible from the data as yet.

Interestingly, individual Ig chain loss—of either the mouse or the human chains—has been frequently observed. Examples of this can be seen in Fig. 1, where the secreted products of several individual hybridomas from a single lymphoma patient are shown. Note that either the human or the mouse light chain can be lost. It is the mouse light-chain-loss hybrids that have been among the most stable for human Ig production.

III. Characterization of the Secreted Human Immunoglobulin

The secreted products of one (CLL) × (P3/X63-Ag8) hybrid were analyzed by sequential immunoabsorption and polyacrylamide gel electrophoresis (PAGE) in SDS (Fig. 2) (Levy and Dilley, 1978). It was found that a variety of molecules were secreted. Many of them involved shuffled mouse and human Ig chains, including full IgG (mouse γ chains) molecules containing one human and one mouse light chain and full IgM molecules (human μ chains) containing some human as well as some mouse light chains. No molecules containing both human μ chains and mouse γ chains were formed. The complexity of this situation was greatly reduced when NS-1 was used instead of P3/X63-Ag8 as the mouse partner. The mouse plasmacytoma contributed only a light chain to the mixed chain products (Fig. 1). One hybrid, K6H6, which had lost the production

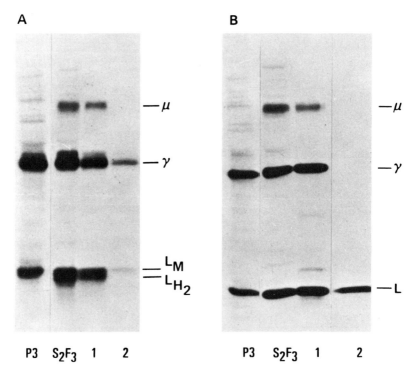

FIGURE 2. Analysis of secreted Ig molecules of hybrid S_2F_3. ^{14}C-labeled products of hybrid S_2F_3 (P3/X63-Ag8 × CLL) were analyzed by SDS-PAGE in 10% acrylamide under reducing conditions. Samples are compared before and after immunoabsorption and elution from sequential anti-Ig columns. (A) Anti-human column first, anti-mouse column second. (B) Anti-mouse column first, anti-human column second. Note that molecules containing both mouse and human light chains are absorbed by either an anti-mouse column or an anti-human column; molecules containing human μ and molecules containing mouse γ are absorbed by either column.

of the mouse light chain, was selected for an extensive analysis. This hybrid secreted only the human μ heavy chain and λ light chain. No free, unassembled chains were secreted, since removal of all the light chains also removed all the heavy chains and vice versa (Fig. 3). Furthermore, these heavy and light chains were assembled into full IgM pentamers as revealed by electrophoresis in 4% acrylamide (Ziegler and Hengartner, 1977) under nonreducing conditions (Fig. 4). IgM pentamers were excised from the 4% gel and electrophoresed in a second dimension in 15% acrylamide after complete reduction, revealing a μ heavy chain, a homogeneous light chain, but no evidence of a J chain (gel not shown). Thus, the secreted Ig of hybrid K6H6 was a homogeneous human IgM pentamer containing no J chain. Hybrid K6H6 has persisted in secreting both human heavy and light chains after twelve months of continuous culture. No subclones have been obtainable that have lost production of either of these Ig chains.

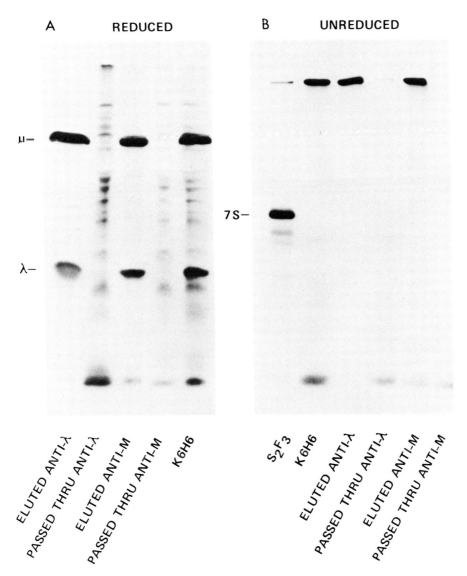

FIGURE 3. Analysis of secreted Ig molecules of hybrid K6H6. ^{14}C-labeled products of hybrid K6H6 [NS-1 × lymphoma cells (Ka)] were electrophoresed in SDS in a 10% acrylamide gel under reducing conditions (A) or in a 5% gel under nonreducing conditions (B) after absorption either to anti-human·λ columns or to anti-human μ columns. Note that all molecules containing μ are absorbed to anti-λ columns and all molecules containing λ chains are absorbed to anti-μ columns. Thus, no free chains are secreted. Also, all secreted Ig molecules of hybrid K6H6 are of high molecular weight— too large to enter the 5% gel, whereas the hybrid S_2F_3 secreted both high-molecular-weight molecules as well as 7 S IgG molecules.

FIGURE 4. Further analysis of size of secreted hybridoma IgM molecules. ^{14}C-Labeled S$_2$F$_3$ and K6H6 were electrophoresed under nonreducing conditions in 4% acrylamide with 0.7% DATD, a system allowing entry of 19 S IgM molecules. All the molecules secreted by K6H6 are 19 S, whereas S$_2$F$_3$ secreted both 7 S and 19 S molecules.

IV. Relationship between Secreted μ Chains and Membrane μ Chains

Immunoglobulins (Ig) produced by B cells are destined to be either secreted or deposited on the cell membrane. It is conceivable that the difference in function between membrane Ig and secreted Ig would be reflected in differences in the structure of these two Ig types. A number of studies have shown that the chain of spleen cell-surface IgM is different from the μ chain of normally secreted IgM molecules (Lisowksa-Bernstein and Vassali, 1975; Melcher and Uhr, 1976). An example of the same phenomenon from a different cell source is shown in Fig. 5, where the membrane μ chain of the original CLL cells is compared to the μ chain of a secreted IgM. The membrane μ chain clearly migrated

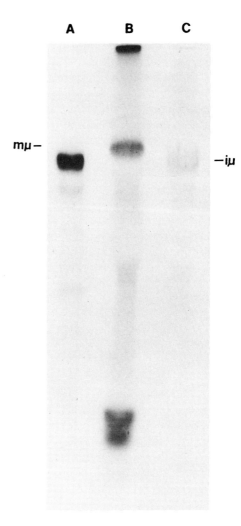

FIGURE 5. Relationship between μ chain of secreted IgM and membrane IgM. Ka lymphoma cells were surface iodinated with ^{125}I and lactoperoxidase or internally labeled with [14C]leucine. Detergent-solubilized extracts were immunoprecipitated with anti-human μ antiserum and analyzed by SDS-PAGE in 20-cm-long 12% gels. Lane A contains an ^{125}I-labeled, secreted human IgM as a marker. Lane B contains the ^{125}I-labeled material from Ka membranes and Lane C contains the [14C]-labeled material from Ka internal proteins. The μ chain of the membrane IgM (mμ) has a slower mobility than either the μ chain of the secreted IgM or the μ chain of the internal IgM (iμ).

more slowly than the secreted μ chain on the SDS gel. A similar difference in apparent molecular weight (AMW) between the membrane μ chain and the secreted μ chain from either a murine B-cell line, 38C-13, or from a lymphoid cell from a leukemic cow, have been reported (Haimovich, 1977; Bergman and Haimovich, 1978). The difference in AMW between the membrane μ chain and the secreted μ chains could be due either to a difference in the carbohydrate moiety with a concomitant alteration in the SDS binding or to a difference in the protein portion, implying the existance of two separate mRNA molecules coding for different μ-chain products. Sequence analysis of the N-terminal portion of membrane and secreted μ chains of murine B lymphoma line 38C-13 suggests that they are identical in the N-terminal positions. Results of carboxypeptidase digestion with either a murine B lymphocytoma, McPc-1748, and with a human lymphocyte B cell line, Bristol-8 (McIlhinney *et al.,* 1978), as well as with the murine lymphoma 38C-13, indicated that both membrane and secreted μ chains have a C-terminal tyrosine residue. In direct contrast to these reports, the data obtained with a human B cell line, Daudi (Williams *et al.,* 1978), indicate that the C-terminal region of Daudi μ chains differs from that of the secreted μ chain. Recent peptide mapping analysis suggest that there is a difference in the peptide composition between the secreted and the membrane μ chain (Yuan *et al.,* 1979; L. Hood, personal communication, 1979). Thus, although membrane and secreted μ chain may differ in part of their constant regions, no conclusion is yet possible to the exact nature of the structural difference.

Since our CLL cells have a relatively large amount of membrane IgM and lack the capacity to secrete IgM, it was of interest to determine which form of μ chain appeared in the secreted product of the hybridomas. In Fig. 6, the μ chain of the ^{14}C-labeled secreted IgM from hybrid K6H6 is compared to the μ chain of the ^{125}I-labeled membrane IgM of the CLL parent. The hybrid cells themselves contained no cell surface Ig; however, the IgM molecule they secreted was composed of μ chains with a mobility identical to that of the original membrane μ chain. Large quantities of the rescued membrane μ chain are now available for structure studies.

V. Relationship between Production of μ Chain and the Presence of μ Chain mRNA

A number of the mouse × human hybridomas produce the human Ig chains but fail to secrete them. An example of this is hybrid K6D11. In Figure 1, it can be seen that no μ or λ chains are secreted, yet by immunofluorescence 65% of the hybrid cells contained intracellular human λ (but not μ chains). Conversely, mouse Ig secretion can occur in some of these interspecies hybrids without the production of human Ig. An example of this is shown in Fig. 7, where complementation of the secretory defect of the NS-1 cell was accom-

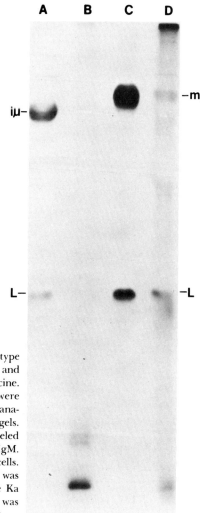

FIGURE 6. Hybrid cells secrete IgM with membrane type μ chains. K6H6 cells were surface iodinated with ^{125}I and lactoperoxidase or internally labelled with [14C]leucine. Secreted and detergent-solubilized cellular materials were immunoprecipitated with anti-human μ antiserum and analyzed by SDS-PAGE on 20-cm-long 12% acrylamide gels. Lane A: 14C-labeled intracellular IgM. Lane B: 125I-labeled membrane material. Lane C: 14C-labeled secreted IgM. Lane D: 125I-labeled membrane IgM from Ka parent cells. Note that the mobility of the μ chain of the secreted IgM was identical to that of the original membrane IgM of the Ka parent cell and not that of the internal IgM (which was identical to a normally secreted IgM molecule; see Fig. 5).

plished by the human partner without the production of human Ig. Clearly the processes of Ig production and Ig secretion can be separately studied in these hybrids.

When no human Ig production occurs in these hybrids a number of explanations are possible, from defects as proximal as a missing chromosome to defects as distal as an unstable protein product. We have asked the question whether or not the production of human μ chain by these hybrid cells can be correlated with the presence of functional μ mRNA. Total poly-A-containing RNA was prepared from producing and nonproducing hybridomas and used to stimulate protein synthesis *in vitro* in a rabbit reticulocyte lysate system. The

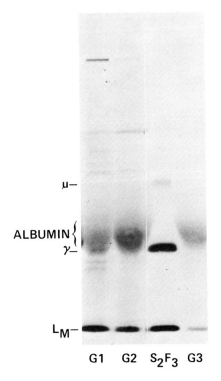

FIGURE 7. Complementation for mouse Ig secretion by human cells. The ¹⁴C-labeled products of several hybridomas between NS-1 and the same human lymphoma cells are shown on SDS-PAGE 7% acrylamide, under reducing conditions. Note that mouse light secretion occurs in all these hybrids without secretion of any human chain. An artifact due to overloading by albumin from the culture medium is also present on the gel.

radiolabeled protein products were immunoprecipitated with an anti-human μ-chain antiserum and analyzed by SDS-PAGE (Fig. 8). It can be seen that translatable μ-chain mRNA was easily detectable in the μ-chain-producing cell lines K6B8 and K5D5, whereas it was undetectable in the nonproducing line K5D11. These results indicate that the production defect in this nonproducing hybrid is due to absence of the specific mRNA and not to a defect in its translation or the stability of the protein product. The results also indicate that the human × mouse hybrids that do produce human Ig chains should be good sources of mRNA for the production of human Ig cDNA, since most of the mRNA in these hybrid cells is the product of the mouse genome.

FIGURE 8. Human μ-chain production correlates with the presence of μ chain mRNA. In gel A the secretion products from three hybridomas are shown: two IgM secretors (K6B8 and K5D5) and one nonsecretor (K6D11). In gel B, anti-μ immunoprecipitates of the reticulocyte cell-free translation products of poly-A-containing RNA from these three hybridomas are shown. The control was an immunoprecipitate from the reticulocyte system with no RNA added. A clear μ-chain product is seen from the translation of RNA from the producing hybrids. Actually, two closely spaced bands are seen, one of which may represent a precursor of the mature μ chain. No μ chain is seen when RNA from the nonproducer K6D11 was used.

A   **K6B8 K5D5 K6D11**

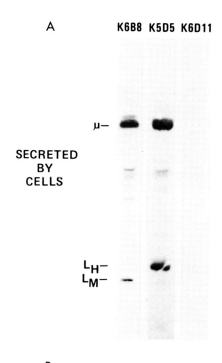

SECRETED
BY
CELLS

μ—

L H—
L M—

B   **K6B8 K5D5 K6D11 CONT**

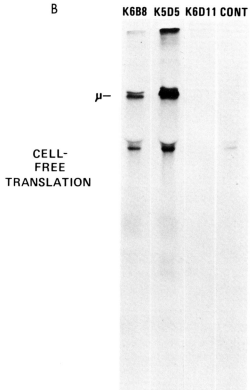

μ—

CELL-
FREE
TRANSLATION

VI. Production of an Antiidiotype Reagent against the Rescued Human Immunoglobulin

Our original objective for making secreting hybridomas from human malignant B cells was to obtain the monoclonal Ig from these cells for use as a tumor specific marker (Stevenson and Stevenson, 1975). Since we know that the input human cell populations as well as the resulting hybridomas produced a homogeneous Ig of identical light-chain type, we could predict that the idiotype of the secreted product would be a specific marker for the original malignant clone. Among the series of hyrids produced from the cells of one patient (Ka) we chose K6H6 as a source of the Ka idiotype because it had lost secretion of the mouse light chain (Fig. 1). Thus, only a single homogeneous V_L-V_H combination defined by the secreted human μ and λ chains was present. The cell line was grown in low-protein medium and the Ka protein was purified by ammonium sulfate precipitation followed by affinity chromatography on an anti-human μ chain column. The product was analyzed by radioimmunoassay and SDS-PAGE and

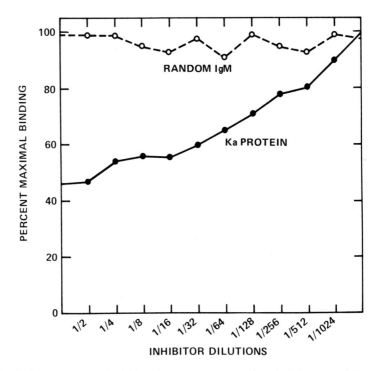

FIGURE 9. Antiidiotype assay. A rabbit antiserum was prepared against the rescued Ka protein from hybrid K6H6 and absorbed to make it idiotype specific. The globulin fraction of the antiserum was used at a dilution of 1/800 to coat the wells of polyvinyl plates. [^{125}I]Ka protein was added (30,000 cpm/well) and its binding was competed by either unlabeled Ka protein or an unrelated human IgM(λ).

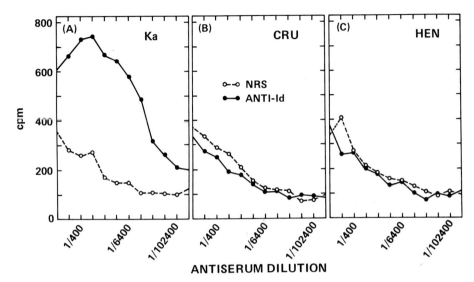

FIGURE 10. Individual specificity of the anit-Ka idiotype. The rabbit anti-Ka idiotype or normal rabbit serum was added in a volume of 25 μl to an equal volume of 10⁵ glutaraldehyde-fixed cells in suspension, incubated for 6 hr at room temperature, and washed. Cell-bound antibody was detected by the addition of ^{125}I-labeled, purified goat anti-rabbit Ig. Specific binding of the anti-Ka idiotype occurred only with cells from patient Ka and not with cells from two other patients (Cru and Hen) with B-cell malignancies.

found to contain relatively pure human IgM, with a trace of albumin. A rabbit was immunized and boosted with 30 μg of the purified Ka protein in complete Freund's adjuvant. Antiserum was rendered idiotype specific by solid-phase absorption on fetal calf serum, pooled human IgG, and an unrelated human IgM(λ).

The anti-Ka idiotype was tested for specificity first in a protein competition assay (Fig. 9). Flexible vinyl 96-well plates were coated with the antiidiotype antiserum. The binding of ^{125}I-labeled Ka protein to these plates was successfully competed with unlabeled Ka protein, but not by unrelated human IgM(λ), nor by normal human serum (not shown). Thus, the absorbed antiserum was Ka-protein-specific. Next, the antiserum was tested for cell specificity by a binding assay (Levy and Dilley, 1977) using glutaraldehyde-fixed target cells and an ^{125}I-labeled, purified goat anti-rabbit detecting reagent. Target cells were derived from three patients with B-cell malignancy: Cru, cell-surface IgM(κ); Hen, cell-surface IgM(λ); and Ka, cell-surface IgM(λ). Figure 10 shows that the absorbed anti-Ka idiotype gave specific binding only to Ka cells, and not to Cru or Hen, nor to random normal lymphocytes (not shown). With this anti-Ka idiotype serum, it should now be possible to ask a number of questions relating to the immunobiology of human B-cell malignancy.

VII. Summary

Human × mouse hybridomas can be made using either the secreting or the nonsecreting myeloma cell lines. These hybridomas can synthesize and secrete human Ig chains, either as mixed mouse–human molecules or as fully assembled homogeneous human molecules. Human Ig production, while frequently lost as human chromosomes are segregated, can be a stable property of these hybrid cells. A variety of types of human B cells, represented by various human malignant B-cell populations, can serve as hybridization partners and can lead to human Ig-secreting hybridomas. Thus nonsecreting human cells can be caused to switch on secretion of Ig after hybridization. In at least one case, the secreted μ chain from the hybridoma is structurally similar to parental membrane μ chain. In one hybrid clone the absence of μ-chain production has been shown to be a result of the lack of the appropriate mRNA.

These human × mouse hybridomas should be extremely useful in the future for chromosomal mapping of human Ig genes, the production of human Ig mRNA and cDNA probes, the elucidation of the structure of membrane μ chain, and investigating the immunobiology of human B-cell neoplasms. The availability of rescued Ig from nonsecreting human B-cell tumors provides an approach to these tumors through the production of specific antiidiotype reagents. Furthermore, the successful and stable production of human Ig by these hybridomas indicates that specific monoclonal human antibodies are obtainable if human B cells with the appropriate specificities are used for hybridization.

ACKNOWLEDGMENTS

This work was supported by grants from NIH (CA 21223-03) and the American Cancer Society (IM-114-A). R. Levy is an investigator of the Howard Hughes Medical Institute.

References

Bergman, Y., and Haimovich, J., 1978, B lymphocytes contain three species of μ chains, Eur. J. Immunol. 8:876.

Eshhar, Z., Blatt, C., Bergman, Y., and Haimovich, J., 1979, Induction of IgM secretion from B-cells by fusion, J. Immunol. 122:2430.

Filippa, D., Lieberman, P., Erlandson, R., Koziner, B., Siegal, F., Turnbull, A., Zimring, A., and Good, R., 1978, A study of malignant lymphomas using light and ultramicroscopic, cytochemical and immunologic techniques, Am. J. Med. 64:259.

Haimovich, J., 1977, Membrane immunoglobulins of bovine leukemic lymphocytes, Immunochemistry 14:337.

Laskov, R., Kim, K., and Asofsky, R., 1979, Induction of amplified synthesis and secretion of IgM by fusion of murine B lymphoma with myeloma cells, Proc. Natl. Acad. Sci. USA 76:915.

Levy, R., and Dilley, J., 1977, The *in vitro* antibody response to cell surface antigens. I. The xenogenic response to human leukemia cells, *J. Immunol.* **119:**387.

Levy, R. and Dilley, J., 1978, Rescue of immunoglobulin secretion of human neoplastic lymphoid cells by somatic cell hybridization, *Proc. Natl. Acad. Sci. USA* **75:**2411.

Levy, R., and Kaplan, H., eds., 1978, *Malignant lymphoma: A Series of Workshops on the Biology of Human Cancer, Report No. 7,* International Union Against Cancer, Geneva.

Levy, R., Dilley, J., Sikora, K., and Kucherlapati, R., 1978, Hybrids of normal and malignant T and B lymphocytes, *Curr. Top. Microbiol. Immunol.* **81:**170.

Lisowska-Bernstein, B., and Vassalli, P., 1975, The surface immunoglobulins of mouse spleen B lymphocytes. Radioiodination, biosynthetic labeling and immunofluourescent studies, in: *Membrane Receptors of Lymphocytes* (J. L. Preud'homme and F. N. Kowilsky, eds.), North-Holland Publishing Co., Amsterdam, p. 39.

McIlhinney, R., Richardson, N., and Feinstein, A., 1978, Evidence for a C-terminal tyrosine residue in human and mouse B-lymphocyte membrane μ chains, *Nature* **272:**555.

Melcher, U., and Uhr, J., 1976, Cell surface immunoglobulin. XVI. Polypeptide chain structure of mouse IgM and IgD-like molecule, *J. Immunol.* **116:**409.

Salmon, S., and Seligmann, M., 1974, B cell neoplasia in man, *Lancet* **ii:**1230.

Schwaber, J., 1975, Immunoglobulin production by a human–mouse somatic cell hybrid, *Exp. Cell Res.* **93:**343.

Schwaber, S., and Rosen, F., 1978, Induction of human immunoglobulin synthesis and secretion in somatic cell hybrids of mouse myeloma and human B lymphocytes from patients with agammaglobulinemia, *J. Exp. Med.* **148:**974.

Stevenson, G., and Stevenson, F., 1975, Antibody to a molecularly-defined antigen confined to a tumor cell surface, *Nature* **254:**714.

Williams, B., Kubo, R., and Howard, M., 1978, μ Chains from a nonsecretor B cell line differ from secreted μ chains at the C-terminal end, *J. Immunol.* **121:**2435.

Yuan, D., Uhr, J., Knapp, M., Slavin, S., Strober, S., and Vitetta, E., 1979. Structural difference between the μ chains of cell associated and secreted IgM, in: *Scottsdale Symposium of B Lymphocytes and the Immune Response* (M. Cooper, D. Mosier, I. Scher, and E. Vitetta, eds.), Elsevier North-Holland, Amsterdam, p. 23.

Ziegler, A., and Hengartner, H., 1977, Sodium dodecyl sulfate electrophoresis of high molecular weight proteins in N,N'-diallyltrartardiamide-cross-linked polyacrylamide slab gels, *Eur. J. Immunol.* **7:**690.

10
Monoclonal Antibodies against Human Tumor-Associated Antigens

ROGER H. KENNETT, ZDENKA L. JONAK, AND
KATHLEEN B. BECHTOL

I. Introduction

It is now well established that certain tumor cells express surface antigens that are not present on cells in the tissue from which the tumor was initially derived (Ruddon, 1978; Greaves and Janossy, 1978). Such antigens have several possible origins: (1) new genetic information resulting from either mutation or oncogenic viral infection, (2) expression of normal genetic information out of temporal or cellular context, such as the expression of fetal antigens on cells in an adult, (3) rearrangement or modification of normal cell surface structures by mechanisms such as glycosylation, protease activity, or intermolecular interactions due to changes in membrane structure or fluidity. The production of specific antibody reagents against these antigens would facilitate analysis of their structure and genetic origin and also provide a means of detection and perhaps even selective destruction of tumor cells (Table I).

II. Tumor-Specific Antigens and Tumor-Associated Antigens

It is, in practice, difficult to assign an antigen detected on a tumor cell to category (1) in Section I, i.e., to being a truly "tumor-specific" antigen. The

ROGER H. KENNETT • Department of Human Genetics, University of Pennsylvania, School of Medicine, Philadelphia, Pennsylvania 19104. ZDENKA L. JONAK AND KATHLEEN B. BECHTOL • Wistar Institute of Anatomy and Biology, Philadelphia, Pennsylvania 19104.

TABLE I

Potential Uses of Monoclonal Antibodies against Tumor-Associated Antigens

1. Isolation of tumor-associated antigens by affinity chromatography
2. Detection of the expression of portions of the gene in bacterial colonies or phage plaques containing a cloning vector with a part of the "tumor antigen" gene incorporated
3. Tumor identification
   a. Diagnosis
   b. Detection of metastasis
4. Specific delivery of covalently bound cytotoxic drugs to tumor cells
5. Cytolysis of tumor cells

antigen could, for example, also be present on a small subpopulation of normal cells from which the tumor was derived or could be expressed on fetal cells as well as tumor cells. Nevertheless, a differentiation antigen or a fetal antigen present on only a small number of normal adult cells may for some purposes be treated as a "tumor-specific" antigen. It may, for example, be possible to use an antibody against such an antigen to detect tumor cells in blood or bone marrow because the number of normal cells expressing the antigen is not sufficient to interfere with the assay. Such an antigen would thus be operationally "tumor-specific."

As an example, human chronic lymphocytic leukemia (CLL) cells of B-cell origin express on their surface immunoglobulin (Ig) molecules that have a variable region characteristic of the particular B-cell clone from which the tumor was derived. Lampson and Levy (1978) have discussed the possible use of antibodies that react with the specific variable region (idiotype; see Clevinger *et al.,* this volume) of the tumor cells of one CLL patient, but do not react with the patient's normal cells lacking the idiotype. Such antiidiotype antibodies would therefore be operationally "tumor-specific."

III. Human Tumor Antigens—Detection by Monoclonal Antibodies

For investigators examining human tumor-associated antigens, who are therefore limited to heterospecific immunizations, the possibility of obtaining monoclonal antibodies against these antigens provides a major technical advantage. By eliminating the problem of antibodies against human species antigens that must be removed from standard antisera by absorptions, Köhler and Milstein's (1976) contribution brings the analysis of the genetics and biochemistry of human tumor-associated antigens into the realm of the practical.

At the first hybridoma workshop Levy *et al.* (1978) described attempts to produce monoclonal antibodies against human leukemia cells in spleen fragment cultures and from hybridomas. Although they obtained antibodies reacting with subpopulations of lymphocytes and others that apparently react with polymorphic determinants, they found no antibodies that reacted specifically with leukemia cells. Binding of the antibodies to the immunizing leukemia cells was much higher than to peripheral blood lymphocytes, but there was significant binding to normal cells in the patient and in his parents. Whether or not this lower level binding was actually due to specific binding by the Fab portion of the monoclonal antibody was not established.

Two groups have reported production of monoclonal antibodies that react with human melanomas and not with the other types of human cells tested. Koprowski et al. (1978) isolated monoclonal antibodies reacting with melanomas. Nude mice injected with the hybridoma lines secreting these antibodies exhibited suppression of the growth of melanoma tumors. The antibodies react with melanomas from several individuals but do not react with nonmalignant cells from the same patient or with cells from a giant hairy nevus or cells from tumors of other tissue origins (Steplewski et al., 1979).

Yeh et al. (1979) reported monoclonal antibodies that react strongly with the melanoma cells used for immunization, weakly with 2 of 11 other melanomas, and showed no binding on several other types of normal cells or tumor cells. In neither of these cases is there an indication of whether the antibodies bind to a small proportion of normal melanocytes or with fetal cells such as melanoblasts or other melanocyte precursors. It is also possible that some of them may be against differentiation antigens such as the Ia-like antigens shown to be expressed on melanomas (Winchester et al., 1978). In any case these antibodies are potentially useful for many of the applications listed in Table I.

Antibodies that react with human colorectal carcinoma and not with normal colonic mucosa or other normal and malignant human cells have been reported by Herlyn et al. (1979). The antibodies react with cultured tumor cells and with tumor cells freshly isolated from patients. They do not react with carcinoembryonic antigen secreted by the cells. Whether they react with a specific tumor antigen is not determined, but it is likely that these antibodies will be useful in characterization of colorectal carcinomas and may prove useful for immunodiagnosis of this common form of cancer.

IV. Antibodies to Human Neuroblastoma

We describe here the production, characterization, and use of a monoclonal antibody against human neuroblastoma (Kennett and Gilbert, 1979). Our experimental methods are given in detail in the Appendix. Prior to the production of hybridomas we were using several immunization protocols designed to minimize antispecies reactivity resulting from injection of human cells into mice (Table II). These protocols were used to reduce the response to human antigens common to most human cells and result in a more specific response to tumor-specific or cell-type-specific antigens. We have continued to use these protocols with the intention of reducing the number of hybridomas making antispecies antibodies

TABLE II

Methods of Restricting the Immune Response to Human Cell-Surface Antigens

Method	Reference
Immunization with membrane fractions containing a limited number of membrane components	Goodfellow et al. (1976)
Immunization with one cell type coated with antibodies made against another cell type	Brown et al. (1975); Kennett and Gilbert (1979)
Immunization with solubilized cell membrane that has been passed through an affinity column to remove immunodominant antigens	Springer (this volume)
Immunization with mouse × human hybrids having a few human chromosomes and thus expressing a limited number of human antigens	Buck and Bodmer (1975)
Immunization with cell-culture supernatant containing a restricted selection of cell-surface antigens, which are shed or secreted and remain stable in significant amounts	Kennett et al. (1978)

and thus increase the proportion against the antigens specific for the cells injected.

For production of antineuroblastoma antibodies we used spleen cells from a C57B1/6J mouse immunized twice with a cultured human neuroblastoma, IMR6, that had been coated with a mouse antiserum against a human lymphoblastoid line, 8866. The spleen cells were fused to the plasmacytoma line P3/X63-Ag8 (Köhler and Milstein, 1976). Hybrids grew in all 576 wells of six microtiter plates. Supernatants from 88 of 200 wells tested were cytolytic for IMR6. However, 59 of these 88 were not cytolytic for the lymphoblastoid line 8866.

We then tested the binding of these antibodies to IMR6 and 8866, detecting bound monoclonal antibody with a second ^{125}I-labeled antibody, rabbit antimouse Fab. We chose two monoclonal antibodies that bind to IMR6 but not to 8866 for further analysis. The binding of these two antibodies was tested against a panel of human cell types, including homogenized human fetal brain and adult brain (Fig. 1). The antibody PI153/3 reacts with neuroblastomas, retinoblastomas, and a glioblastoma, which are all tumors derived from neuroectoderm (Knudson and Meadows, 1978), and also with fetal brain, but does not react with the other human cell types tested. Absorption analysis (Fig. 2) showed a significant amount of antigen on fetal brain and neuroblastoma but none detectable on adult brain or a lymphoblastoid line. Binding of the antibody to fetal tissues (Fig. 3) showed no significant binding to tissues other than brain, with the exception of a low level to adrenal gland; this is of interest because neuroblastomas frequently are found in the adrenal medulla, which is derived embryologically from the neuroectoderm. There was no binding to mouse fetal or adult brain or the mouse neuroblastoma C1300. Thus PI153/3 defines a human oncofetal neural antigen.

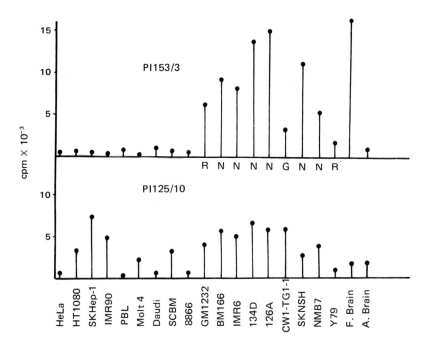

FIGURE 1. Binding of PI153/3 and PI125/10 antibodies to human cells. Between 0.5×10^6 of each cell type or an equivalent packed cell volume of homogenized brain was incubated for 1 hr at 4°C with $25 \mu l$ of supernatant or diluted ascites fluid. The cells were washed, and ^{125}I-labeled anti-Fab was added (100,000 cpm). After incubation the tubes were washed twice and counted. Samples were done in duplicate. The neuroblastomas (N) tested were 134D, IMR6, 126A, BM166, SKNSH, and NMB7; the retinoblastomas (R) were GM1232 and Y79; and the glioblastoma (G) was CW1-TG1-1 (A. McMorris, Wistar Institute). Other cell lines were fibrosarcoma HT1080 (C. Croce, Wistar Institute); hepatoma SKHep-1 (J. Fogh, Sloan-Kettering); fibroblast IMR90 (Institute for Medical Research, Camden); B-lymphoblastoid lines Daudi, SCBM, 8866; T-cell line Molt 4; peripheral blood lymphocytes (PBL); and HeLa cells D98-AH/2. The same background binding was found with whole adult human brain (A.Brain) or with separate preparations of gray or white matter from cerebellum or cerebrum. F. Brain, fetal brain from 20-week fetus autopsied after spontaneous abortion at Children's Hospital of Philadelphia. [From Kennett and Gilbert (1979). Copyright by the American Association for the Advancement of Science. Reproduced with permission.]

The other antibody, PI125, reacts with several different types of cell and may detect an antigen that is present on more than one type of cell, or alternatively may detect one form of a polymorphic determinant that is present in another form(s) on the other cells in the panel. Because PI153/3 is more restricted in its distribution, further work concentrated on this antibody and the corresponding cell-surface antigen. Analysis by immunodiffusion and by sodium dodecyl sulfate (SDS) electrophoresis of the Ig chains produce by PI153/3 in addition to the Υ1 κ of the parental myeloma indicated that the heavy chain from the lymphocyte parent of PI153/3 is of the IgM class (Fig. 4).

Affinity chromatography on a PI153/3 column of enzymatically solubilized cell-surface molecules (Momoi et al., 1980) indicated that the antigenic determinant recognized by the antibody is probably the carbohydrate portion of a cell-

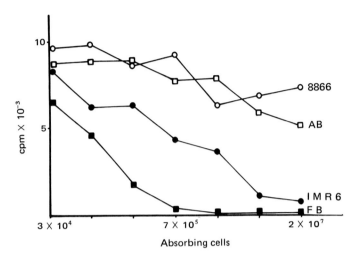

FIGURE 2. Absorption of PI153/3 ascites. PI153/3 ascites (diluted to 1:1000) was absorbed with 8866, a B-lymphoblastoid line; IMR6, a neuroblastoma; and packed-cell equivalents of homogenized human adult brain (AB) and fetal brain (FB); and the binding of the absorbed antibody solution was tested against IMR6. The indicated number of cells at a 1:3 dilution, suspended in a final volume of $50 \mu l$, was incubated with $50 \mu l$ of ascites fluid at a dilution of 1:1000 for 1 hr at 4°C. The cells were removed by centrifugation, and the antibody remaining in the supernatant was detected by binding to IMR6, using the binding assay described in Fig. 1. The ratio of packed-cell volume to liquid at the highest concentration of cells was 1:2. [From Kennett and Gilbert (1979). Copyright by the American Association for the Advancement of Science. Reproduced with permission.]

surface glycoprotein. Further analysis of additional malignant cell types has indicated that the PI153/3 antibody reacts with some B-cell and null-cell leukemias including the cell line REH derived from a null-cell acute lymphoblastic leukemia (Kennett et al., 1980). Determination of whether the antigen detected on neuroblastomas is the same in molecular weight and structure as that detected on leukemias must await further analysis of detergent-solubilized antigens from both cell types. One must certainly keep in mind that monoclonal antibodies react with a single antigenic determinant and that it is possible that as a result of structural homology the same or a very similar antigenic determinant may appear on two different molecules. Thus unless identity of the antigens is determined biochemically, reactivity of a monoclonal antibody with two different cell types does not necessarily mean that the same gene product is expressed on both.

V. Detection of Metastatic Neuroblastoma

Reacting the PI153/3 antibody with bone marrow cells followed by a rabbit anti-mouse Ig linked to peroxidase plus diaminobenzidine, H_2O_2, and osmium tetroxide allows detection of cells expressing the PI153/3 antigen (Kennett et al.,

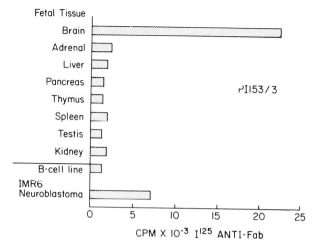

FIGURE 3. Reaction of PI153/3 antibody with human fetal tissues. Tissues were dispersed gently and equivalent packed cell volumes incubated with PI153/3 supernatant. Bound antibody was detected with [^{125}I]-anti-mouse Fab. No background counts have been subtracted.

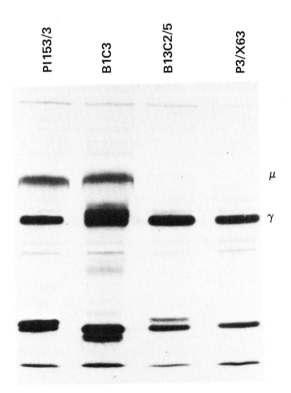

FIGURE 4. SDS–polyacrylamide gel electrophoresis of Ig produced by parental plasmacytoma line P3/X63-Ag8 (γ1κ) and hybridomas made with this line. The cells were labeled for 18 hr with [^{35}S]methionine in medium designed to optimize Ig production. When 20 μl of medium was added to SDS sample buffer, the chains separated by reduction with mercaptoethanol, and the samples applied to the gel. The dried gel was exposed to X-ray film for 2 days and developed. PI153/3 secretes the γ1 κ of P3/X63-Ag8 plus a new light chain and a new heavy chain of the μ class, as determined by its higher molecular weight and confirmed by immunodiffusion.

1980). There are no cells labeled by this procedure in normal bone marrow, but neuroblastoma cells can be detected in patients where metastasis has taken place (Fig. 5). Using this procedure it has been possible to observe tumor cells in marrows where they were undetectable by conventional procedures, which depend on finding clumps of the large tumor cells. It is possible that the PI153/3 antibody, which is IgM and thus cytolytic, could be used to remove neuroblastoma cells from marrow taken prior to treatment of the patient with drugs or radiation. Such treated autologous marrow could then be stored frozen and reinjected after treatment of the patient.

With the expression of the PI153/3 antigen on leukemia cells in mind (see Section IV), one must consider the possibility that the antigenic determinant defined by the antibody may be expressed on immature lymphoblasts. For example, following a course of chemotherapy neuroblastoma patients generally exhibit an abnormally high proportion of immature marrow elements, some of which are morphologically similar to small neuroblastoma cells (Evans and Hummeler, 1973). Though normal bone marrow does not have PI153/3-reactive cells, the reactivity of the immature repopulating cells with the antibody is not yet known. One must, therefore, be hesitant to make a diagnosis based solely on the presence or absence of a single antigenic determinant detected by a single monoclonal antibody in tissues such as regenerating bone marrow.

There are various ways to approach this problem to assure that one is identifying a specific cell type among a heterogeneous population rather than detecting related antigenic determinants or expressions of a single determinant on two different antigens.

1. One can use the first monoclonal antibody to isolate the antigen and make more monoclonal antibodies against other determinants on the same molecule. These antibodies may then be used in combination to confirm the presence of that specific molecule. For example, one monoclonal antibody could be reacted with the cells and be detected using peroxidase-labeled anti-mouse Ig, and then a second monoclonal antibody conjugated to biotin could be reacted with the preparation and its binding detected with fluorescein-labeled avidin (Heitzman and Richards, 1974; S. J. Singer, personal communication). This assay procedure would indicate whether all the cells detected expressed both "tumor-specific" determinants.

2. Additional tumor-specific antibodies against other antigens could be isolated. In addition to the PI153/3 antibody, which reacts with human, but not mouse, neuroblastoma, we have now isolated other monoclonal antibodies that react with human neuroblastomas. These antibodies were made in mice against mouse neuroblastoma C1300 and react with human neuroblastomas (Bechtol *et al.*, this volume). These antibodies, which are against different antigen(s), can be used in conjunction with the PI153/3 antibody to confirm the identification of neuroblastoma in marrow.

3. To show that the cells in marrow detected with PI153/3 are not immature B cells or null-cell blasts we can use a second monoclonal antibody against

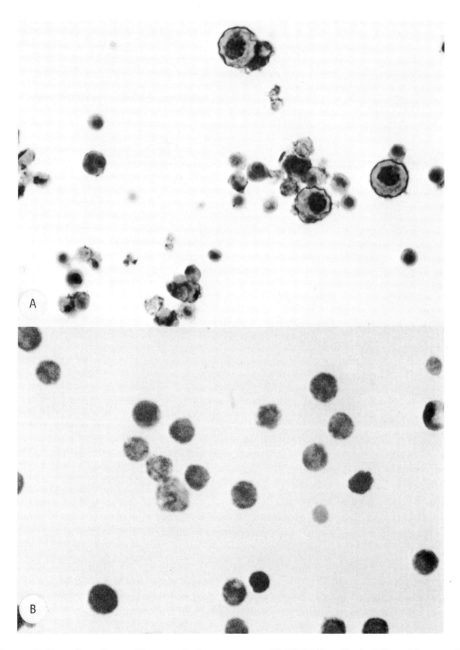

FIGURE 5. Detection of neuroblastomas in bone marrow with PI153/3 antibody followed by peroxidase-labeled anti-mouse Ig, H_2O_2 deaminobenzidine, and OsO_4. Cells expressing the antigen show a dark precipitate around the cell (A). Controls without PI153/3 or with another antibody of the same class (IgM) show no precipitates (B). Normal control bone marrow from marrow donors shows no labeled cells.

human Ia antigens that reacts with all the leukemic lymphocytes detected by PI153/3 but does not react with neuroblastomas (Kennett *et al.*, 1980). In this case the second monoclonal antibody allows one to demonstrate that the first is reacting with one type of cell but not another and thus confirm the presence of neuroblastoma in the patient's marrow.

It is clear that as a bank of monoclonal antibodies with well-defined reactivity against specific cell types is derived, it will be possible to identify specific tumor cells and specific subpopulations of normal cells with increased confidence and in ways that will make the above applications possible.

In addition to the detection of tumor cells and specific lysis of tumor cells by antibody there is one other practical application of tumor-specific monoclonal antibodies that may turn out to be particularly useful. Several investigators have suggested that tumor-specific antisera could be used as a means of delivering cytotoxic drugs, lectins, or radiation specifically to tumor cells (Davies and O'Neill, 1975). With the availability of monoclonal antibodies that are truly tumor-specific and lack the background binding often present in antisera this means of killing tumor cells specifically *in vivo* becomes a real possibility.

VI. *Monoclonal Antibodies and Genetics of Human Tumor Antigens*

In addition to providing new ways to identify and isolate tumor-associated antigens, monoclonal antibodies also facilitate two different approaches to the study of the genetics of human tumor-associated antigens, one at the chromosome level and one at the level of the DNA. As antibodies against tumor-associated antigens are produced, it will be useful to make mouse × human hybrids using human tumor cells expressing the antigens and closely related mouse tumor lines. These mouse × human hybrids can then be screened for expression of the human tumor antigen. Each clone of mouse × human hybrids usually maintains the mouse chromosomes of the parental cell plus a nearly random assortment of a few human chromosomes (Ruddle, 1973; Solomon and Jones, this volume). If the chromosome containing the gene for the human tumor antigen is present and the hybrid has been made with a mouse cell line that permits expression of the antigen, then the human tumor antigen can be detected on the hybrid cells. By correlating the expression of the antigen with the presence of a specific human chromosome, one may define the chromosomal location of the gene for the tumor antigen. Certain tumor-associated antigens may be in the category of differentiation antigens and for this reason it is probably wise to choose for fusion a mouse cell line that is closely related in cellular origin to the human tumor being studied. This will maximize the chances for expression of the human gene product (Davidson, 1974). In preliminary studies using a set of mouse × human hybrids made between P3/X63-Ag8 and human

B-CLL cells that express the determinant detected by PI153/3, and another set of hybrids made between human neuroblastoma and mouse fibroblasts, we have been able to show that the gene for the PI153/3 antigen is not on the same chromosome (6) as the human HLA major histocompatibility antigens (Table III). Mouse × human hybrids expressing a human antigen and containing a limited number of human chromosomes will also be a useful source of mRNA specific for the tumor antigen gene.

A second potentially useful application of monoclonal antibodies is to detect the expression of genes cloned in bacterial plasmids. This technique provides a way to isolate the gene for the antigen and analyze the tumor-associated antigen at the level of the genetic material. With the stipulation that the antigenic determinant is protein in nature and there is therefore a direct relationship between the gene structure and the structure of the antigen, analysis of the molecular weight of the antigen isolated by the antibody would provide a reasonable estimate of the size of the corresponding mRNA. By taking the appropriate fractions of mRNA and making cDNA and cloning it in a plasmid such as pBR322 we could obtain clones of recombinant DNA containing portions of the gene for the antigen. Using a similar procedure Villa-Komaroff et al. (1978) cloned the gene for proinsulin and obtained clones of X1776 infected with the plasmids

TABLE III

Expression of Differentiation Antigens Detected by Monoclonal Antibodies on Mouse × Human Hybrids[a]

Cell line	PI153/3 oncofetal antigen	P3B13C2 anti-B-cell	H76A2 anti-B-cell	W6/32 HLA
IMR6 (neuroblastoma)	+			+
8866 (B-cell line)		+	+	+
D-CLL (chronic lymphocytic leukemia)	+	+	+	+
Neuroblastoma × fibroblast hybrids				
NRSTP-4M				
NRSTP-76	+			
N4BTP-8				
Leukemia × plasmacytoma hybrids				
P3D 13			+	+
P3D 18	+		+	+
P3D 19			+	+
P3D 20				
P39 30		+	+	+
P3D 32	+		+	+

[a]The expression of antigens identified by four monoclonal antibodies were detected on mouse × human hybrids by cytotoxicity and immunofluorescence. PI153/3 reacts with neuroblastomas, fetal brain, and some leukemias; P3B13C2 with human B cells, H76A2 with human, mouse, and rat B cells (Gasser et al., 1979) and W6/32 against HLA (Parham and Bodmer, 1978). The H76A2 and W6/32 (HLA) antigens are on the same chromosome (6), while the other two antigens are on two other chromosomes.

that synthesized immunoprecipitable portions of the proinsulin gene product. Several laboratories have reported the use of standard antisera in radioimmunoassay to detect specific translation products in bacterial colonies or phage plaques containing recombinant DNA (Broome and Gilbert, 1978; Erlich et al., 1978). Monoclonal antibodies provide an advantage over antisera, since they are highly specific and can be obtained free of other immunoglobulins which produce a significant amount of nonspecific background binding. They can also be labeled metabolically in culture with radioactive amino acids. The one disadvantage is that they react with only a single antigenic determinant, and the methods so far described require binding to a number of determinants on the same molecule. This problem can be easily overcome by using the first monoclonal antibody to isolate the antigen so that it can be used for specific immunization and production of monoclonal antibodies against other determinants on the molecule. By producing monoclonal antibodies against as many determinants on a given molecule as possible, and using them in specific combinations, one could maximize the chances of picking up clones of bacteria expressing various portions of the total antigen molecule. The use of monoclonal antibodies as probes in this way in conjunction with methods designed to maximize expression of cloned genes (Roberts et al., 1979) makes it likely that in the near future we will see the genes for several cell-surface antigens, including tumor-associated antigens, isolated and characterized. Once this has been accomplished, it is but a matter of time before it is determined whether the genes for each tumor antigen present in the tumor cells are present in the normal human germline genome and if so whether for each antigen the difference in normal cells and corresponding tumor cells is at the level of gene structure or regulation.

Monoclonal antibodies against differentiation antigens will certainly also play a significant role in the classification and diagnosis of heterogeneous groups of tumors such as leukemias. Leukemia cells have already been classified into subtypes to some extent by using antisera against differentiation antigens and by using the presence of various cell-surface receptors and enzymes (Greaves and Janossy, 1978). We have attempted several times to produce antibodies against leukemia-specific antigens by immunizing with whole leukemia cells (ALL and CLL). Upon careful analysis we find, as Levy et al. (1978) reported, that the antibodies react with certain tumors and with various subpopulations of normal lymphocytes. These antibodies and others against lymphocyte surface markers will become valuable tools for classification of leukemias prior to selection of therapy regimen and also as a means of monitoring the effectiveness of treatment.

We are now in the process of using the immunization protocols listed in Table II to make monoclonal antibodies against antigens that are truly leukemia-specific.

It is clear that we have only begun to see the effects that Kohler and Milstein's initial observations of proliferating hybrids making monoclonal anti-sheep red blood cell antibodies will have on developments in cell biology, human genetics, and tumor immunology.

ACKNOWLEDGMENTS

This work was supported by NIH grants CA-24263 and CA-14489 and NSF grant PCM76-82997. We are thankful for the excellent technical assistance of Jeannie B. Haas, Barbara Meyer, and Harriet Hopkins-Davis.

References

Broome, S., and Gilbert, W., 1978, Immunological screening method to detect specific translation products, *Proc. Natl. Acad. Sci. USA* **75**:2746.
Brown, G., Capellaro, D., and Greaves, M., 1975, Leukemia-associated antigens in man, *J. Natl. Cancer Inst.* **55**:1281.
Buck, D., and Bodmer, W. F., 1975, The human species antigen on chromosome 11, *Birth Defects Orig. Artic. Ser.* **11**:87.
Davidson, R. L., 1974, Gene expression in somatic cell hybrids, *Annu. Rev. Genet.* **8**:195.
Davies, D. A. L., and O'Neill, G. J., 1975, Methods of cancer immunochemotherapy (DRAB and DRAC) using antisera against tumor specific membrane antigens, in: *Proceedings International Cancer Congress XI, Florence, 1974* (P. Bacalussi, U. Veeronesi, and N. Cascinelli, eds.), Elsevier, Amsterdam, pp. 218–221.
Erlich, H. A., Cohen, S. N., and McDevitt, H. O., 1978, A sensitive radioimmunoassay for detecting products translated from cloned DNA fragments, *Cell* **13**:681.
Evans, A. E., and Hummeler, K., 1973, The significance of primative cells in narrow aspirates of children with neuroblastoma, *Cancer* **4**:906.
Gasser, D. L., Winters, B. A., Haas, J. B., McKearn, T. J., and Kennett, R. H., 1979, Monoclonal antibody directed to a B cell antigen present on rats, mice, and humans, *Proc. Natl. Acad. Sci. USA* **76**:4636.
Goodfellow, P., Barnstable, C., Jones, E., Bodmer, W., Crumpton, M., and Snary, D., 1976, Production of specific antisera to human B lymphocytes, *Tissue Antigens* **7**:105.
Greaves, M., and Janossy, G., 1978, Patterns of gene expression and the cellular origins of human leukemias, *Biochim. Biophys. Acta* **516**:193.
Heitzmann, H., and Richards, F. M., 1974, Use of the avidin–biotin complex for specific staining of biological membranes in electron microscopy, *Proc. Natl. Acad. Sci. USA* **71**:3537.
Herlyn, M., Steplewski, Z., Herlyn, D., and Koprowski, H., 1979, Colorectal carcinoma-specific antigen: Detection by means of monoclonal antibodies, *Proc. Natl. Acad. Sci. USA* **76**:1438.
Kennett, R. H., and Gilbert, F., 1979, Hybrid myelomas producing antibodies against a human neuroblastoma antigen present on fetal brain, *Science* **203**:1120.
Kennett, R. H., Denis, K. A., Tung, A. S., and Klinman, N. R., 1978, Hybrid plasmacytoma production: Fusions with adult spleen cells, monoclonal spleen fragments, neonatal spleen cells and human spleen cells, *Curr. Top. Microbiol. Immunol.* **81**:77.
Kennett, R. H., Jonak, Z. L., and Bechtol, K. B., 1980, Characterization of antigens with monoclonal antibodies, in: *Advances in Neuroblastoma Research* (A. Evans, ed.), Raven Press, New York, pp. 209–219.
Knudson, A. G., and Meadows, A. T., 1978, Developmental genetics of neural tumors in man, in: *Cell Differentiation and Neoplasia* (G. F. Saunders, ed.), Raven Press, New York, pp. 83–92.
Köhler, G., and Milstein, C., 1976, Derivation of specific antibody-producing tissue culture and tumor lines by cell fusion, *Eur. J. Immunol.* **6**:5.
Koprowski, H., Steplewski, Z., Herlyn, D., and Herlyn, M., 1978, Study of antibodies against human melanoma produced by somatic cell hybrids, *Proc. Natl. Acad. Sci. USA* **75**:3405.
Lampson, L., and Levy, R., 1978, A role for clonal antigens in cancer diagnosis and therapy, *J. Natl. Cancer Inst.* **62**:217.

Levy, R., Dilley, J., and Lampson, L. A., 1978, Human normal and leukemia cell surface antigens. Mouse monoclonal antibodies as probes, *Curr. Top. Microbiol. Immunol.* **81:**164.

Momoi, M., Kennett, R. H., and Glick, M. C., 1980, A surface glycoprotein as a human neuroblastoma antigen detected by monoclonal antibody, in: *Advances in Neuroblastoma Research* (A. Evans, ed.), Raven Press, New York, pp. 177–181.

Parham, P., and Bodmer, W. F., 1978, Monoclonal antibody to a human histocompatibility alloantigen, HLA-A2, *Nature* **276:**397.

Roberts, T. M., Kacich, R., and Ptashne, M., 1979, A general method for maximizing expression of a cloned gene, *Proc. Natl. Acad. Sci. USA* **76:**760.

Ruddle, F., 1973, Linkage analysis in man by somatic cell genetics, *Nature* **242:**165.

Ruddon, R. W., ed., 1978, *Biological Markers of Neoplasia: Basic and Applied Aspects,* Elsevier/North-Holland, New York.

Steplewski, Z., Herlyn, M., Herlyn, D., Clark, W. H., and Koprowski, H., 1979, Reactivity of monoclonal anti-melanoma antibodies with melanoma cells freshly isolated from primary and metastatic melanoma, *Eur. J. Immunol.* **9:**94.

Villa-Komaroff, L., Efstratiadis, S., Broome, S., Lomedico, P., Tizard, R., Naber, S. P., Shick, W. L., and Gilbert, W., 1978, A bacterial clone synthesizing proinsulin, *Proc. Natl. Acad. Sci. USA* **75:**3727.

Winchester, R. J., Wang, C., Gibofsky, A., Kinkel, H., Lloyd, K. O., and Old, L. J., 1978, Expression of Ia-like antigens on cultured human malignant melanoma cell lines, *Proc. Natl. Acad. Sci. USA* **75:**6235.

Yeh, M., Hellstrom, I., Brown, J. P., Warner, G. A., Hansen, J. A., and Hellstrom, K. E., 1979, Cell surface antigens of human melanoma identified by monoclonal antibody, *Proc. Natl. Acad. Sci. USA* **76:**2927.

Part IV
Monoclonal Antibodies as Probes in the Study of Cellular Differentiation and Immunogenetics

11

Germ-Cell-Related and Nervous-System-Related Differentiation and Tumor Antigens

KATHLEEN B. BECHTOL, ZDENKA L. JONAK, AND ROGER H. KENNETT

I. Introduction

In recent years increasing attention has been given to the cell surface as an important functional part of the cell. Its component molecular structure and the mechanisms for its involvement in the interactions of cells with their environment are currently the subject of intensive study. Considerable evidence suggests that important aspects of many complex cell–environment interactions involve specific components of the cell surface. A graphic example of this is the species-specific aggregation factors of sponge (Frazier and Glaser, 1979). The factor (molecule), eluted from the sponge cells in Ca^{2+}, Mg^{2+}-free seawater, will cause species-specific aggregation of dissociated sponge cells. While the role of this molecule in the intact sponge is unknown, it may function as one part of the complex system that maintains the cellular associations of the live sponge. Examples of specific surface function in higher organisms are tissue-specific aggregation of cells (Culp, 1978), the sorting out of cells from different tissues (e.g., mesonephric and chondrogenic cells) in cultures (Steinberg, 1978), and the requirement in kidney tubule induction for cell-surface contact between metanephrogenic mesenchyme and ureteric bud cells (Wartiovaara et al., 1974; Lehtonen et al., 1975). Several mechanisms for cell-surface interactions have been proposed, but few of the interactions are well understood.

KATHLEEN B. BECHTOL AND ZDENKA L. JONAK • Wistar Institute of Anatomy and Biology, Philadelphia, Pennsylvania 19104. ROGER H. KENNETT • Department of Human Genetics, University of Pennsylvania, School of Medicine, Philadelphia, Pennsylvania 19104.

Cell-surface composition clearly does differ between cells of differing function (e.g., lymphocytes and neurons), between the same cell in distinct stages of its maturity (e.g., an erythroblast and an erythrocyte), and between different surface regions of a single specialized cell (e.g., a neuron's presynaptic region and cell body). The molecular complexity of the cell surface as displayed on differentiating cells and on tumor cells presumably reflects the complex role of the cell surface in cellular behavior (e.g., receptors), nutrition (e.g., transport proteins), and so on.

A few naturally occurring probes, such as toxins and lectins, have been used to study surface components. However, such naturally occurring probes are rare and, more frequently, reagents specific for surface components have been generated through immunization (i.e., production of specific antisera). A number of cell-surface antigens (determinants on molecules) have been defined in this way, though few outside of those related to the immune system have been studied extensively.

Recently, however, the production of monoclonal antibodies from immune lymphocytes fused with myeloma cells (Köhler and Milstein, 1976) has provided an unprecedented opportunity for defining cell-surface components through the use of monospecific antibodies that can be produced almost at will by appropriate immunization and screening procedures. We, like many others, have taken advantage of this opportunity. In this chapter we will discuss our experiments and show examples of the resulting hybridomas that are producing monoclonal antibodies to cells in various steps on germ-cell differentiation or to differentiation and/or tumor antigens of the nervous system.

II. Immunizations

Most surface molecules relevant to cell differentiation and tumor phenotype have not yet been identified, and their tissue and temporal distributions are therefore not yet known. Nevertheless, a simplifying constraint can be put on the initial monoclonal antibody assault on these "differentiation molecules." One can rule out markers with widespread or ubiquitous tissue distribution and focus on tissue-, cell type-, and/or time-limited determinants. Operationally, this focusing can be accomplished in part at the time of lymphocyte stimulation by restricting the set of antigenic determinants presented to the immune system. The limited but complex response is then broken down into its monoclonal components by hybridoma formation. The response can be focused on a single molecule if that molecule is used in partially or extensively purified form. More importantly, restriction of the response can also be accomplished using whole cells and using complex populations of cells.

Tumor-related molecules and cell-surface components of many differentiating systems [viz., early embryo; central nervous system (CNS)] are not normally available to the immune system. Many of the antigenic determinants on these molecules are, therefore, "foreign" or "non-self" and the animal is able to respond to these antigens by producing specific antibody. In contrast, an animal does not generally respond if challenged with its own adult and/or ubiquitous "self" antigens. For this reason, syngeneic immunization focuses the response on the "non-self" subset of the antigens present on the immunizing cells.

A similar effect of diminishing or blocking the response to a subset of determinants on the cell can be obtained by precoating the immunizing cells with antibodies to the unwanted determinants (see Kennett *et al.*, 1978, and this volume). This approach can be applied to many systems which could be studied by xenogeneic antibodies, viz., mouse anti-*Drosophila* or slime mold differentiation antigens. Moreover, it can be applied using monoclonal antibodies in the precoating, thus directing the production of additional monoclonal antibodies toward new determinants. It is important to recognize that by limiting the antigen subset presented at the time of immunization, thus providing a prescreening of the resulting hybridoma crop, allowing the suppression of response to major immunogens and enhancing detection of the response to more minor ones, one can to some degree control the specificity of hybridomas that will be recovered.

III. Use of Monoclonal Antibodies to Study Spermatogenesis

Spermatogenesis is an interesting developmental system that involves the differentiation of the germ cells, through a series of complex changes, to form the adult spermatozoa. Spermatogenesis begins after birth when the primitive germ cells mature into the permanent stem cells of cyclic spermatogenesis. The permanent stem cells undergo mitosis throughout the rest of the life of the animal, renewing themselves and producing daughter cells that differentiate to spermatozoa. The daughter cells (spermatogonia) first enter into a period of mitosis with incomplete cytokinesis, thus producing a series of cells in identical steps of differentiation and linked by cytoplasmic bridges. This mitotic period lasts approximately 6 days in mouse. The cells then enter meiotic prophase.

In the juvenile testis some of the germ cells enter meiotic prophase as early as 8 to 10 days of postnatal life. Some of these cells degenerate, but others progress through meiotic prophase and into meiotic divisions I and II by 19 days of age. Following meiosis the haploid cells (spermatids) undergo a number of structural changes, including nuclear condensation and acrosome and flagellum formation. The entire sequence from stem cell to released testicular spermatozoon requires 34.5 days in the adult mouse. Within each section of testis tubule new generations of spermatogenesis are initiated every 8.6 days in the mouse. Looking at the tubule in cross section, the sequential generations of differentiating germ cells are arranged in concentric rings in the tubule epithelium (except in man where the generations are intermixed). The younger generations lie closer to the basement membrane, and the older generations lie progressively nearer the lumen of the tubule. In the juvenile testis, the number of generations increases to four to five as the testis matures. This number is then maintained in the adult by regular initiation of new generations and the release of completed spermatozoa. Because of the precise time interval between initiations of spermatogenesis and the regular timing of the progression of cells through the spermatogenic sequence cross sections of testis tubules display a series of highly regular associations of differentiation steps. Each section of tubule epithelium cycles through this series of cell-type associations (stages), and in general sequential segments of seminiferous tubule are in sequential stages of spermatogenesis, so that there appear to be waves of spermatogenesis down the tubule. The sum of events in the cycling epithelium is continuous spermatogenesis by the testis. During this series of developmental changes, the germ cells are surrounded by the epithelial element of the spermatogenic tubules, the Sertoli cells.

Spermatocytes (meiotic cells) and spermatids are sequestered from the immune system by the "blood–testis barrier" which consists of a basal lamina and specialized junctions between the Sertoli cells near the periphery of the seminiferous tubules (Gilula et al., 1976; Nagato and Suzuki, 1976). The network of tight junctions prevents the passage of cells and macromolecules from the blood into the inner portion of the tubule. Spermatogonia and preleptotene spermatocytes lie on the basal side of the Sertoli-cell junctions (Dym, 1973), whereas leptotene and later spermatocytes and spermatids are located within the inner, sequestered compartment of the tubule. The antigens of these cells are therefore not normally presented to the immune system of the animal as "self" antigens.

Taking advantage of the immunologically privileged location of these cells, we have used syngeneic immunization to focus on tissue-related surface molecules. Because the juvenile testis progressively becomes populated with successive steps of spermatogenesis, it provides a series of ever widening windows on the component cell types of spermatogenesis. By choosing the age of juvenile testis to be used as donor cells for immunization, one can choose the subset of cell types observed. Thus, a younger testis provides a small, early subset of the cell types in spermatogenesis; an older testis displays a larger, more complete subset.

For the first fusion (Table I), the recipient 129 strain female was immunized with a heterogeneous suspension of cells derived from adult 129 strain testis by mechanical disruption of the testis tubules. To avoid modification of the surface antigens no enzymes were added to aid in release of the cells from the tubules. Cells for the secondary immunization of this mouse were from immature, 26-day-old testis and were prepared in the same way as the previous cells. Because of the age of the donor, the second inoculum contained germ cells only through midspermatid stages and did not include late spermatids or formed testicular sperm. For both the donor cell populations used in the above immunizations, cells in early phases of spermatogenesis were present in the donor testes, but the more mature cells present in these testes provided the major part of the immunizing inoculum. The reason for this is as follows: (1) as the result of mitotic and meiotic divisions during the maturation sequence the more mature cells make up a larger proportion of the cells in the tubules, and (2) the more mature cells are more easily released from the tubule epithelium. Fusion I thus largely concentrated on immunization with spermatocytes and early- to mid-

TABLE I
Anti-Testis Immunizations

Donor cells for immunization			Number of hybrids		
Primary	Secondary	Myeloma	Total	Testis binding[a]	% Positive
1. Adult[b]	26-day	P3/X63-Ag8	264	31	12
2. 18-day, precoated[c]	20-day, precoated	SP2/0-Ag14	43	8	19

[a]Number of hybrids with supernatants showing binding activity above background, to suspension of testis cells of the immunizating donor age, in radioimmunoassay (see Appendix).
[b]Age of strain 129 donors of testis cells.
[c]Cells were precoated with monoclonal antibodies XT-I and XT-II at saturating concentrations for 1 hr on ice, spun down, resuspended in phosphate-buffered saline (PBS) and used for immunization.

development spermatids. The reactivity of three of the resulting hybridomas will be described in Section V.

For the second fusion (Table I), cells from 18- and 20-day-old testes were used for the primary and secondary immunizations, respectively. These donor testes contained a small number of early spermatids, but the majority of cells were in various stages of meiosis (Nebel *et al.*, 1961). These latter cells were therefore quantitatively the major component of the immunizing inoculum. It was known at the time of these immunizations that two of the monoclonal antibodies from fusion I, XT-I and XT-II (see Section V), showed their peak binding activity to testes of about 19 days. Therefore to decrease or avoid the possibility of producing major immunization against these same determinants again the donor cells for both primary and secondary immunizations were precoated with these two antibodies before being used in the immunizations. Three of the hybridomas resulting from these immunizations will be described in Section V.

IV. Use of Monoclonal Antibodies to Study Differentiation and Tumors of the Nervous System

Cells and macromolecules of the blood and lymph are prevented from entering the central nervous system by the "blood–brain barrier." Thus, as in the testis, antigens of central nervous system cells exist in an immunologically privileged site, so that the host animal remains immunologically reactive to them and can respond if they are presented to the immune system through injury, disease, or deliberate experimental immunization. Some of the nervous-system-related surface molecules also exist on cells of the peripheral nervous system. In this location some of the antigens may be more accessible to the immune system and the animal may be tolerant to them. However, the syndrome of experimental allergic encephalomyelitis suggests that there are nervous system antigens to which the normal intact animal is not tolerant. To focus on some of these antigens we have immunized syngeneically with the mouse neuroblastoma C1300. The C1300 cell line was chosen as a model for tumor- and nervous-system-related surface antigens.

In general A/J-strain mice inoculated with the syngeneic C1300 neuroblastoma rapidly develop tumors and die within a few weeks. We therefore investigated several alternative protocols for immunization (Table II). For short-term immunizations with live cells (I, II, and III) the splenic lymphocytes were taken for fusion several days prior to the expected death of the animal from tumor. Longer immunization protocols were possible using gluteraldehyde-fixed cells,

TABLE II

Immunizations for Anti-Mouse Neuroblastoma C1300

Fusion no.	Immunization protocol[a]	Myeloma parent	Total	Positive on C1300[b]	%(+)
Ia,b	i.p. 5×10^6 live 7 d → i.v. 5×10^6 live 3 d → fusion[c]	× SP-2 NS-1	37 39	0 0	
II	s.c. 2×10^6 live 11 d → i.v. 5×10^6 live 3 d → fusion[d] (actively growing solid tumor)	× SP-2	49	6	12
III	1/2 of splenic lymphocytes from II[d] cultured 24 hr *in vitro* prior to fusion	× SP-2	99	1?[e]	
IV	s.c. 2×10^6 Glut 3 d → s.c. 2×10^6 Glut 7 d → i.v. 5×10^6 Glut 3 d → fusion	× SP-2	5	0	
V	s.c. 2×10^6 Glut 3 d → s.c. 2×10^6 Glut 38 d → i.v. 5×10^6 Glut 3 d → fusion	× 8653	12	0	
VI	s.c. 2×10^6 Glut 3 d → s.c. 2×10^6 Glut 7 d → i.v. 5×10^6 Glut 31 d → i.v. 5×10^6 Live 3 d → fusion	× 8653	21	0	
VII	s.c. 2×10^6 Glut 3 d → s.c. 2×10^6 Glut 38 d → i.v. 5×10^6 Glut 33 d → s.c. 4×10^6 Live 16 d → fusion (actively growing solid tumor)	× SP-2	102	18	17

[a]Inoculation method (i.p., intraperitoneal; s.c., subcutaneous; i.v., intravenous); number of cells in inoculum; cells used live or fixed with 0.123% glutaraldehyde (Glut) for 5 min at 25°C and washed with PBS before injection; days (d) to subsequent procedure.
[b]Binding of supernatant to C1300 as detected in indirect radioimmunoassay using [^{125}I]rabbit anti-mouse Fab.
[c]Two spleens pooled and one half used for fusion with SP-2, one half with NS-1.
[d]Two spleens pooled and one half of cells used in fusion II, one half in fusion III.
[e]Clone lost and could not be confirmed.

in some cases followed by a final immunization with live cells. While this allowed for more repeated immunizations, the immunogenicity of fixed cells may differ from that of live cells, and, moreover, some of the surface antigens may be modified by the fixation process. Various combinations of intraperitoneal, intravenous and subcutaneous immunizations were used. However, as seen in Table II, only those mice with actively growing subcutaneous tumors at the time of fusion (II, III, and VII) produced clones secreting C1300-binding activity. The frequency of positive clones in fusions II and VII was 12% and 17%, respectively, which is consistent with the frequencies of positive clones found using other immunogens (Köhler and Shulman, 1978). Maintaining the immunized splenic lymphocytes in tissue culture for 24 hr prior to fusion (III) decreased rather than enhanced the recovery of C1300-binding hybrids.

V. Reactivity of Anti-Testis and Anti-C1300 Hybridomas

Following fusion by the method of Kennett et al. (1978), the cell suspensions were distributed into 500 to 600 microtiter wells. When macroscopically visible colonies appeared 2 to 3 weeks later, the binding activity present in the medium of these wells was assayed by indirect radioimmunoassay, using the immunizing cell type as target and [^{125}I]rabbit anti-mouse Ig or Fab as detecting reagent. In general, all wells showing binding activity above background were kept for further analysis.

The dilution binding curves for supernatants from six anti-testis hybridomas and one anti-C1300 hybridoma, using adult testis cells as targets in the assay, are shown in Fig. 1. The anti-C1300, II2B9, shows no detectable binding activity on testis cells. Under the given assay conditions three of the anti-testis antibodies, XT-I, XT-II, and XT-IV, which are IgG2a, IgG2b, and IgM, respectively, fail to reach concentrations that saturate the available antigenic sites on the testis cells. The slope of the binding curve for XT-IV is less than that for XT-I or XT-II, suggesting that (1) XT-IV has lower avidity for the testis cells than do XT-I and XT-II, and/or (2) the radioiodinated anti-Ig reagent has greater avidity for IgG than for IgM antibodies. It would appear that the first explanation is at least in part correct as two other IgM monoclonal antibodies, ST-V and ST-VI, show steeper binding slopes under the same conditions. Resolution of this question will await more precise quantitation of the avidities of these antibodies (Frankel and Gerhard, 1979; see also Appendix).

Three of the anti-testis monoclonal antibodies, ST-V, ST-VI, and ST-VII, show a plateau of binding, apparently at saturation of the available target sites. The radiolabeled rabbit anti-mouse immunoglobulin (Ig) is nonlimiting in these assays. Each of these plateaus shows a prozone with increasing supernatant concentration. The cause of this prozone effect is unknown, though possibilities include (1) stripping of antigen–antibody complexes from the surface of the cell, which could be prevented in some cases by target-cell fixation, or (2) increased monovalent binding and consequent lower avidity of the antibody for the target

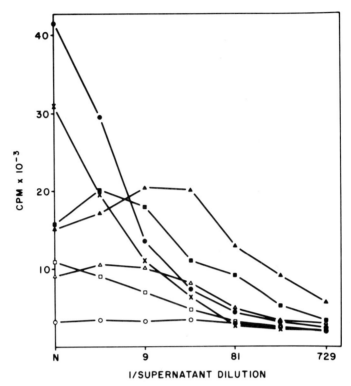

FIGURE 1. Binding of serial dilutions of XT-I (●), XT-II (×), XT-IV (□), ST-V (■), ST-VI (▲), ST-VII(△), and II2B9 (○) to testis cells in a two-step radioimmunoassay using nonlimiting amounts of [^{125}I]rabbit anti-mouse Ig as the second step. N, neat, undiluted supernatant.

cell. Whatever the cause, the effect can be quite striking and has on occasion led to lack of detection of a secreted antibody during spot checks of highly concentrated supernatants.

The distribution of bound antibodies among the complex population of testis cells can be visualized by an indirect binding assay using horseradish peroxidase-coupled anti-mouse Ig. Figure 2 shows a suspension of cells from 19-day old testis treated with either peroxidase-coupled anti-mouse Ig (Fig. 2A) or with monoclonal antibody XT-I followed by peroxidase-coupled anti-mouse Ig (Fig. 2B). Both slides were developed with diaminobenzidine and peroxide followed by OsO$_4$. The very dark small cells in both photographs are red cells which possess endogenous peroxidase activity. The several larger cells of uniform darkness are dead cells that have internally trapped the reagents. In the population treated with XT-I (Fig. 2B), several cells show positive staining, which appears in the photographed focal plane as a dark ring of reaction product at the surface of the cell. Focusing at different levels on the cells reveals that they are labeled over their entire surface. Many of the labeled cells appear to be in stages of meiosis, based on their size and their morphology, following counterstaining with hematoxyline and eosin (not shown). However, positive identification of the

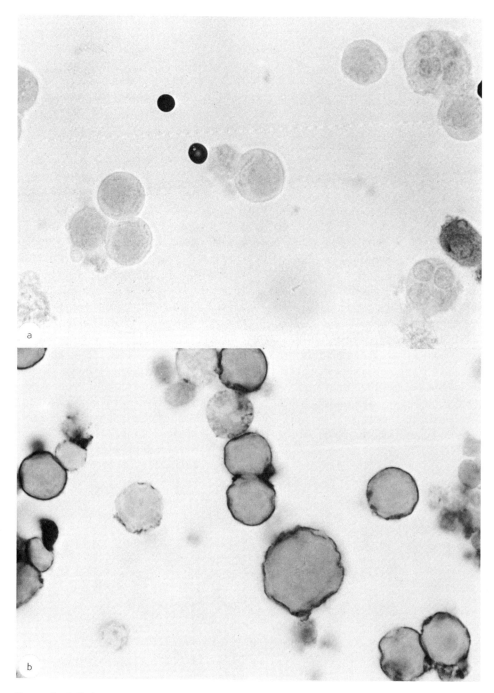

FIGURE 2. Cells from 19-day-old 129-strain testis treated with (a) peroxidase-coupled anti-mouse Ig
or (b) monoclonal antibody XT-I followed by peroxidase-coupled anti-mouse Ig. Antibody localization is visualized by addition of peroxide and diaminobenzidine, followed by addition of OsO$_4$.

precise set of germ-cell-differentiation steps binding ST-I and analysis of quantitative variations in binding await further studies at the electron-microscope level and/or on intact tubule sections.

An overall view of the expression of antigen ST-I can be obtained by quantitative absorption of ST-I supernatant with the total population of testis cells at various juvenile ages. These populations contain germ cells only through specific steps of differentiation, and the total-testis preparations, following gentle disruption in a loose homogenizer, includes all of the cells present in the testes. As seen in Fig. 3, the concentrations of the antigen detected by XT-I changes as the juvenile testis matures. It is undetectable at eight days under the given assay conditions, can be found by 13 days and increases in concentration in the whole testis until the animal approaches maturity, when its concentration declines slightly. The XT-I antigen is also present, though in much smaller amounts, on epididymal sperm (Bechtol *et al.,* 1979). Also shown in Fig. 3 is the quantitation of another antigen, recognized by monoclonal antibody XT-II. The XT-2 antigen also increases during development; however, this antigen, in contrast to XT-1, is detectable at 8 days of age and is not found on epididymal sperm. Thus by implication from the various subsets of differentiating gametes present in the juvenile testes used for absorption, the two antigens XT-1 and XT-2 would appear to be expressed on overlapping subsets of the gametogenic sequence.

The tissue distribution of binding activity for the anti-testis antibodies from Fig. 1 is shown in Table III. Four of the antibodies, XT-I, XT-II, ST-V, and ST-VI, show testis-related binding activity, and the recognized determinants do not appear to be present on related species, such as rat, hamster, and guinea pig. Neither of the two antibodies tested, XT-I and XT-II, was found to react significantly with F9 teratocarcinoma cells or with preimplantation embryos (D. Solter, personal communication). In contrast, the remaining two antibodies, XT-IV and ST-VII, each appear to bind a determinant or family of determinants with wide tissue and species distribution. Antigens detected by XT-IV and ST-VII are present on both male and female brain.

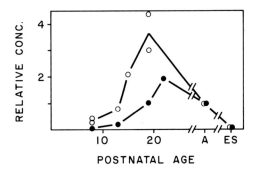

FIGURE 3. Absorbing capacity of juvenile testis and epididymal sperm relative to absorbing capacity of adult testis (defined as 1) for XT-I (●) and XT-II (○) supernatants. A, adult; ES, epididymal sperm. Each point represents a separate determination. [Reproduced from Bechtol *et al.* (1979) with permission.]

TABLE III
Anti-Testis Hybridomas

	Hybridomas[a]					
	XT-I	XT-II	XT-IV	ST-V	ST-VI	ST-VII
Fusion No. (Table I)	1	1	1	2	2	2
Ig chains	γ2a	γ2b	μ	μ,κ	μ,κ	α,κ
Binding to						
Testis						
Mouse	+	+	+	+	+	+
Rat	−	−	+	−	−	+
Hamster	−	−				
Guinea pig				−	−	+
Mouse						
Epidermal sperm	+	−		+	+	
F9[b]	−	−				
Whole ovary	−	−				
Preimplantation embryos[c]	−	−				
Spleen	−	−		−	−	+
Liver	−	−	+	−	−	
Kidney	−	−		−	−	+
Brain	−	−	+	−	−	+
C1300[d]			+			
Rat						
Brain			+			
Human						
IMR6[e]			+			

[a]+, positive by quantitative absorption, −, undetectable by quantitative absorption.
[b]F9, mouse teratocarcinoma.
[c]Davor Solter (personal communication), determined by indirect immunofluorescence and by cytotoxicity.
[d]C1300, mouse neuroblastoma.
[e]IMR6, human neuroblastoma.

The tissue distribution of seven anti-C1300 monoclonal antibodies is shown in Table IV. Semiquantitative analysis of the binding of these seven IgM antibodies shows tissue-related variations in their binding. These differences are being exploited by using some of these antibodies to detect the presence of antigen-bearing metastatic neuroblastoma cells among the antigen-negative cells of the blood and bone marrow. Several anti-neuroblastoma monoclonal antibodies, including anti-IMR6 human neuroblastoma (Kennett and Gilbert, 1979), and the anti-C1300 antibodies II2B9 and VII5G9, both of which react with human neuroblastoma, are currently being used in a study to determine their specificity for detecting neuroblastoma metastasis in human bone marrow. From the data in Table IV it appears that the same two anti-C1300 antibodies might also be suitable for detecting neuroblastoma metastasis in the liver (at least in mouse); however, they appear less appropriate for detecting metastases in the kidney. The distribution of binding of the anti-C1300 antibodies within the nervous system has not yet been extensively investigated. However, preliminary

TABLE IV
Anti-C1300 Hybridomas

	Hybridomas[a]						
	II-2B9	II-1H2	II-1F4	VII-1G9	VII-1G3	VII-5G9	VII-2D2
Fusion no. (Table II)	II	II	II	VII	VII	VII	VII
Ig chains	μ	μ	μ	μ	μ	μ	μ
Binding to							
C1300[b]	++++	+++	+++	+	++	+++++	++++
IMR6[c]	++	+++	++	±	++	++++	±
A/J adult brain	++++	+++	+++	+	++	++++	++
A/J testis	−	++	+	−	+	+++	−
A/J spleen	−	+	−	−	−	±	−
A/J liver	−	++++	−	−	++++	−	−
A/J kidney	+	+	+	±	+	+++	±

[a]Semiquantitative tissue distribution of antibody binding in radioimmunoassay using target cells as listed and [^{125}I]rabbit anti-mouse Fab as detecting reagent. Number of +'s is based on counts per minute bound above background to equal volumes of the target tissues.
[b]C1300, mouse neuroblastoma.
[c]IMR6, human neuroblastoma.

results suggest that at least some show a restricted cell-type distribution within the nervous system. Thus, the same antibodies can be exploited to investigate two very different questions, one involving the distribution of binding specificity in the whole organism, the other within the CNS.

VI. Conclusion

Detailed analysis of both gametogenesis and nervous system development will depend on the ability to identify the cell types and their degree of differentiation. Monoclonal antibodies such as those described in this chapter can be used to analyze cell populations in terms of their composition by cell-sorting techniques or by visual techniques *in situ* such as fluoresceninated or peroxidase-coupled antibody. The function of the antigenic molecules themselves can be explored by determining the effect of the antibody on the differentiating cells. Several instances of cell-surface glycoprotein receptors are currently known, the biology of which is affected by antibodies in various disease states. These include autoantibodies to the insulin receptor (Kahn, 1979), to thyroid-stimulating hormone receptor in Graves's disease (Volpé, 1979), and to the acetylcholine receptor in myasthenia gravis (Drachman, 1979). Some antibodies to the first two receptors have been shown to mimic the effects of adding insulin or thyroid-stimulating hormone themselves. Production of these effects requires that the antibodies be bivalent; Fab fragments do not elicit the biological response (Kahn, 1979; Volpé, 1979). Though such effects have been produced by polyclonal antibodies, similar perturbations should be possible using monoclonal reagents or groups of monoclonal reagents capable of causing sufficient cross-linking.

Monoclonal antibodies binding to tumor cells can be used to detect primary and metastatic tumors and potentially can be used for the destruction *in vivo* of tumor cells through targeting cytotoxic drugs to the tumor cells using covalently coupled drug–antibody complexes. The function of the recognized antigen on the tumor cell can also be explored as described above for differentiation antigens.

A large number of systems, including those described in this section and in the introduction to this chapter, can now be explored in greater detail, using chemically pure monoclonal antibody reagents as probes for the molecular components of the system. Such studies should bring to light details of cell-surface composition, which will provide further insights into cell-surface function.

ACKNOWLEDGMENTS

This research was supported by USPHS Grants GM23892, NS15427, CA18930, CA09140, CA24263, and CA14489 and NSF Grant PCM76-82997.

References

Bechtol, K. B., Brown, S. C., and Kennett, R. H., 1979, Recognition of differentiation antigens of spermatogenesis in the mouse by using antibodies from spleen cell–myeloma hybrids after syngeneic immunization, *Proc. Natl. Acad. Sci. USA* **76:**363.

Culp, L. A., 1978, Biochemical determinants of cell adhesion, *Curr. Top. Membranes Transport* **11:**327.

Drachman, D. B., 1979, Immunopathology of myasthenia gravis, *Fed. Proc.* **38:**2613.

Dym, M., 1973, The fine structure of the monkey *(Macaca)* Sertoli cell and its role in maintaining the blood–testis barrier, *Anat. Rec.* **175:**639.

Frankel, M. E., and Gerhard, W., 1979, The rapid determination of binding constants for anti-viral antibodies by radioimmune assay. An analysis of the interaction between hybridoma proteins and influenza virus, *Mol. Immunol.* **16:**101.

Frazier, W., and Glaser, L., 1979, Surface components and cell recognition, *Annu. Rev. Biochem.* **48:**491.

Gilula, N. B., Fawcett, D. W., and Aoki, A., 1976, The Sertoli cell occluding junctions and gap junctions in mature and developing mammalian testis, *Dev. Biol.* **50:**142.

Kahn, C. R., 1979, Autoantibodies to the insulin receptor: Clinical and molecular aspects, *Fed. Proc.* **38:**2607.

Kennett, R. H., and Gilbert, F., 1979, Hybrid myelomas producing antibodies against a human neuroblastoma antigen present on fetal brain, *Science* **203:**1120.

Kennett, R. H., Denis, K. A., Tung, A. S., and Klinman, N. R., 1978, Hybrid plasmacytoma production: Fusions with adult spleen cells, monoclonal spleen fragments, neonatal spleen cells and human spleen cells, *Curr. Top. Microbiol. Immunol.* **81:**77.

Köhler, G., and Milstein, C., 1976, Derivation of specific antibody-producing tissue culture and tumor lines by cell fusion, *Eur. J. Immunol.* **6:**511.

Köhler, G., and Shulman, M. J., 1978, Cellular and molecular restrictions of the lymphocyte fusion, *Curr. Top. Microbiol. Immunol.* **81**:143.

Lehtonen, E., Wartiovaara, J., Nordling, S., and Saxén, L., 1975, Demonstration of cytoplasmic processes in Millipore filters permitting kidney tubule induction, *J. Embryol. Exp. Morphol.* **33**:187.

Nagato, T., and Suzuki, F., 1976, Freeze-fracture observations on the intercellular junctions of Sertoli cells and of Leydig cells in the human testis, *Cell Tissue Res.* **166**:37.

Nebel, B. R., Amarose, A. P., and Hackett, E. H., 1961, Calendar of gametogenic development in the prepubertal male mouse, *Science* **134**:832.

Steinberg, M. S., 1978, Specific cell ligands and the differential adhesion hypothesis: How do they fit together? in: *Specificity of Embryological Interactions* (D. R. Garrod, ed.), Chapman and Hall, London, pp. 97–130.

Volpé, R., 1979, Immunopathology of Graves' disease, *Fed. Proc.* **38**:2611.

Wartiovaara, J., Nordling, S., Lehtonen, E., and Saxen, L., 1974, Transfilter induction of kidney tubules: Correlation with cytoplasmic penetration into Nucleopore filters, *J. Embryol. Exp. Morphol.* **33**:187.

12
Cell-Surface Differentiation in the Mouse

Characterization of "Jumping" and "Lineage" Antigens Using Xenogeneic Rat Monoclonal Antibodies

TIMOTHY A. SPRINGER

I. Introduction

Differentiation is the process whereby indifferent cells give rise to specialized tissues and cellular subpopulations with distinctive characteristics. This involves the coordinated control of many different genes, some of which affect the expression of molecules at the cell surface. Those molecules that can be identified with antibodies and are expressed on some but not all tissues are called differentiation antigens (Boyse and Old, 1969). Both qualitative and quantitative variations occur in the expression of differentiation antigens.

A salient advantage of probing surface, as opposed to intracellular differentiation antigens, is that various methodologies involving antibodies bound to the surface allow intact cells to be separated on the basis of their state of differentiation. Functional capacity may then be related to cell-surface phenotype. Furthermore, antibodies are versatile probes that may also be used to inhibit or modify the activity of molecules in their native cell-surface environment or for the isolation and biochemical characterization of surface molecules.

The richness of the cell surface in terms of the great variety of different antigens displayed, even on a single type of cell, has in the past been a considerable obstacle to analysis. The Köhler and Milstein (1976) hybrid technique has therefore been of tremendous importance for developments in this field. We

---

TIMOTHY A. SPRINGER • Pathology Department, Harvard Medical School, Boston, Massachusetts 02115.

have explored the use of the myeloma-hybrid technique for the xenogeneic analysis of differentiation antigens in the mouse, with particular emphasis on leukocyte antigens (Springer *et al.*, 1978a,b; see Milstein *et al.*, 1979, and Milstein and Lennox, 1980, for a review of studies in both the rat and mouse). Probably more surface antigens have been defined in the mouse than in any other species, and thus one question was with what frequency the myeloma-hybrid method would allow discovery of novel surface antigens. Most previously defined surface antigens in the mouse had been identified by alloimmunization of one strain with another, in which congenic strains were used to restrict the immunizing stimulus to the polymorphic products of a short chromosomal segment. In contrast, our object was to study differentiation in the broadest sense and thus to elicit strong antibodies to as wide a range of surface molecules as possible. Xenoimmunization, of rats with mouse spleen cells, was therefore chosen. The resultant multispecific response to a large array of different cell-surface molecules was then resolved by cloning into a set of hybrid lines each recognizing an individual determinant on an individual cell-surface molecule.

II. Techniques for Obtaining and Characterizing Monoclonal Antibodies to Differentiation Antigens

A. Immunization and Hybridization

Most procedures have previously been described in detail (Springer *et al.*, 1978b). Briefly, rats were primed two times with mouse spleen cells enriched for T lymphocytes by nylon-wool filtration or by concanavalin A (Con A) stimulation and depleted of red blood cells (RBC) by Isopaque–Ficoll sedimentation. An intravenous boost was given 3 days prior to the hybridization experiment. Fusion with polyethyleneglycol (PEG) was as described (Galfré *et al.*, 1977), except the PEG solution (~50% w/w) was made by autoclaving 10 g PEG, allowing it to cool partially, and while still liquid, adding 10 ml Dulbecco's Modified Eagle's Medium (DMEM). After fusion of 2×10^8 rat spleen cells with 2×10^7 P3-NSI/1-Ag4-1 (NSI) nonsecretor myeloma cells, the cells were aliquoted into $96\times$ 2-ml wells and grown in hypoxanthine–aminopterin–thymidine (HAT) medium (Littlefield, 1964). These cultures were designated M1/1-M1/96. Clones derived from these cultures by agar cloning are designated with a second number, e.g., M1/9.3, and if recloned, a third, e.g., M1/9.3.4. All lines described here have been subcloned at least once. For brevity, clone designations have been omitted except to distinguish clones recognizing different antigens isolated from the same culture.

B. Identification of Positive Cultures

After 2 weeks of growth positive clones were tested in an indirect ^{125}I-anti-rat immunoglobulin (Ig) cell binding assay as previously described (Springer *et al.*, 1978b). In this assay rat antibodies secreted into tissue-culture supernatants were first incubated with target cells at 4°C for 45 min in microtiter plates, washed, then incubated with ^{125}I-rabbit F(ab')$_2$ anti-rat IgG or Fab for a further 45 min at 4°C, washed, and counted in a γ spectrometer. Xenogeneic antibodies are much more convenient to assay than allogeneic ones because ^{125}I-anti-rat Ig absorbed with mouse IgG can be used, preventing cross-reaction with mouse Ig on B lymphocytes or absorbed onto Fc receptors. Of 94 cultures 92 contained specific antibody-secreting hybrids. From the Poisson distribution it was estimated that each culture contained an average of four independently fused, successful, specific antibody-secreting cells. These were in addition to an undetermined number of negative hybrids. After further growth over a 7-week period, faster-growing clones became dominant, and some cultures became negative. Then 17 of the cultures were cloned in soft agar. A total of 500 clones were transferred to liquid culture, and their culture supernatants were tested in the indirect ^{125}I-anti-rat Ig-binding assay. From 7 of the cultures 47 clones were identified as positive. The fraction positive ranged from 2/48 for M1/9 to 19/19 for M1/89. Multiple clones from the same culture were compared for reactivity with different cells, such as thymocytes, spleen white cells, and mouse RBC and sheep RBC, and by titration of clonal supernatants (Springer *et al.*, 1978b) or of spleen target cells (Springer *et al.*, 1978a) in ^{125}I-anti-rat Ig indirect binding assays. In the case of multiple identical clones, two representatives, generally with the highest titer in the binding assay, were saved. From each of three cultures, two different clones with distinct antigenic specificities were isolated, i.e., M1/9.3 and M1/9.47, M1/22.25 and M1/22.54, and M1/89.1 and M1/89.18. A single type of clone was isolated from four cultures.

Since these clones (the first 10 listed in Table I) were selected for no criteria other than reactivity in the indirect binding assay, they represent a random collection of monoclonal antibodies directed against surface antigens. They recognize five types of antigens, some of which had been previously identified by alloantisera. One, the Forssman antigen, had previously been identified by relatively monospecific xenoantisera (Boyd, 1966). The common leukocyte antigen (CLA) had previously been precipitated by one component of polyspecific anti-lymphocyte sera (Trowbridge and Mazauskas, 1976), but monspecific sera had not been previously obtainable, even by absorption. The M1/69, M1/75, and M1/70 antigens (Table I) had not been previously identified by any means. The small degree of overlap between these antigens and those previously identified and the ease with which further novel antigens could be identified (see Section IV) suggests that currently known antigens only represent the tip of the iceberg, and that the vast majority of antigens are still lurking on the cell surface awaiting identification.

C. Stability

When lines are grown continuously for long periods in culture, antibody activity is periodically monitored and recloning is carried out every 6 months. After each cloning aliquots of cells are frozen in liquid N$_2$. After the first subcloning the lines appear quite stable, e.g., variants with loss of either the specific

TABLE I

Mouse Differentiation Antigens Identified by Rat Monoclonal Antibodies

Clones	Cellular recognition	Antigen	Designation
M1/22.25 M1/87	Early embryos,[a] germinal tissue, erythroblasts, sheep RBC but not mouse RBC	Heat-stable,[b] Forssman glycosphingolipid	Forssman
M1/9.47, M1/22.54 M1/69, M1/89.1	Mouse RBC, granulocytes, monocytes, B lymphocytes, thymocytes but not peripheral T lymphocytes	Heat-stable, no iodinated or [^{35}S]methionine-labeled component	Heat-stable antigen (HSA)[c]
M1/75	Mouse RBC, not on thymocytes or lymphocytes	Heat-stable, no iodinated or [^{35}S]methionine-labeled component	Heat-stable antigen (HSA)[c]
M1/9.3 M1/89.18	Leukocytes	MW ~ 200,000[d]	Common leukocyte antigen (CLA)
M1/42	Almost all cells	MW 46,000 and 12,000	H-2
M1/84	Leukocytes, mast-nucleated bone marrow cells, others?	MW 46,000	?
M1/70	Granulocytes and mononuclear phagocytes[e]	MW 190,000 and 105,000	Mac-1
M3/31, M3/38	Mononuclear phagocytes	MW 32,000	Mac-2
M3/84	Mononuclear phagocytes	MW 110,000	Mac-3

[a]Stern *et al.* (1978); Willison and Stern (1978).
[b]Stable at 120°C for 15 min.
[c]This group of antibodies competes between themselves for binding to mouse red blood cells.
[d]The molecular weight of this antigen depends on the source from which it is isolated: molecular weight 230,000 from B lymphocytes or molecular weights 200,000 and 180,000 from T lymphocytes.
[e]Springer *et al.* (1979).

or myeloma light chain are found at a frequency of slightly less than 10^{-2} several months later. However, it is extremely important to clone the initial cultures, even if derived from a single hybrid cell, since chromosome losses leading to specific heavy- or light-chain losses are particularly frequent in the early stages of growth. Using the procedures described above no lines have ever been lost subsequent to obtaining the first positive clone.

D. Immunoprecipitation

Antigen specificity was investigated by immunoprecipitation and sodium dodecyl sulfate–polyacrylamide gel electrophoresis (SDS-PAGE) of radioactively labeled cell-surface molecules (Fig. 1). An extremely heterogeneous mixture of proteins was precipitated by the serum antibodies from the rat contributing the spleen for the fusion. The monoclonal pattern was much simpler. Two mono-

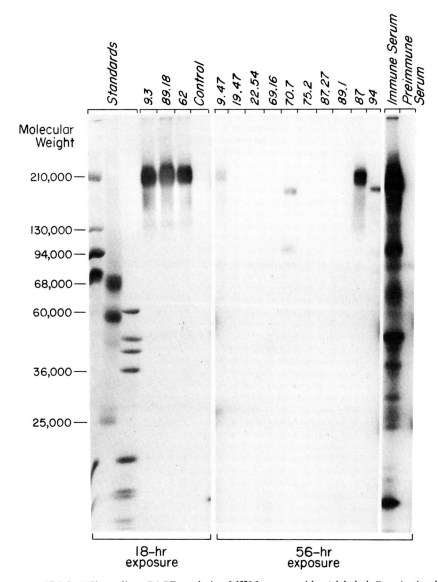

FIGURE 1. SDS 7–15% gradient PAGE analysis of ^{125}I(lactoperoxidase)-labeled Con A-stimulated spleen cell surface, Triton X-100-solubilized molecules precipitated by M1 clone antibodies and rabbit anti-rat IgG.

clonal antibodies precipitated a polypeptide of molecular weight 210,000, while another, M1/70, precipitated two polypeptides of molecular weights 190,000 and 105,000. It was also important to note that a number of monoclonal antibodies did not precipitate any material which could be labeled with ^{125}I. All these react with antigenic determinants that are stable to autoclaving (Table I) and are thus likely to be carbohydrate.

The precipitation experiments illustrate the most important advantage of the monoclonal technique: the ability to use a "dirty" immunogen but to obtain monoclonal antibodies recognizing only a single component of the total mixture. The lack of background precipitation demonstrates the extraordinary specificity of monoclonal antibodies and their utility in protein purification. Because they are pure, monoclonal antibodies are also much more potent than classical antisera. For example, 100 ng of M1/70 antibody, which is obtained in 1 µl of spent culture medium, is sufficient to precipitate maximally its antigen from a lysate of 5×10^5 peritoneal exudate cells. The comparable quantity of alloantiserum normally used to effect precipitation is about 10 µl, containing approximately 100 µg of IgG or 1000-fold more.

E. Strain Distributions

The clones listed in Table I have been tested on 6–20 inbred mouse strains of different H-2 types and backgrounds. None show any allospecificity, suggesting that only a small minority of cell-surface antigenic determinants are subject to polymorphic variation. Similarly Parham and Bodmer (1978) immunized mice with human HLA-A2 antigen and found that only 4 of 13 lines that reacted with the highly polymorphic HLA heavy chain recognized polymorphic determinants.

F. Tumor-Cell Panels

Tumor-cell lines are useful models for studying differentiation antigens, since each line is usually a homogeneous population of cells arrested in a particular stage of differentiation. Screening of tumor-cell panels proved to be particularly important in the study of two clones, M1/70 and M1/22.25, which gave weak binding to spleen cells. M1/70 gave specific binding of only 2 times background binding, considered barely significant. However, binding plateaued out to a 1000-fold dilution of supernatant, suggesting limitation by the antigen concentration in spleen, rather than antibody concentration. To quantitatively compare the amounts of antigen expressed on a number of tumor lines as well as normal cells the indirect ^{125}I-anti-Ig binding assay was conducted with serial dilutions of cells. For each monoclonal antibody similarly shaped titration curves, plateauing at a characteristic level, were obtained for all positive lines. Antigen concentration was expressed as (cells/ml giving half-maximal binding)$^{-1} \times 10^9$, or "antigen titer," which is proportional to antigen site number. M1/70 antigen is expressed on the P338D$_1$ macrophagelike tumor line in 100 times greater quantity than on spleen cells but not on T or B lymphomas or the NSI myeloma line (Table II). Further work has confirmed that M1/70 antigen (Mac-1) is a marker of the granulocytic–monocytic line of differentiation.

Similar, though less quantitative, experiments showed that the M1/22.25 Forssman antibody specifically labels embryonal carcinoma cell lines but not thymoma, mastocytoma, myeloma, Abelson or Moloney lymphoma, Friend leukemia, neuroblastoma, fibroblast, or methylcholanthrene-induced sarcoma lines (Stern et al., 1978). Subsequent work demonstrated the presence of M1/22.25 antigen on germinal tissue and temporally and topographically limited expression on early mouse embryos (Willison and Stern, 1978). Thus tumor-cell panel screening is a particularly useful means of characterizing monoclonal antibodies that recognize small subpopulations. Of 12 clones recovered from the M1 hybridization (the anti-HSA, Mac-1, and Forssman clones) 8 recognize antigens present on 25% or less of the nylon-wool, Ficoll–Isopaque purified cells used in priming (see Table IV).

Tumor-cell typing also provided information about the relationship between different antigens. Similarity between M1/9.3 and M1/89.18 antigen was suggested by their identical tumor cell distributions (Table II). This was confirmed by immunoprecipitation of the same antigen of molecular weight 210,000 and competition for the same cell-surface site in antibody cross-inhibition experiments. Differences were suggested between M1/69 and M1/75, both of which recognize an HSA on mouse RBC. M1/69 but not M1/75 antigen is expressed on thymocytes, splenic white cells, and B- and T-lymphoma lines (Table II). The differences were confirmed in cross-inhibition experiments (see Section IV.B).

TABLE II
Antigen Titers on Tumor Lines and Normal Cells[a]

	M1/9.3	M1/89.18	M1/69	M1/75	M1/70
Red blood cells	<0.2	<0.2	150	110	<0.02
Spleen Ficoll–Isopaque pellet	37	40	90	20	(5)
Spleen Ficoll–Isopaque band	170	125	67	<0.4	(3)
Thymocytes	150	130	60	<0.4	<0.8
SIA T lymphoma	950	650	2500	<2	<4
S49 T lymphoma	1100	770	1700	<2	<4
BW 5147 T lymphoma	2900	2000	270	<2	<0.8
R8 CL7 Abelson lymphoma	650	500	570	<10	<4
NSI myeloma	<6	<6	(5)	<2	<0.2
P388D$_1$ macrophagelike line	200	250	(3)	<2	480

[a]Titer = $10^9 \times$(cells/ml giving half-maximal ^{125}I-anti-Ig binding)$^{-1}$. See text for details. Parentheses indicate extrapolated value; weak binding was found at highest cell concentration tested. < Means that binding was negative at highest concentration tested.

G. Fluorescence-Activated Cell Sorter Analysis

Single-cell suspensions were prepared from lymphoid tissues, labeled with monoclonal antibodies, washed, labeled with affinity purified fluoresceinisothiocyanate (FITC)-rabbit F(ab')$_2$ anti-rat IgG absorbed with mouse IgG, again washed, and subjected to fluorescence-activated cell sorter (FACS) analysis

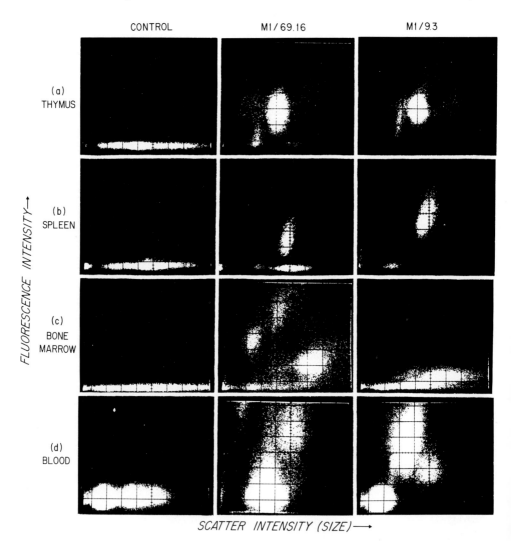

FIGURE 2. FACS two-dimensional resolution of lymphoid tissue cell subpopulations labeled by monoclonal antibodies. Dots mark the intersection of the fluorescence and scatter intensities of individual cells. Cells were purified by Ficoll–Isopaque sedimentation and labeled as described in the text. Some remaining RBC were apparent in bone marrow and blood. An irrelevant rat monoclonal supernatant, R4/18.2, was used as the control. Fluorescence and scatter gains were identical within each tissue but differed between tissues. (a) Thymocytes; (b) spleen cells; (c) bone marrow; (d) blood cells. Populations in increasing order of scatter intensity are RBC, lymphocytes, and monocytes.

(Loken and Herzenberg, 1975). As each cell passes through the FACS laser beam, two parameters are measured: fluorescence emission and light scattering. Fluorescence intensity is directly proportional to the number of FITC molecules bound per cell (and hence in saturating conditions, to the number of antigenic sites); light-scattering intensity is related to cell size but is also influenced by other factors such as cell density and shape. The information from the analysis of 40,000–200,000 cells is displayed in the form of dot plots on a cathode-ray tube of the FACS in Fig. 2. Each cell is displayed as a dot at the intersection of its fluorescence (y axis) and scatter (x axis) intensities. The combination of these two parameters, together with the extraordinary specificity of the monoclonal reagents, resolves in many cases discrete cellular subpopulations. These two dimensional displays or cellular fingerprints are characteristic for each combination of tissue and monoclonal antibody, much in the way that peptide fingerprints are characteristic for each combination of protein and protease. Moreover, just in the way that a subpopulation of pure molecules may be eluted from an area of a chromatogram and chemically characterized, subpopulations of pure cells may be "eluted" from any rectangular subdivision of the dot plot by the selection of appropriate fluorescence and scatter "windows" during sorting. The subpopulations may then be characterized by functional or morphologic criteria. For example, Wright–Giemsa staining of sorted subpopulations from bone marrow shows that M1/69.16 can separate granulocytes from small and large lymphocytes and that M1/9.3 (at higher fluorescence gain) can separate small, mature lymphocytes from immature lymphocytes and granulocytic precursors. Furthermore, it now seems possible to assess the purity of sorted cellular subpopulations by labeling with different monoclonal antibodies and fluorochromes, just as molecular purity is usually checked using analytical separation conditions differing from the preparative conditions.

Even when monoclonal antibodies do not completely resolve cell populations, they can give information about their relative heterogeneity or homogeneity. For example, the quite uniform labeling of blood monocytes, the population with highest scatter in Fig. 2d, supports the idea that during transport from bone marrow to the tissues, monocytes are arrested in a uniform state of differentiation, and that diversification occurs only after crossing the endothelium and encountering particular tissues and levels of inflammation. In contrast, while all lymphocytes are labeled by M1/9.3, it is clear that blood lymphocytes differ in the quantitative amount of M1/9.3 antigen that they express (Fig. 2d), supporting the known heterogeneity of these cells.

III. Properties of Rat Monoclonal Antibodies

A. Quantitation of Immunoglobulin Chains

Large quantities of monoclonal antibodies can be obtained by growth of rat–mouse hybrid lines in tissue culture (Table III). Quantitation is by Mancini single

Table III
Properties of Rat Monoclonal Antibodies[a]

Monoclonal antibody	Class or subclass	Complement-mediated lysis[b]	Staph A[d] binding	Active antibody concentration (range, μg/ml)	Chain composition of subclones
M1/22.25	μ	+	−	30–44	HL
M1/87	μ	+	−	62–88	HLK
M3/31	μ	N.D.[c]	−	22–36	HLK
M3/84	γ1	N.D.	+	20–25	HL
M1/9.3	γ2a	−?	−	58–235	HLK, HL
M1/42	γ2a	−?	−	90–106	HLK
M1/84	γ2a	−?	−	51	HL
M3/38	γ2a	N.D.	−	101	HLK
M1/70	γ2b	+	−	50–118	HL
M1/89.18	γ2b	+	N.D.	—[e]	HK?
M1/9.47	γ2b	+	−	98–110	HLK
M1/69	γ2b	+	−	100–252	HLK, HL, HK
M1/89.1	γ2b	+	−	126–174	HLK
M1/22.54	γ2c	+	+	94–119	HLK
M1/75	γ2c	+	+	77–87	HLK

[a]See text for details of determinations.
[b]Springer *et al.* (1978b).
[c]N.D., not determined.
[d]Staph A, protein A-bearing *Staphylococcus aureus*.
[e]The rabbit anti-rat Fab antibody used in single radial immunodiffusion is unreactive with this antibody (see Springer *et al.*, 1978b).

radial immunodiffusion (Ouchterlony and Nilsson, 1978) against rabbit anti-rat Fab. This antibody does not react with the NSI myeloma κ chain or H chain in combination with it (e.g., M1/89.18), and thus the values in Table III reflect the concentration of active half-molecules containing heavy chains associated with specific rat light chains. The presence of either γ or μ specific heavy (H) chains and specific light (L) or myeloma kappa (κ) chains have been investigated by SDS gel electrophoresis, isoelectric focusing (IEF) (Springer *et al.*, 1978b), and a radioimmunoassay detecting κ chain V_L determinants (Springer, submitted for publication). Chain compositions of the subclones and of light-chain loss variants isolated from them are listed in Table III. M1/89.18 appears to be an unusual example of an HK hybrid molecule which retains antigen-binding activity, since specific L chain cannot be detected in either SDS-PAGE or IEF, or by reaction with rabbit anti-rat Fab.

B. Purification

Most lines secrete 50–100 μg/ml of antibody, and purification of large quantities is obtained by growth in 5% fetal calf serum (FCS), precipitation with $(NH_4)_2SO_4$ and diethylaminoethyl (DEAE) cellulose and G-200 chromatography. This yields homogeneous material, as shown by SDS-PAGE (Fig. 3) and

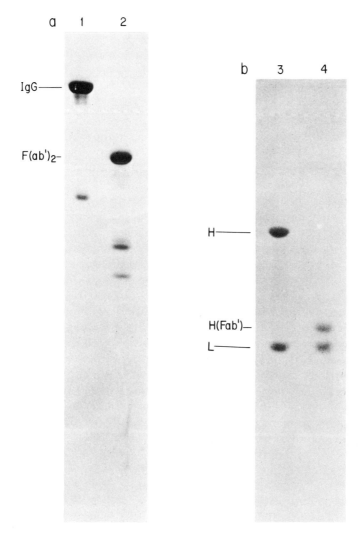

FIGURE 3. SDS–PAGE of purified M1/70 IgG, before and after pepsin digestion. (a) Nonreduced: 1, M1/70 IgG (20 µg); 2, M1/70 F(ab')₂ (20 µg). (b) Reduced: 3, M1/70 IgG (10 µg); 4, M1/70 F(ab')₂ (8 µg). Samples were prepared in SDS buffer containing 50 mM iodoacetamide (nonreduced) or 5% 2-mercaptoethanol (reduced), subjected to SDS 5–15% PAGE, and stained with coomassie blue. The two gels in (a) and (b) were run on separate occasions. The position of calibration proteins established the identity of bands noted in the figures.

agreement between assays for protein and for rat IgG by Mancini immunodiffusion. F(ab')₂ fragments can also readily be obtained (Fig. 3) using standard pH 4 pepsin digestion conditions (Stanworth and Turner, 1978). The inability to grow mouse–rat tumors in normal animals is therefore not a serious drawback of this approach. Athymic nude rats (Festing et al., 1978) present a possible alternative method for large-scale antibody production. Rat myeloma lines suitable for use in cell hybridization have also recently been described (Galfré et al., 1979).

C. Subclass Properties

Rat Ig classes and subclasses were defined by Bazin and co-workers (1974) through the use of a large collection of Ig-secreting ileocecal immunocytomas. Using commercially available typing sera (Miles Laboratories) each of the monoclonal antibodies described here could clearly be placed in one of these subclasses (Table III), confirming the idea that all extant Y subclasses were identified in the Bazin collection. Concentrations of most of the monoclonal antibodies in tissue culture supernatants were sufficiently high to allow typing by direct visualization of precipitin lines in Ouchterlony double immunodiffusion, and the remainder could be typed using 10-fold concentrates.

Monoclonal antibodies offer considerable advantages over myeloma proteins of unknown antibody specificity in assessing the biological properties of Ig classes and subclasses. For example, antibody- and complement-dependent lysis of ^{51}Cr target cells has been used to test for complement fixation (Table III). Antibodies of IgM, IgG2b, and IgG2c classes were clearly lytic in the presence of guinea pig complement. So far no lysis has been observed by three IgG2a subclass antibodies, and the IgG1 antibody has not been tested. Comparison of five antibodies that recognize the same HSA on mouse RBC showed that the three IgG2b's more efficiently utilized complement than the two IgG2c's. The observation that IgG2c's fix complement is in disagreement with the report of Medgyesi *et al.* (1978), who did not have the advantage of using antigen-binding antibodies. It is possible that the 0.5% boric acid purification step used by Medgyesi *et al.* destroyed IgG2c complement-fixing activity, or that heat aggregation does not induce fixation by this subclass.

An interesting property of the IgG2c monoclonals, M1/22.54 and M1/75.21, is their extreme potency in direct hemagglutination. Large clumps of RBCs, several millimeters in diameter, are formed. After unit gravity sedimentation, highly purified splenic white blood cells can be obtained. In contrast, three other monoclonals of the IgG2b subclass that recognize the same HSA on mouse RBC give weak or no agglutination unless anti-rat IgG is added. Strength in agglutination does not correlate with avidity or fine specificity. This suggests that IgG2c's have a more flexible hinge region than IgG2b's.

Another interesting property of the IgG2c subclass is that rats injected with streptococci, a carbohydrate antigen, make almost exclusively antibodies of this subclass (Leslie, 1979). In the case of the HSA, which also appears to be carbohydrate, 2 of 5 clones are IgG2c, compared to 0 of 8 for the anti-protein clones.

Staphylococcus aureus binding properties of all of the rat monoclonals were studied by absorbing neat or 10× supernatants with an equal volume of a 50% suspension of *S. aureus* cowan I strain bacteria in pH 8 buffer (Ey *et al.*, 1978), followed by Mancini immunodiffusion against rabbit anti-rat Fab. Antibodies of the IgG1 and IgG2c subclasses bind, while IgG2a, IgG2b subclasses, and IgM do not. This is in agreement with the results of Medgyesi *et al.* (1978), with the exception that they found 2 of 3 IgM myeloma proteins reactive. ^{125}I-*S. aureus* protein A binding assays have been used to screen for mouse monoclonal antibodies (Oi *et al.*, 1978), but the finding that only 3 of 15 rat monoclonals are *S. aureus*-reactive demonstrates the limitation of the technique in this species.

IV. Murine Differentiation Antigens Identified by Rat Monoclonal Antibodies

A. Forssman Antigen

The Forssman antigen is widely distributed among animal species and bacteria but not in a phylogenetically ordered manner (Boyd, 1966). Rats are Forssman-negative, while mice and guinea pigs are Forssman-positive. The tissue and species distribution of the antigen recognized by M1/22.25 and M1/87 monoclonal antibodies identify it as Forssman. Absorption by autoclaved guinea pig kidney but not ox RBC distinguishes the heterophile activity from that shown by Paul-Bunnell antibodies, which are found in infectious mononucleosis. Moreover, rabbit antiserum to sheep RBC ("hemolysin"), which classically defines this antigen, competitively inhibits the binding of M1/22.25 and M1/87 to sheep RBC (Springer et al., 1978b). Classically, anti-Forssman antibodies are of the IgM class, as are M1/22.25 and M1/87. The Forssman hapten structure from mammalian species including horse, sheep, goat, dog, and guinea pig is N-acetylgalactosaminosyl-(α1-3)-N-acetylgalactosaminosyl-(β1-3)-galactosyl-(α1-4)-galactosyl-(β1-4)-glucosyl)(β1-1)-ceramide (Ziolkowski et al., 1975). The findings that the antigen identified by M1/22.25 on murine embryonal carcinoma cells is stable at 100°C, is absent from cells after methanol treatment, and can be labeled by [^{14}C]galactose but not ^{125}I(lactoperoxidase) or [^{35}S]methionine, are consistent with the above glycolipid structure (Stern et al., 1978).

The distribution of the Forssman antigen in spleen was studied by autoradiography of Wright–Giemsa-stained cytocentrifuge preparations. Polychromatophilic erythroblasts are labeled, while mature erythrocytes and cells of the granulocytic and lymphoid lineages are negative (Springer, Secher, Galfré, and Milstein, manuscript in preparation).

The presence of the Forssman antigen on murine germinal tissues was suggested by tumor-cell panel screening (Stern et al., 1978). Only embryonal carcinoma cell lines are positive. Both nullipotent and pluripotent, undifferentiated teratocarcinoma-derived lines are positive. Under appropriate culture conditions, pluripotent lines differentiate into embryoid bodies, which are considered equivalent to the inner cell mass portion of the mouse embryo around the time of implantation. The outer endodermal layer of the embryoid bodies are Forssman-negative, while the inner core of embryonal carcinoma remains positive. Further differentiation of the embryoid bodies occur if they are allowed to attach to a substrate. Multilayered cell cultures with a variety of differentiated cell types are obtained after 2 weeks of growth, less than 1% of which are Forssman-positive. It therefore appears that most of the differentiated derivatives of teratocarcinoma stem cells do not express the antigen. In the adult male mouse, germinal tissues contain the greatest concentration of Forssman antigen. Brain, kidney, spleen, and lymph nodes but not liver or thymus are also positive.

The expression of the Forssman antigen during development of the normal preimplantation mouse embryo has also been studied, using M1/22.25 monoclonal antibody (Willison and Stern, 1978). The fertilized egg and embryos up to the 8-cell stage are negative. Antigen is first expressed on trophectodermal cells at the time of blastocoel formation (early blastocyst) but disappears after hatching from the zona pellucida, that is, just before implantation into the uterine wall. The trophectoderm of the blastocyst encloses a fluid-filled cavity called the blastocoel, at one end of which lies the inner cell mass, which gives rise to the embryo proper. The inner cell mass is Forssman–positive, as is its first differentiated product, endoderm, at least soon after its formation. This is in contrast to the endoderm formed by teratocarcinoma cells in culture, which is negative. This latter endoderm may represent a type (parietal) that is different from that on the blastocoelic surface of the inner cell mass (visceral).

B. Heat-Stable Antigen

Another antigen that is expressed in highly specific fashion, yet is found on diverse tissues, was also identified in these studies. This antigen is stable at 120°C and cannot be labeled with ^{125}I using lactoperoxidase or with [^{35}S]methionine. These properties suggest a carbohydrate antigenic determinant present in a moiety devoid of methionines or accessible tyrosines, i.e., a glycolipid. However, since definitive structural characterization of this molecule has not yet been pursued, it will be referred to as heat-stable antigen (HSA).

To investigate whether five different monoclonal antibodies identifying a HSA on mouse red blood cells all recognized the same cell-surface antigenic site, cross-inhibition experiments were carried out (Fig. 4). After preincubating target cells with serial dilutions of unlabeled monoclonal antibodies, binding was measured of added [^{3}H]lysine internally labeled monoclonal Ig. All five monoclonals recognizing a HSA on mouse RBC cross-inhibited binding of the two members of this group that were tested, M1/69 and M1/75, confirming recognition of the same site on these cells. However, differences in inhibitory titers and the slopes of inhibition suggested considerable variation among the clones in avidity. None of the other monoclonals, including the anti-Forssmans, were inhibitory. Despite the fact that all five of these antibodies appeared to recognize the same site on mouse RBC, striking differences between them were noted when inhibition of binding to thymocytes was tested. The most dramatic differences were found between M1/69 and M1/75, with the other three being intermediate. The inhibitory titer of the homologous M1/69 supernatant was the same for RBC and thymocytes, while the other clones gave very shallow inhibitory slopes and much lower inhibitory titers on thymocytes. M1/75 did not appear inhibitory at all. The concentrations of the antibodies employed in these experiments were very similar, between 80 and 120 μg/ml in neat culture supernatants. The results thus reflect true differences in antibody avidity and specificity.

These differences were also noted in two other assay systems. (1) While all five clones are lytic for RBC, M1/69 alone lyses thymocytes (Springer et al., 1978b). (2) M1/69 antigen is expressed on splenic lymphocytes, thymocytes, and T and B lymphomas, while M1/75 antigen is not (Table II).

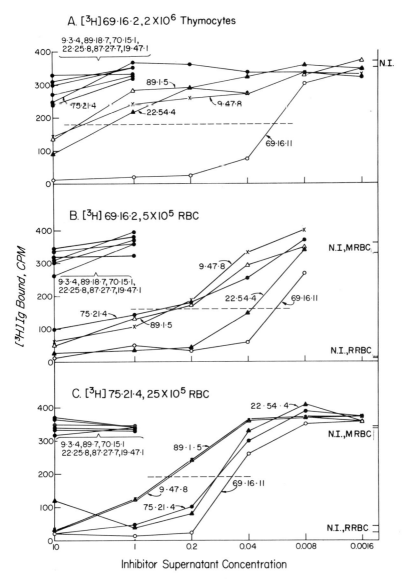

FIGURE 4. Cross-inhibition of binding of [³H]lysine-labeled M1 antibodies by unlabeled clonal supernatants. Target cells were incubated with unlabeled supernatants at various concentrations, then
with supernatants from [³H]lysine internally labeled cells, and the amount of cell-bound radioactivity
was determined. N.I., no inhibition, DMEM 10% FCS substituted for supernatant, MRBC, RRBC,
mouse and rat RBC, respectively.

The working hypothesis is that these clones bind to slightly different (and
perhaps overlapping) portions of a carbohydrate that has a common core structure but also some heterogeneity in its glycosylation both on RBC and particularly when dealing with different tissues. Heterogeneity would affect the affinity
of each antibody differently, depending on the exact subset of carbohydrate
residues recognized, thus giving rise to differences in specificity.

The tissue distribution of M1/69 is RBC > spleen = liver = kidney> lymph nodes = brain (Springer, Secher, Galfré, and Milstein, manuscript in preparation). These results could at least partially be explained by presence of RBC in the tissues. Both mature granulocytes in bone marrow and 16-hr peritoneal exudates and their precursors in bone marrow are strongly positive (Springer *et al.*, 1979). Blood monocytes are also strongly positive (Fig. 2d), but expression is greatly reduced in thioglycollate-induced peritoneal macrophages and is also absent from the macrophagelike line P388D$_1$ (Table II).

M1/69-positive and -negative lymphoid populations are found in spleen (Fig. 2b). Positive and negative lymphoid populations are also seen in blood (Fig. 2d) (though less well resolved), lymph nodes, and by staining with other clones recognizing HSA: M1/9.47, M1/22.54, and M1/89. The nature of these subpopulations was investigated in nylon wool depletion experiments (Table IV). M1/69$^+$ cells were depleted in parallel with Ig$^+$ cells. Furthermore, double labeling experiments show that M1/69 + FITC ā-rat IgG or FITC ā-mouse Fab used either separately or together label almost exactly the same percentage of cells. These experiments show that HSA is expressed on peripheral B lymphocytes but not on any appreciable percentage of peripheral T lymphocytes. The situation on thymocytes is quite different, however. Thymocytes are 95% M1/69-positive (Fig. 2a). Thus thymocytes lose HSA expression upon maturation and entry into the peripheral lymphoid circulation. Apparently changes in the expression of a number of different antigens, including the thymus leukemia antigen (Konda *et al.*, 1973) occur at this stage of thymocyte development.

C. Common Leukocyte Antigen (CLA)

Two clones, M1/9.3 and M1/89.18, precipitate an antigen of molecular weight 200,000 from spleen cells. The antibodies cross-inhibit one another and thus react with identical or proximal determinants on the same molecule. The antigenic determinant is heat-labile and therefore appears to involve protein.

TABLE IV

Nylon-Wool Depletion of Ig and Heat-Stable Antigen-Bearing Spleen Cells[a]

	Ig	Heat-stable antigen			Mac-1	CLA
	ā - Fab (%)	M1/69 (%)	M1/9.47 (%)	M1/89.1 (%)	M1/70 (%)	M1/9.3 (%)
Untreated	54	62	59	57	5	96
Nylon–wool passed						
Exp. 1	14	17	15	15	4	99
Exp. 2	19	24	n.d.	n.d.	5	99

[a]Cells in the lymphocyte scatter peak and slightly larger were counted in this analysis. Somewhat higher values for M1/70 positive cells are obtained by including all larger cells. n.d., No data.

The CLA is bound to *Lens culinaris* lectin affinity columns, suggesting it contains carbohydrate; ^{125}I(lactoperoxidase) and [^{35}S]methionine labeling show it contains protein.

When CLA is precipitated from spleen cells, three bands of molecular weights ~230,000, 200,000, and 180,000 are seen (see Fig. 8); only the smaller two of these bands are precipitated from Con-A-stimulated T lymphocytes (Fig. 1). The larger-molecular-weight form may therefore be derived from B lymphocytes. The same phenomenon had previously been described by Trowbridge and Mazauskas (1976), using polyspecific antisera to precipitate what appears to be the same antigen. Trowbridge (1978) has also derived a hybridoma recognizing this antigen, which he calls T200. All hybrids thus far obtained to this protein recognize all three different molecular weight forms. Furthermore, absorption experiments using classical antisera suggest antigenic identity between the molecules on B and T lymphocytes (Trowbridge and Mazauskas, 1976). Thus the difference in molecular weight of the antigen isolated from different sources could reflect a difference in posttranslational modification such as glycosylation, rather than a difference in amino acid sequence.

Tissue absorption studies show that antigen is present on lymph node and spleen cells, but not on brain, kidney, liver, or RBC. T and B lymphomas and a macrophagelike line are positive (Table II). The P815 mastocytoma and Moloney lymphomas bear the antigen, but a Friend erythroleukemia line, a normal fibroblast line, a methylcholanthrene-induced sarcoma, and an embryonal carcinoma line are negative (Stern *et al.*, 1978). The absence of this antigen on fibroblasts and its presence on lymphocytes distinguishes it from the LETS protein, or fibronectin, which has a similar molecular weight (Yamada and Olden, 1978). In fact, CLA and LETS appear to have mutually exclusive tissue distributions. FACS studies show CLA is present on 96–100% of thymocytes, spleen white cells, blood lymphocytes and monocytes (Fig. 2), thioglycollate-induced 18-hr PEC (neutrophilic granulocytes) and 4-d PEC (macrophages). It labels 77% of nucleated bone marrow cells, and sorting studies suggest these include lymphocytes and granulocytes and their precursors but not erythroid precursors. RBC are negative. Since this antigen is common to all lines of leukocyte differentiation, the designation CLA seems preferable to T200 (thymus-dependent 200,000-molecular-weight polypeptide).

D. M1/42 (H-2K) Antigen

Two clones were identified by immunoprecipitation screening of supernatants from M1 cultures that had been stored in liquid N_2 for 1 year (Fig. 5). Culture M1/42 precipitated two polypeptides of molecular weights 46,000 and 12,000, while M1/84 precipitated much smaller amounts of a polypeptide of molecular weight 46,000. Each line was then thawed and has been successfully cloned and recloned.

The antigen precipitated by M1/42 from C57BL/6J spleen cells has been preliminarily identified as H-2K^b in coprecipitation experiments. Preprecipita-

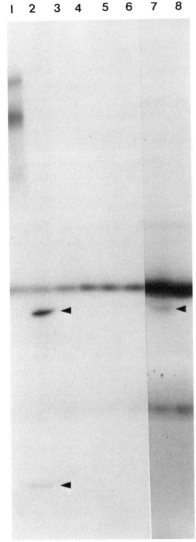

FIGURE 5. SDS 7–15% gradient PAGE of ^{125}I-labeled surface proteins precipitated by frozen M1 culture supernatants. Equal quantities of [125]I(lactoperoxidase)-labeled spleen cells and 4-day thiglycollate-induced PEC that had been solubilized with Triton X-100 were mixed together and immunoprecipitated with 100 μl of clonal supernatants and rabbit anti-rat IgG, reduced, prepared for PAGE, and autoradiographed, as described previously (Springer *et al.*, 1978b). 1, M1/9.3.4; 2, M1/42; 3, M1/81; 4, M1/94; 5, M1/7; 6, M1/79; 7, M1/84; 8, M1/55. Lanes 7 and 8 were exposed 4× longer to emphasize the band precipitated by M1/84. Bands appearing in all lanes are FC-receptor-bound mouse IgG H and L chains that cross-react with the rabbit anti-rat IgG sandwich reagent.

tion with M1/42 removed material reactive with anti-H-2K[b] but not anti-H-2D[b] allosera. Thus M1/42 appears specific for the K end of H-2[b]. M1/42 does not recognize an allodeterminant because ^{125}I-indirect binding assays and immunoprecipitation show it is equally reactive with mice of *b, k, d,* and *s* haplotypes. It is thus possible that the M1/42 antigen is a general marker of H-2K-ness; confirmation of this idea must await mapping of the reactivity in a number of different strains. While alloreagents were essential for the identification of histocompatibility antigens, it seems that xenoreagents may actually offer several practical advantages. For example, a single reagent could be used to isolate H-2K for biochemical analysis from a number of different haplotypes. Preliminary results

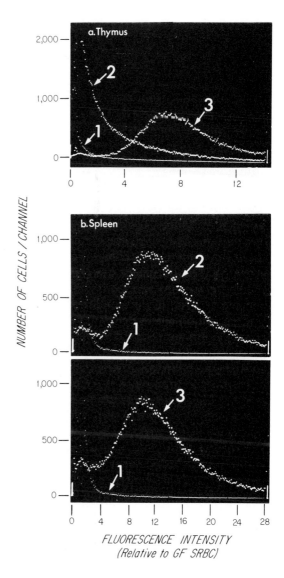

FIGURE 6. FACS analysis of M1/42 and M1/84 antigen expression on thymus and spleen cells. Cells were labeled with monoclonal antibodies and then with FITC anti-rat IgG as described in the text. Fluorescence intensity was standardized with gluteraldehyde-fixed sheep RBC (GF SRBC). 1, control (NSI supernatant with 50 μg/ml of added rat IgG); 2, M1/42; 3, M1/84.

suggest that M1/42–Sepharose columns are useful for the preparation of large-scale quantities of immunologically active H-2K molecules (Mescher and Springer, unpublished).

The use of monoclonal xenoantibodies also simplifies procedures for the labeling of cells with fluorochrome-tagged antibodies. The binding of a large number of different rat anti-mouse monoclonal antibodies can be studied, using a single indirect mouse Ig-absorbed FITC anti-rat Ig antibody preparation. The use of indirect anti-mouse Ig reagents is not feasible with mouse alloantisera because of the problem of cross-reaction with B-lymphocyte-surface Ig or Fc-receptor-bound Ig. Alloantibodies must either be individually labeled with fluorochromes or haptenated and used with indirect fluorochrome–antihapten antibodies (Wofsy *et al.*, 1978).

One example of the use of such xenoreagents to alloantigens is in FACS studies of H-2 expression on T lymphocytes in the thymus and spleen (Fig. 6). H-2 is expressed by 88% of thymocytes. By far the majority of thymocytes express only small quantities while a small proportion of cells express varying amounts up to about 20 times more. In contrast, spleen cells have a quantity of H-2 antigen that is similar to the highest amount seen on thymocytes, and the distribution is much more uniform. H-2 expression increases during thymocyte maturation (Konda *et al.*, 1973, Beller and Unanue, 1978), and thus the distribution of thymocyte H-2 fluorescence intensity probably represents a maturation gradient.

E. M1/84 Antigen

In contrast to M1/42 antigen, the quantity of M1/84 antigen on thymocytes and spleen cells is very similar (Fig. 6), and the distribution is quite uniform in both tissues. The M1/84 polypeptide of molecular weight 46,000 is not identical to that of M1/42 antigen, H-2K^b, or H-2D^b, as shown by coprecipitation experiments. M1/84 labels a smaller proportion (80%) of nucleated bone marrow cells (Fig. 7) than M1/42 (97%) and thus shows some tissue specificity. It is present on all lymphocytes, granulocytes, and monocytes.

F. Mac-1 Antigen

Screening of a tumor-cell panel revealed that M1/70 monoclonal antibody reacts with a macrophagelike line, P388D$_1$, but not with B or T lymphomas, thymocytes, or RBC (Table II). Spleen cells contain 100-fold less of the antigen than the P388D$_1$ line. FACS experiments show that M1/70 antigen is expressed on 44% of bone marrow cells, on peritoneal exudate macrophages (Fig. 7), on blood monocytes, granulocytes, and 8% of spleen cells (Springer *et al.*, 1979). No expression is found on lymphocytes, thymocytes, or nonlymphoid tissues. The specificity of M1/70 for macrophages in peritoneal exudates is demonstrated by comparison to M1/84 (Fig. 7), which stains the smaller lymphocytes and polymorphonuclear cells as well as the larger macrophages. Differentiation from blood monocyte to thioglycollate-induced macrophage is accompanied by a large increase in M1/70 expression in parallel with a large decrease in M1/69 expression. Peritoneal exudate cells (PEC) express 8-fold more M1/70 than positive cells isolated in single-cell suspension from spleens, and about 5- to 10-fold more M1/70 than the 44% of positive cells in marrow (Fig. 7). The latter cells are granulocytic precursors. Monocytic precursors constitute only 0.3% of nucleated bone marrow cells (Van Furth, 1975). Because of its specificity for granulocytes and mononuclear phagocytes and because macrophages are its richest source M1/70 antigen has been designated Mac-1. Mac-1 is the first discrete molecule to be described that is specific to phagocytes.

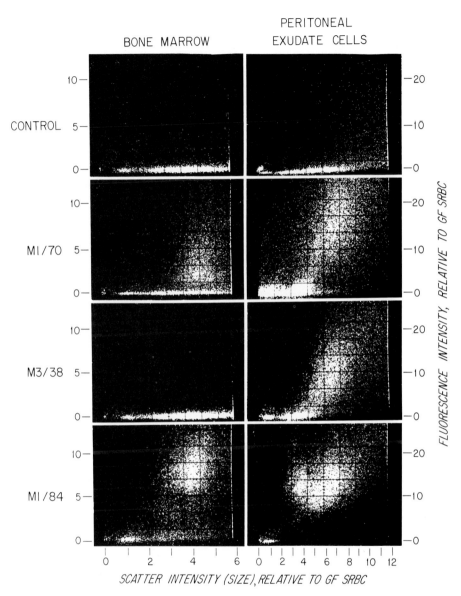

FIGURE 7. FACS dot plot analysis of Mac-1 (M1/70), Mac-2 (M3/38), and M1/84 antigen expression in bone marrow and thioglycollate-induced 4-day PEC populations. Scatter and fluorescence are scaled relative to gluteraldehyde-fixed sheep RBC (GF SRBC). Mouse RBC and macrophages appear at scatter intensities of 1 and 7, respectively. See text for labeling procedures.

The reactivity of M1/70 is not an artifactual association with the avid Fc receptor of macrophages, since (1) indirect ^{125}I-anti-Ig binding is highly specific, 34× the background level of normal rat IgG as control, (2) it cannot be inhibited by high concentrations of normal or heat-aggregated IgG, (3) [^{3}H]lysine-labeled M1/70 antibody binds to mouse but not rat PEC, and (4) M1/70 F(ab')$_2$ frag-

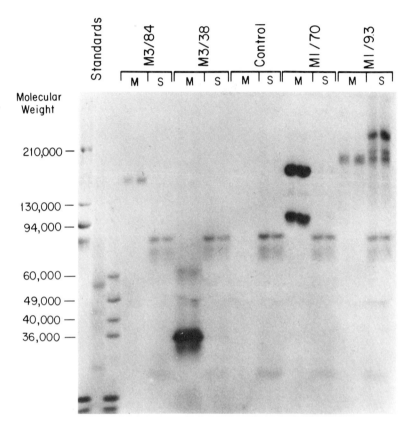

FIGURE 8. SDS 5–12% PAGE autoradiograph of immunoprecipitates from [125]I(lactoperoxidase) spleen cells and 4-day thioglycollate-induced macrophages. Equal quantities of spleen (S) and macrophage (M) Triton X-100-solubilized antigens were indirectly precipitated using monoclonal supernatants or NSI supernatant +50 µg/ml rat IgG as control. Two different concentrations of antibodies were employed in each experimental group: 30 or 100 µl of clonal supernatant and 10 or 33 µl of rabbit anti-rat IgG, electrophoresed in left or right gel lanes, respectively. Samples were reduced with 5% 2-mercaptoethanol. In addition to bands specifically precipitated from spleen cells, μ, δ, and light chains were precipitated by cross-reaction with the rabbit anti-rat IgG. Preclearing with the mouse IgG cross-reactive fraction of rabbit anti-rat IgG coupled to Sepharose had removed IgG bound to macrophages but not sIgD or sIgM.

ments (Fig. 3) titrate to the same endpoint as M1/70 IgG in labeling and antigen-precipitation experiments.

Precipitation experiments confirm that Mac-1 is present in much larger quantities on PEC than on spleen cells (Fig. 8). The same polypeptides are precipitated from spleen cells, but in amounts only visible on prolonged exposure of the autoradiogram. Mac-1 contains two polypeptides of molecular weights 190,000 and 105,000. The same results are obtained using either [125]I(lactoperoxidase) or [35S]methionione labeling of adherent cells, showing that both chains are exposed to the exterior and are synthesized by the macrophage. The amounts of radiolabel incorporated are consistent with equimolar amounts of each chain. The two chains are not linked by disulfide bonds. The working hypothesis that the two chains are noncovalently associated is currently being tested. At least one chain contains carbohydrate because Mac-1 antigen is retained by *L. culinaris* lectin columns. The antigenic determinant recognized by M1/70 appears to involve protein because it is labile to heating.

G. Never Repeating the Past: A Cascade Procedure for Successive Generations of Novel Clones

The discovery of a macrophage-specific clone in the M1 hybridization was serendipitous and probably largely due to chance, since spleen cells purified similarly to those used in the immunization, by nylon wool filtration, contain only 4–8% of M1/70[+] cells (Table IV). In recent experiments (Springer, submitted for publication) we attempted to deliberately elicit and screen for further macrophage-specific hybridomas using a novel cascade procedure (Fig. 9). Rats were immunized with thioglycollate-induced murine macrophage detergent-solubilized membrane proteins that had been purified by the following procedures. Since most if not all surface proteins are glycosylated, the immunogen was partially purified by *L. culinaris* lectin affinity chromatography. Then, to direct the response toward macrophage-specific antigens, antigens with wide tissue distributions that had previously been identified in the M1 hybridization experiment were removed from the immunogen by filtration through Sepharose containing covalently attached M1/9.3 and M1/69 monoclonal antibodies. After removal of detergent, priming in complete Freund's adjuvant, and a final intra-

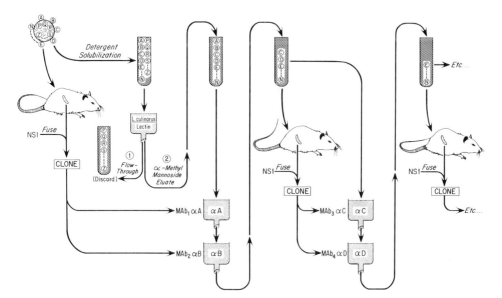

FIGURE 9. Cascade generation of monoclonal antibodies to cell-surface antigens. By combination of cell hybridization and immunoadsorbent techniques, successive generations of novel antibodies may be obtained until finally an entire collection of cell-surface antigens is identified.

venous boost, spleen cells from one rat were fused with NSI myeloma cells and aliquoted into 600 microculture wells. After several weeks the cultures with highest binding activity to PEC in indirect ^{125}I-anti-rat IgG binding assays were chosen for further growth. The specificity of their antibodies was investigated by precipitation of ^{125}I-PEC cell-surface proteins followed by SDS-PAGE analysis. Supernatants from five of the M3 cultures precipitated polypeptides of molecular weights 190,000 and 105,000 and thus demonstrated the same specificity as M1/70. Other supernatants showed specificity for quite different polypeptides. A polypeptide of molecular weight 32,000 was precipitated by 11 cultures, two of which, M3/31 and M3/38, have been isolated as stable subclones. An antigen of molecular weight 110,000 was recognized by one culture, M3/84, which has also been cloned. However, none of the clones recognized the CLA polypeptide of molecular weight 210,000 despite the fact that this antigen appears to be highly immunodominant and is present on macrophage surfaces. This suggested that the cascade purification procedure successfully subtracted this antigen from the mixture of molecules used in immunization. Radioimmunoassays also demonstrated removal of the antigen by the immunoadsorbent column.

The cascade procedure described here eliminates the problem of immunodominant antigens. It should allow continual successive generations of novel monoclonal antibodies to be obtained until finally, the last (and probably most weakly immunogenic) cell-surface antigen is identified. This procedure is also proposed for the identification of all intracellular antigens (Milstein and Lennox, 1979).

H. Mac-2 and Mac-3 Antigens

The antigen of molecular weight 32,000 precipitated by M3/31 and M3/38, designated Mac-2, and the antigen of molecular weight 110,000 precipitated by M3/84, designated Mac-3 are precipitated in much greater quantities from PEC than from spleen cells (Fig. 8). The same polypeptides are seen after labeling with either ^{125}I(lactoperoxidase) or [^{35}S]methionine. The L. culinaris experiments show that these antigens contain carbohydrate, and thus they are glycoproteins. Mac-2 (and Mac-3), in contrast to Mac-1, are not expressed on bone marrow cells (0–1% positive) (Fig. 7). These results rule out expression on granulocyte precursors, but not on promonocytes, which constitute only 0.3% of nucleated bone marrow cells. Mac-2 and Mac-3 appear to be expressed on the monocytic line of differentiation at some stage after divergence from the granulocytic line, while Mac-1 is found on both branches. Mac-2 and Mac-3 antibodies label 6–9% of spleen cells and 0–2% of thymocytes. In peritoneal exudates, macrophages but not smaller cells such as polymorphs or lymphocytes are labeled (Fig. 7). Peritoneal exudate macrophages are stained much more brightly than positive cells in spleen or blood. Thus, as in the case of Mac-1, expression is greatly increased during differentiation of monocytes to stimulated peritoneal macrophages.

V. Patterns of Differentiation Antigen Expression

A. "Jumping" Differentiation Antigens

In considering the antigens that have been identified in these studies, two strikingly different types of tissue distribution patterns emerge. "Lineage" antigens, exemplified by CLA, Mac-1, Mac-2, and Mac-3, are expressed in an ontogenetically or functionally orderly fashion. "Jumping" antigens (Milstein and Lennox, 1980), exemplified by the Forssman and HSA antigens are not. Distantly related tissues often will share expression of a jumping antigen while more closely related tissues do not. These two classes should perhaps be thought of as extremes in a continuum, with some antigens such as H-2 lying somewhere in between. However, as will be discussed below, it appears that jumping antigens share other properties besides their occurrence on disparate tissues. They thus may constitute a truly distinct class of surface antigens with different functional properties than lineage antigens.

A number of jumping antigens have previously been described. Perhaps the best known is Thy-1 antigen, which has been thoroughly characterized with allo- and xenoantisera and to which both rat anti-mouse and mouse anti-mouse monoclonal antibodies have been obtained (Hämmerling et al., 1978; Marshak-Rothstein et al., 1979). Thy-1 expression in the mouse is shared by disparate tissues such as fibroblasts, brain cells, and lymphocytes. Subclasses of lymphocytes differ in expression, with T but not B cells being positive. Dramatic changes in Thy-1 expression occur during brain cell development. Thy-1 is not found on 19-day fetal brain cells but is well expressed on a subpopulation of brain cells 10 days after birth or after cultivation of fetal cells in vitro (Mirsky and Thompson, 1975). Another example of a jumping antigen is asialo-GM_1 ganglioside. This glycosphinogolipid is found on peripheral T lymphocytes but not on thymocytes or peripheral B lymphocytes (Stein et al., 1978). This is exactly the reverse of the situation for the HSA. A number of jumping antigens have also been identified by monoclonal antibodies in the rat. W3/13, a glycoprotein of molecular weight 95,000, is found on T lymphocytes and plaque-forming cells but is absent from B lymphocytes (Williams et al., 1977, Milstein and Lennox, 1980). MRC 0×2, a glycoprotein of molecular weight 60,000, is found on brain, thymocytes, and B but not T lymphocytes (Milstein and Lennox, 1980). Solter and Knowles (1978) identified a jumping antigen by syngeneic immunization of mice with teratocarcinoma cell lines. An IgM monoclonal antibody was obtained which recognizes a stage-specific embryonic glycolipid, distinct from the Forssman specificity. Its topographic distribution on pre-implantation embryos resembles that of the Forssman antigen, although the time of first appearance, at the 8-cell stage, is earlier. It is found on mouse brain and kidney and mouse and human sperm and teratocarcinomas, but not on sheep RBC. Similarly, the peanut agglutinin, which is specific for terminal D-galactose residues, reacts with preimplantation em-

TABLE V
Jumping Antigens Can Have Wide Tissue Distributions Yet within a Given Line of Differentiation Mark a Specific Developmental Stage

Line of differentiation	Antigen	Negative stage	Positive stage	Negative stage
Erythroid	Forssman	?	Polychromatophilic erythroblast	Erythrocyte
Embryonic trophectoderm	Forssman	Morula	Early blastocyst	Late blastocyst
T lymphocyte	Heat-stable	?	Thymocyte	Peripheral T lymphocyte

bryos, cells of the spermatogenic series, and embryonal carcinoma cells but not on their differentiated derivatives (Reisner *et al.*, 1977). This lectin is also reactive with 80–90% of thymic but not peripheral lymphocytes or RBC (London *et al.*, 1978). While perhaps broader, the specificity of this lectin might include that of the Forssman and/or the Solter and Knowles (1978) antibodies.

A striking property of jumping antigens is that within a given line of differentiation, change in antigen expression is often correlated with cellular migration to a different tissue (Table V). Loss of Forssman antigen expression in the mouse erythroblast precedes exit from hematopoietic tissue into the circulation and in the trophectoderm precedes implantation in the uterus. A decrease in HSA occurs after blood monocytes cross the endothelium and differentiate into stimulated macrophages. Loss of HSA from thymocytes occurs slightly before or concomitantly with entry into the peripheral lymphoid circulation. Appearance of asialo-GM_1 ganglioside occurs at the same time (Stein *et al.*, 1978).

Adhesive properties also change during thymocyte maturation. Stamper and Woodruff (1976) have demonstrated selective adhesion of recirculating lymphocytes during emigration from blood to lymph nodes. Migration to lymph nodes occurs via specialized high endothelial venules and not through other vascular endothelia in lymph nodes. In experiments measuring binding of lymphocytes to fixed sections of lymph nodes, avid binding to the specialized venule endothelia was observed for lymphocytes from thoracic duct, spleen, and lymph nodes, but not for thymocytes. Thoracic duct lymphocytes were found to adhere about 100 times more frequently to specialized venule endothelia than to normal vascular endothelia. Adhesive interactions appear to play a particularly important role in guiding the migration of individual cells in embryogenesis and in hematopoietic and lymphoid systems (see Marchase *et al.*, 1976, for a review). While there is no direct evidence that jumping antigens are involved in the control of adhesive specificity, the numerous correlations between changes in jumping antigen expression and cellular migration make this an intriguing possibility.

All the glycolipid antigens identified here belong to the jumping antigen category. Glycoproteins may be expressed as either jumping or lineage antigens. Whether carbohydrate plays in general a more important role in the function of jumping antigens than of lineage antigens is unknown. It is interesting, however, that the most thoroughly studied example of a glycoprotein jumping antigen, Thy-1, is a small glycoprotein with a high percentage of carbohydrate, 30% (Williams *et al.*, 1976), and that certain pleiotrophic mutations in carbohydrate biosynthesis prevent the surface expression of Thy-1 but not a number of other cell-surface glycoproteins (Trowbridge *et al.*, 1978).

The different ways in which lineage antigens and jumping antigens appear to be deployed during development is schematically summarized in Fig. 10. Combinatorial use of lineage and jumping antigens allows a very economical means for achieving cell-surface diversity. Jumping antigens, perhaps in different combinations, might fulfill similar functions in quite different tissues. This economy would have important consequences for host defense. The probability of cross-reaction between viral or bacterial and host cell surface antigens would be reduced, as would the probability that an appropriate receptor for virus would be expressed.

A common characteristic of Thy-1 antigen and the Forssman antigen, and perhaps of jumping antigens in general, is species variation in the tissue distribution patterns. In the mouse Thy-1 is expressed on thymocytes and on T but not B lymphocytes, while in the rat it is found on 40% of bone marrow cells and is expressed on thymocytes but not on most peripheral T lymphocytes (Williams *et al.*, 1976). Expression of the dog Thy-1 homologue is similar to that of the mouse except that kidney is strongly positive. The human homologue is present on kidney, absent from thymus and lymphoid compartments, and as in the mouse, rat, and dog, is present on brain (Dalchau and Fabre, 1979). It has long been known that Forssman antigen distributions vary considerably among species. In the guinea pig Forssman antigen is found on nearly all tissues but not on erythrocytes, while exactly the opposite type of distribution is found in the sheep and goat (Boyd, 1966). This suggests considerable flexibility in the manner in which jumping antigens are employed. Perhaps this is allowed by redundancy in the antigens that regulate any particular function, such as adhesion. If so, evolutionary changes in their expression could have subtle and potentially important effects on organismal development.

Jumping antigens have been identified with monoclonal antibodies, both in

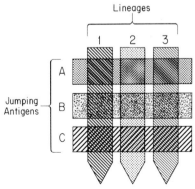

FIGURE 10. Combinatorial use of lineage and jumping antigens helps generate cell-surface diversity. The course of development is portrayed as occurring from the top to the bottom of the figure.

the mouse and in the rat, with a surprisingly high frequency. This is probably explained by the very wide window through which the cell surface is seen using the monoclonal approach in conjunction with xenogeneic immunization and the indirect ^{125}I-anti-Ig binding assay. By comparison, alloimmunization selects for polymorphic antigens and xenoimmunization with one tissue and absorption with others selects for lineage antigens. Identification of antibodies by their ability to precipitate ^{125}I- or [^{35}S]methionine-labeled antigens selects against glycolipids.

The possibility of chemical dissimilarity between jumping (or lineage) antigens isolated from different tissues must always be considered, especially since monoclonal antibodies recognize only one out of many possible determinants on a molecule. Gross dissimilarity between the antigens recognized in different tissues has not been found, such as would be predicted by the multiple recognition theory of Richards et al. (1975). However, some smaller differences have been noted. For example, the HSA on RBC bears both the M1/69 and M1/75 determinants, while the HSA on white blood cells bears only the former. Furthermore, the CLAs on T cells and B cells all bear both M1/9.3 and M1/89.18 determinants, but the differing molecular weight of this antigen when isolated from B or T lymphoid sources suggests other differences, perhaps in glycosylation. Moreover, Williams et al. (1976) have found striking differences in the carbohydrate composition of brain as opposed to thymus Thy-1 antigen. This heterogeneity in the antigens themselves introduces a further complexity in the analysis of cell surfaces.

The existence of jumping antigens also demonstrates the pitfalls of assigning ontogenetic relatedness between cells on the basis of a single surface marker. A number of shared antigens should be demonstrated before conclusions are drawn.

B. "Lineage" Differentiation Antigens

The more circumscribed distribution of lineage antigens distinguishes them from jumping antigens and suggests them to be important in the unique functions of the cells on which they are expressed. Unlike jumping antigens, species variation in pattern of expression would not be expected. In this regard it is of interest that Mac-1 cross-reacts with human cells and exhibits the same specificity for monocytes in humans as found in the mouse (Ault and Springer, manuscript in preparation). Breadth of expression of lineage antigens appears to approximately reflect different levels of specialization during differentiation (Fig. 11). Thus the expression of CLA is restricted to leukocytes, Mac-1 to "professional" phagocytes (granulocytes and mononuclear phagocytes) and Mac-2 and Mac-3 to mononuclear phagocytes. Sometimes closely related sublines do not all express an antigen. For example, erythrocytes, granulocytes, monocytes, and megakaryocytes share a pluripotent stem cell, which differs from the lymphocyte stem cell, and both of these stem cells are in turn derived from a more primitive progenitor cell (Cline, 1975). Yet all leukocytes share the CLA, whereas erythrocytes and

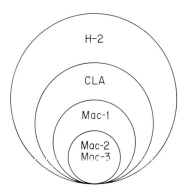

FIGURE 11. Expression of lineage antigens correlates with specialization during differentiation.

their immediate precursors do not. The pattern of expression does not exactly recapitulate ontogeny, but is closer to what would be expected on the basis of functional relatedness. Similarly, monocytes and B but not T lymphocytes share expression of Ia antigens and trypsin-resistant Fc receptors for aggregated IgG (FcRII). Unkeless (1979) has prepared a rat monoclonal antibody that blocks the macrophage FcRII but not FcRI site, and also the FcRII site on B cells. Quantitative changes in expression or even complete loss may also occur during development of the lineage. For example, the absence of CLA from certain myeloma lines but its expression on B cells and B lymphomas suggests that in differentiation of B cells to plasma cells, expression of this antigen may be lost.

In the rat a number of lineage antigens have also been identified using monoclonal antibodies. MRC OX1 recognizes a CLA, which in molecular weight and tissue distribution appears similar to the CLA in the mouse (Sunderland *et al.*, 1979). W3/25 is specific for a T-lymphocyte functional subset (White *et al.*, 1978). Cells mediating help for B cells and graft-vs.-host reactivity are contained within the W3/25-positive subpopulation of 80% of thoracic duct lymphocytes. The 10% subpopulation of unlabeled T lymphocytes contains the allogeneic suppressor cells. This and similar reagents should be of great value in the study of T-lymphocyte subsets.

The value of monoclonal reagents in the study of differentiation is also well illustrated by the derivation of antibodies to Mac-1, -2, and -3. This is the first time that individual molecules marking the phagocyte (Mac-1) and mononuclear phagocyte (Mac-2 and -3) lines of differentiation have been identified. Mononuclear phagocytes are a very interesting system for studying differentiation. Their precursors are formed in bone marrow and are transported to tissues in the blood, where they have a half-life of about 22 hr. Upon crossing the endothelium, they differentiate into cells with diverse functional and morphological characteristics, such as alveolar macrophages, peritoneal macrophages, thymic macrophages, liver Kupffer cells, bone osteoclasts, and epidermal Langerhans cells (Hobart and McConnell, 1975). Differentiation to "activated" tumoricidal and microbicidal macrophages may occur in response to inflammatory stimuli such as mediators released by T lymphocytes (Bianco and Edelson, 1977). The possibility is being tested whether mononuclear phagocytes localized in certain tissues lack Mac-1, -2, -3 expression. If so, this would provide further evidence for the diversity of these cells. In peritoneal exudates, all macrophages express Mac-1, -2, and -3 antigens. Ia antisera, however, define peritoneal exudate macrophage subpopulations (Cowing *et al.*, 1978), and it remains possible that further Mac antigens identifying these subpopulations will be found.

VI. Concluding Remarks

Studies utilizing monoclonal antibodies are beginning to reveal interesting patterns of antigen expression on developing cell surfaces. Two extremely different types of antigen distributions, with perhaps also some intermediate types, were noted in this study. "Jumping" antigens have tissue distributions which are patchy and widely scattered, often undergo change during cellular migration, and are often different for the homologues in other species. Carbohydrate often appears to be a prominent structural component. Their distribution suggests a role in modulation of generalized membrane phenomena such as intercellular adhesion. "Lineage" antigens have tissue distributions which are much more restricted, may undergo changes in expression during maturation and are similar for the homologues in different species. Their distribution suggests participation in the specialized functions of the cells on which they are expressed. It will be interesting to learn whether these generalizations can be extended as more antigens on leukocytes and other types of cells are studied.

The ease with which novel surface antigens have been identified up to now strongly suggests that only a small fraction of the total are presently identified. The ultimate goal of identifying the entire array of cell-surface antigens seems possible in the next few decades, particularly with the availability of cascade schemes for the production of antibodies against antigens of successively lower immunodominance. Using a complete set of monoclonal antibodies, the total ebb and flow of antigen expression during differentiation and development could be quantitatively described.

The study of differentiation is just one of the many uses of monoclonal antibodies. Analysis of tissue distribution is an important step in assessing the likely functional importance of a particular antigen before more detailed chemical and functional characterization is carried out. Monoclonal antibodies appear particularly well suited for studying the structure and function of membrane molecules. This is because unlike enzymes or Fc receptors, most cell-surface molecules may not retain biological activity after isolation. For example, in the macrophage, many functions such as phagocytosis, chemotaxis, tumor killing, or induction of immune responsiveness no doubt require the interactions of a number of different molecules in the context of the whole cell. Monoclonal antibodies should therefore be highly valuable not only for the isolation of individual cell-surface molecules but also to probe or modify the activity of these molecules in their native environment on the cell surface. In this regard, Mac-1, -2, and -3 antibodies are currently being tested for inhibition of a panel of macrophage-specific, surface-associated activities. Parallel studies on the structure and membrane integration of Mac-1, -2, and -3 antigens are also being carried out.

ACKNOWLEDGMENTS

I thank G. Galfrè, E. Lennox, C. Milstein, D. Secher, P. Stern, K. Willison, and A. Ziegler for stimulating collaboration in portions of the work summarized here; A. Munro for providing encouragement and laboratory facilities during the early part of this work; B. Benacerraf and other members of the Pathology Department at Harvard Medical School for advice and encouragement; D. Gubbins for expert technical assistance; E. Adams and J. Davis for skillful operation of the FACS; T. Greenberg for superb assistance in preparing the manuscript; and M. Mescher for critically reading the manuscript. This work was supported in part by NIH grant AI-14732.

References

Bazin, H., Beckers, A., and Querinjean, P., 1974, Three classes and four (sub)classes of rat immunoglobulins: IgM, IgA, IgE and IgG$_1$, IgG$_{2a}$, IgG$_{2b}$, IgG$_{2c}$, Eur. J. Immunol. **4**:44.

Beller, D. I., and Unanue, E. R., 1978, Thymic macrophages modulate one stage of T cell differentiation in vitro, J. Immunol. **121**:1861.

Bianco, C., and Edelson, P. J., 1977, Characteristics of the activated macrophage, in: Immune Effector Mechanisms in Disease (M. Weksler, S. Litwin, R. Riggio, and G. Siskind, eds.), Grune and Stratton, New York, pp. 1–9.

Boyd, W. C., 1966, Fundamentals of Immunology, Wiley, New York, p. 195.

Boyse, E. A., and Old, L. J., 1969, Some aspects of normal and abnormal cell surface genetics, Annu. Rev. Genet. **3**:269.

Cline, M. J., 1975, The White Cell, Harvard University Press, Cambridge, Mass.

Cowing, C., Schwartz, B. D., and Dickler, H. B., 1978, Macrophage populations differ in their expression of Ia antigens, J. Immunol. **120**:378.

Dalchau, R., and Fabre, J. W., 1979, Identification and unusual tissue distribution of the canine and human homologues of Thy-1 (θ), J. Exp. Med. **149**:576.

Ey, P. L., Prowse, S. J., and Jenkin, C. R., 1978, Isolation of pure IgG$_1$, IgG$_{2a}$ and IgG$_{2b}$ immunoglobulins from mouse serum using protein A–Sepharose, Immunochemistry **15**:429.

Festing, M. F. W., May, D., Connors, T. A., Lovell, D., and Sparrow, S., 1978, An athymic nude mutation in the rat, Nature **274**:365.

Galfrè, G., Howe, S. C., Milstein, C., Butcher, G. W., and Howard, J. C., 1977, Antibodies to major histocompatibility antigens produced by hybrid cell lines, Nature **266**:550.

Galfrè, G., Milstein, C., and Wright, B., 1979, Rat × rat hybrid myelomas and a monoclonal anti-Fd portion of mouse IgG, Nature **277**:131.

Hämmerling, G. J., Lemke, H., Hämmerling, U., Höhmann, C., Wallich, R., and Rajewsky, K., 1978, Monoclonal antibodies against murine cell surface antigens: Anti-H-2, anti-Ia, and anti-T cell antibodies, Curr. Top. Microbiol. Immunol. **81**:100.

Hobart, M. J., and McConnell, I., 1975, The Immune System, Blackwell Scientific, Oxford, p. 180.

Köhler, G., and Milstein, C., 1976, Derivation of specific antibody-producing tissue culture and tumour lines by cell fusion, Eur. J. Immunol. **6**:511.

Konda, S., Stockert, E., and Smith, R. T., 1973, Immunologic properties of mouse thymus cells: Membrane antigen patterns associated with various cell subpopulations, *Cell. Immunol.* **7:**275.

Leslie, G. A., 1979, Expression of a cross-reactive idiotype on the IgG$_{2C}$ subclass of rat anti-strepto-coccal carbohydrate antibody, *Mol. Immunol.* **16:**281.

Littlefield, J. W., 1964, Selection of hybrids from matings of fibroblasts *in vitro* and their presumed recombinants, *Science* **145:**709.

Loken, M. R., and Herzenberg, L. A., 1975, Analysis of cell populations with a fluorescence-activated cell sorter, *Ann. NY Acad. Sci.* **254:**163.

London, J., Berrih, S., and Bach, J.-F., 1978, Peanut agglutinin. I. A new tool for studying T lymphocyte subpopulations, *J. Immunol.* **121:**438.

Marchase, R. B., Vosbeck, K., and Roth, S., 1976, Intercellular adhesive specificity, *Biochim. Biophys. Acta* **457:**385.

Marshak-Rothstein, A., Fink, P., Gridley, T., Raulet, D. H., Bevan, M. J., and Gefter, M. L., 1979, Properties and applications of monoclonal antibodies directed against determinants of the Thy-1 locus, *J. Immunol.* **122:**2491.

Medgyesi, G. A., Füst, G., Gergely, J., and Bazin, H., 1978, Classes and subclasses of rat immuno-globulins: Interaction with the complement system and with staphylococcal protein A, *Immuno-chemistry* **15:**125.

Milstein, C., and Lennox, E., 1980, The use of monoclonal antibody techniques in the study of developing cell surfaces, *Curr. Top. Dev. Biol.* (in press).

Milstein, C., Galfrè, G., Secher, D. S., and Springer, T., 1979, Monoclonal antibodies and cell surface antigens in: *Genetics and Human Biology: Possibilities and Realities,* Ciba Foundation Symposium No. 66, Excerpta Medica, Amsterdam. Reprinted in *Cell Biol. Int. Rep.* **3:**1–16.

Mirsky, R., and Thompson, E. J., 1975, Thy 1 (theta) antigen on the surface of morphologically distinct brain cell types, *Cell* **4:**95.

Oi, V. T., Jones, P. P., Goding, J. W., Herzenberg, L. A., and Herzenberg, L. A., 1978, Properties of monoclonal antibodies to mouse Ig allotypes, H-2, and Ia antigens, *Curr. Top. Microbiol. Immunol.* **81:**115.

Ouchterlony, Ö., and Nilsson, L. Å., 1978, Immunodiffusion and immunoelectrophoresis, in: *Hand-book of Experimental Immunology* (D. M. Weir, ed.), Blackwell, Oxford, P. 19.10.

Parham, P., and Bodmer, W. F., 1978, Monoclonal antibody to a human histocompatibility alloanti-gen, HLA-A2, *Nature* **276:**397.

Reisner, Y., Gachelin, G., Dubois, P., Nicolas, J.-F., Sharon, N., and Jacob, F., 1977, Interaction of peanut agglutinin, a lectin specific for nonreducing terminal D-galactosyl residues, with em-bryonal carcinoma cells, *Dev. Biol.* **61:**20.

Richards, F. F., Konigsberg, W. H., Rosenstein, R. W., and Varga, J. M., 1975, On the specificity of antibodies, *Science* **187:**130.

Solter, D., and Knowles, B. B., 1978, Monoclonal antibody defining a stage-specific mouse embryonic antigen (SSEA-1), *Proc. Natl. Acad. Sci. USA* **75:**5565.

Springer, T., Galfrè, G., Secher, D., and Milstein, C., 1978a, Monoclonal xenogeneic antibodies to mouse leukocyte antigens: Identification of macrophage-specific and other differentiation anti-gens, *Curr. Top. Microbiol. Immunol.* **81:**45.

Springer, T., Galfrè, G., Secher, D. S., and Milstein, C., 1978b, Monoclonal xenogeneic antibodies to murine cell surface antigens: Identification of novel leukocyte differentiation antigens, *Eur. J. Immunol.* **8:**539.

Springer, T., Galfrè, G., Secher, D. S., and Milstein, C., 1979, Mac-1: A macrophage differentiation antigen identified by monoclonal antibody, *Eur. J. Immunol.* **9:**301.

Stamper, Jr., H. B., and Woodruff, J. J., 1976, Lymphocyte homing into lymph nodes: *In vitro* demonstration of the selective affinity of recirculating lymphocytes for high-endothelial venules, *J. Exp. Med.* **144:**828.

Stanworth, D. R., and Turner, M. W., 1978, Immunochemical analysis, in: *Handbook of Experimental Immunology* (D. M. Weir, ed.), Blackwell, Oxford, p. 6.25.

Stein, K. E., Schwarting, G. A., and Marcus, D. M., 1978, Glycolipid markers of murine lymphocyte subpopulations, *J. Immunol.* **120:**676.

Stern, P., Willison, K., Lennox, E., Galfrè, G., Milstein, C., Secher, D., Ziegler, A., and Springer, T.,

1978, Monoclonal antibodies as probes for differentiation and tumor associated antigens: A Forssman specificity on teratocarcinoma stem cells, *Cell* **14:**775.

Sunderland, C. A., McMaster, W. R., and Williams, A. R., 1979, Purification with monoclonal antibody of a predominant leukocyte-common antigen and glycoprotein from rat thymocytes, *Eur. J. Immunol.* **9:**155.

Trowbridge, I. S., 1978, Interspecies spleen–myeloma hybrid producing monoclonal antibodies against mouse lymphocyte surface glycoprotein, T200, *J. Exp. Med.* **148:**313.

Trowbridge, I. S., and Mazauskas, C., 1976, Immunological properties of murine thymus-dependent lymphocyte surface glycoproteins, *Eur. J. Immunol.* **6:**557.

Trowbridge, I. S., Hyman, R., and Mazauskas, C., 1978, The synthesis and properties of T25 glycoprotein in Thy-1-negative mutant lymphoma cells, *Cell* **14:**21.

Unkeless, J., 1979, Characterization of a monoclonal antibody directed against mouse macrophage and lymphocyte Fc receptors, *J. Exp. Med.* **150:**580.

Van Furth, R., 1975, Modulation of monocyte production, in: *Mononuclear Phagocytes in Immunity, Infection and Pathology* (R. Van Furth, ed.), Blackwell, Oxford, p. 161.

White, R. A. H., Mason, D. W., Williams, A. F., Galfrè, G., and Milstein, C., 1978, T-lymphocyte heterogeneity in the rat: Separation of functional subpopulations using a monoclonal antibody, *J. Exp. Med.* **148:**664.

Williams, A. F., Barclay, A. N., Letarte-Muirhead, M., and Morris, R. J., 1976, Rat Thy-1 antigens from thymus and brain: Their tissue distribution, purification, and chemical composition, *Cold Spring Harbor Symp. Quant. Biol.* **41:**51.

Williams, A. F., Galfre, G., and Milstein, C., 1977, Analysis of cell surfaces by xenogeneic myeloma-hybrid antibodies: Differentiation antigens of rat lymphocytes, *Cell* **12:**663.

Willison, K. R., and Stern, P. L., 1978, Expression of a Forssman antigenic specificity in the preimplantation mouse embryo, *Cell* **14:**785.

Wofsy, L., Henry, C., and Cammisuli, S., 1978, Hapten-sandwich labeling of cell surface antigens, *Contemp. Top. Mol. Immunol.* **7:**215.

Yamada, K. M., and Olden, K., 1978, Fibronectins—Adhesive glycoproteins of cell surface and blood, *Nature* **275:**179.

Ziolkowski, C. H. J., Fraser, B. S., and Mallette, M. F., 1975, Sheep erythrocyte Forssman hapten, an isohapten system: Composition of the ceramide, *Immunochemistry* **12:**297.

13
Rat–Mouse Hybridomas and Their Application to Studies of the Major Histocompatibility Complex

Thomas J. McKearn, Dawn E. Smilek, and Frank W. Fitch

I. Introduction

This chapter will address two main issues: (1) the general properties of interspecies hybridoma cell lines prepared by fusion of mutant mouse myeloma cells to lymphoid cells from immunized rats, and (2) the application of hybridoma technology to studies involving the structure and function of the major histocompatibility complex in inbred rodents.

II. General Properties of Rat–Mouse Hybridomas

Chapters 12 and 14 also deal with the preparation and properties of rat–mouse hybridomas, and, although we have used somewhat different techniques, our overall experience with rat–mouse hybridomas parallels the general findings

Thomas J. McKearn • Department of Pathology, Divisions of Research Immunology and Laboratory Medicine, University of Pennsylvania, School of Medicine, Philadelphia, Pennsylvania 19104. Dawn E. Smilek • Department of Pathology, Division of Research Immunology, University of Pennsylvania, School of Medicine, Philadelphia, Pennsylvania 19104. Frank W. Fitch • The Committee on Immunology and the Department of Pathology, University of Chicago, Chicago, Illinois 60637.

reported in those studies. During the past two years, we have developed and characterized several hundred rat–mouse hybridomas. In comparing rat–mouse hybridomas, we have reached the following conclusions (Table I).

The two main advantages of the mouse–mouse system are the greater volume of information regarding mouse immunogenetics and the ability to passage intraspecies mouse–mouse hybridomas as tumors in a conventional murine host. Interspecies hybridomas prepared between rats and mice have, in our experience, been invariably rejected by either conventional rats or mice. One must therefore resort to using either athymic animals or conventional animals which have been immunosuppressed using a regimen of antilymphocyte serum and/or total body irradiation in order to achieve growth *in vivo* of these interspecies hybridomas (see Appendix).

Interspecies rat–mouse hybridomas do offer a number of distinct advantages as alternatives to mouse–mouse hybridomas. Over 90% of rat–mouse hybridomas produced between Lewis rats and either P3/X63-Ag8 or SP2/0-Ag14 secrete a rat κ light chain whose allotype is non-cross-reactive with BALB/c κ light chains. This light-chain marker can therefore serve as one useful parameter for quantifying the amount of rat immunglobulin (Ig) in a given culture supernatant. Alternatively, one can prepare rat anti-mouse Ig and mouse anti-

TABLE I

Comparison of Mouse–Mouse Hybridomas with Rat–Mouse Hybridomas

Mouse–mouse more advantageous	Rat–mouse more advantageous	Either combination equally useful
1. Mouse immunoglobulin genetics and antisera are better and defined.	1. Rat κ light chain allotype marker does not cross-react with mouse light chains and is present on >90% of rat–mouse hybridomas.	1. Functional and karyotypic stability of cell lines is equivalent.
2. Hybridomas can be grown in conventional mice.	2. Rat karyotype is easily distinguished from mouse.	2. Fusion efficiency is equivalent.
	3. Degree of H and L chain misassembly is less in rat–mouse hybridomas.	3. Each species may react qualitatively or quantitatively differently than the other in response to a given antigen.
	4. Spleen is the major if not sole site of antibody production after intravenous injection of antigen in the rat.	
	5. Larger size of rats allows repeated sampling of an individual's spleen or lymph nodes over time.	

rat Ig antisera for specific Ig quantification. The specificities of such sera may be directed against either heavy or light Ig chains.

The second point for consideration is the ease with which one may distinguish the karyotype of rat and mouse cells. A normal rat has 42 chromosomes with 14 metacentrics, while the mouse has 40 chromosomes, none of which are metacentric. This difference in karyotype is therefore a useful parameter for assessing the stability of interspecies hybridomas. Our experience in following the karyotype of rat–mouse hybridomas, which have been in continuous culture for 18 months, has shown that the total chromosome count and the number of identifiable rat markers are relatively stable (McKearn *et al.*, 1979a).

One of the major problems of mouse–mouse hybridomas prepared with secretor myelomas is the misassembly of Ig light and heavy chains by such cells. Isoelectric focusing (IEF) patterns of nonreduced biosynthetically labeled proteins from such cells show marked distortion of the parental myeloma spectrotype and generally reveal a multitude of additional bands at various pIs (M. Sarmiento, personal communication). Similar IEF gels of rat–mouse hybridomas show faithful reproduction of the parental myeloma spectrotype and a handful of novel bands that generally show uniform spacing around a heavy central band (McKearn *et al.*, 1979a). Thus, within the limits of resolution of the autoradiographic IEF techniques, rat–mouse hybridomas show minimal amounts of chain misassembly.

Most investigators have used splenic lymphoid cells as fusion partners for hybridoma experiments. One presumes that some portion of the antigen administered to an individual will localize to the spleen and stimulate generation of antibody-forming cells in that organ. It may be of more than passing interest, therefore, to recall experiments in rats by Rowley (1950) in which splenectomy effectively eliminated the serum antibody response to intravenously administered sheep erythrocytes. This effect has been observed with other particulate antigens but is less pronounced with soluble antigens. Similar experiments performed in mice gave much less impressive diminution of the serum antibody response to sheep erythrocytes (J. Sprent, personal communication). The implications of these data are that the rat spleen serves as the site for sequestration and differentiation of the responding lymphoid cells after intravenous injection of particulate antigens.

Finally, the obvious point should be made that rats are bigger than mice. One can therefore repeatedly sample portions of the spleen from an individual rat after antigen challenge in order to determine with time the changing pattern of an immune response within a given animal. Indeed, the prospect of repeated sampling of the B-cell response in an individual should permit for rather rigorous testing of the network hypothesis of immune regulation (Jerne, 1974).

Rat–mouse hybridomas may prove to be more desirable than the intraspecies mouse–mouse hybridomas in some circumstances. The potential utility of rat–mouse hybridomas has of course not been fully realized, but one indication of the general applicability of this approach can be gleaned from a brief summary of the cloned hybridoma cell lines that have been developed in our laboratories (Table II).

TABLE II
Summary of Lewis Rat–Mouse Hybridomas Prepared in Our Laboratories

Immunogen	Responder strain	Specificity of hybridomas
C3H mouse thymocytes	Lewis rat	1. Thy 1.2 2. Murine "T-cell" antigen
Friend virus infected BALB.B cell lysate	Lewis rat	"Virus altered H-2^b"
Calf uterine estrogen receptor	Lewis rat	Estrogen receptor[a]
Acetylcholine receptor from Torpedo california	Lewis rat	Acetylcholine[b] receptor; 4 patterns of reactivity
Hyaluronidase-treated chondroitin sulfate proteoglycan from embryonic chick epiphyses	Lewis rat	Protein of chick[c] proteoglycan; several patterns of reactivity, including one which reacts with cell-free synthesized product
Brown Norway rat lymphoid cells	Lewis rat	Class I determinants of AgB-3
DA rat lymphoid cells	Lewis rat	Class I determinants of AgB-4

[a]See Greene et al. (1980) for details of derivation and characterization of this antibody.
[b]See Gomez et al. (1979) for details of derivation and characterization of this antibody.
[c]See A. Dorfman (1979) for details of derivation and characterization of this antibody.

III. Application of Hybridoma Technology to Studies of the Rat Major Histocompatibility Complex

A. Introduction

The major histocompatibility complex (MHC) is a collection of genes whose products can profoundly affect the immunological responsiveness of an individual. Indeed, some authors have argued that the functions of the immune system and MHC gene products are overlapping and extensively interwoven. Thus in the mouse, where genetic definition is currently most precise, the K/D portions of the $H-2$ complex serve as restriction elements for virus-specific and "hapten-modified self" killer cells (Doherty et al., 1976) and also provide the primary targets for most allogeneic killer cells (Nabholz *et al.*, 1974). Gene products encoded by the *I* region provide strong primary stimuli to allogeneic cells in mixed leukocyte cultures (Bach *et al.*, 1977) or graft-vs.-host reactions (Klein and Park, 1973) and also can serve as restriction elements for certain cell–cell interactions that occur during the course of an immune response (Niederhuber, 1978). Other *I*-region genes are involved in regulation of the overall magnitude of immune responses to selected antigens (Benacerraf and Germain, 1978) and additional *I*-region gene products appear to be involved in production of T-cell factors that may augment or suppress immune responses (Tada *et al.*, 1977; Taussig *et al.*, 1979). The final major category of MHC gene products includes various components of the complement pathway, which for some curious reason happen to be closely linked to MHC loci of both man and mouse.

The serological identification of MHC gene products has traditionally rested on the demonstration of antibody production following alloimmunization or, less frequently, on the presence of residual antibody reactivity in a heterologous immune serum after extensive absorption with cells or tissues from an appropriate individual. Such an approach places certain constraints on the system, i.e., alloimmunization presumably permits detection only of those MHC determinants that are polymorphic within the species, while absorbed heterologous antisera often display only very weak residual reactivity. Hybridoma technology offers the possibility of deriving monoclonal and therefore presumably monospecific antibodies, which may possess strikingly high titers. Moreover, the long lifespan of these hybridoma cell lines would seemingly imply that one could rigorously characterize these biological products and thereby provide materials of reagent quality for use in the analysis of MHC gene products.

We initially chose to derive monoclonal anti-MHC alloantibodies in alloimmunized rats for the following reasons: It is well established in this inbred rat system [Lewis anti-Brown Norway (BN)] that certain alloimmune sera were markedly effective in selectively suppressing both humoral and cell-mediated immunity toward alloantigens (Stuart *et al.*, 1968). Furthermore, in the case of renal allograft enhancement a single injection of an "effective" alloimmune serum could induce a state of suppressed alloreactivity *in vivo*, which would persist for the life of the experimental animal. One major problem with this system, however, has been the failure of various groups to agree on the characteristics of the "enhancing antibodies" (Jones *et al.*, 1972; Davis and Alkins, 1974; Soulillou *et al.*, 1976). Indeed, it can be fairly stated that "enhancing antibodies" have not been adequately characterized in terms of their antigenic specificity(ies), heavy and light chain classes or their idiotypic specificities.

In the rat B and T cells reactive with alloantigens have been reported to share idiotypic specificities. The studies that purported to show such reactivities are potentially flawed in terms of their experimental design. Both McKearn (1974) and Binz and Wigzell (1975) used either purified alloantibody obtained from immune serum or T cells from mixed leukocyte cultures to prepare their antiidiotypic antisera. If one accepts the possibility that T-cell receptors may be shed into immune serum (Ramseier, 1974) or that alloactivated T cells can contain contaminating B cells or antigen–antibody complexes on their surface

(Hudson and Sprent, 1976), then one realizes that the immunogen in neither of the cases cited above is necessarily free of products from the "contaminating" cell type. It follows therefore that some or all of the "shared" idiotypic specificities between B and T cells could represent reactivities against these contaminants. The availability of hybridoma antibodies with anti-MHC specificity now provides starting materials with unambiguous credentials that can be used to examine this question.

The MHC in rats is less well-defined than its H-2 counterpart in the mouse. In large part this is due to a paucity of MHC recombinant rat strains that can be used for classical genetic analysis (Butcher and Howard, 1977; Stark *et al.*, 1977). Anti-MHC hybridomas in the rat could circumvent this problem and may provide additional information that is not predicted by the current genetic analyses of this and other MHC loci. Experiments were therefore undertaken to derive a suitably large collection of rat anti-MHC hybridomas in order to pursue these general issues. The materials and methods used in those experiments have been published elsewhere (McKearn *et al.*, 1978, 1979a,b) so that the following discussion will only briefly deal with such details.

B. Experimental Findings

Ficoll–Hypaque-separated spleen cells from Lewis rats immunized with BN cells were fused to one of several mutant mouse myeloma cells with polyethyleneglycol and the fusion products seeded into microtiter plates (Costar) in medium containing hypoxanthine, aminopterin, and thymidine (HAT). Wells containing proliferating hybridoma cells were screened for cytotoxic antibody using a complement-dependent ^{51}Cr-release assay. In general we have found that the use of concanavalin A (Con A) blast cells as target cells and selected lots of agar-absorbed rabbit sera as complement allows for optimal sensitivity in this screening assay.

The proportion of initially seeded wells that contained cytotoxic antibody has varied from less than 10% to greater than 90% of the total wells seeded despite our best attempts to reproduce faithfully the immunization protocols and culture conditions. Preliminary studies using an indirect binding radioimmunoassay to assess antibody secretion have given higher proportions of positive wells than the cytotoxic screening assay. However, the proportion of wells secreting cytotoxic antibodies has generally been sufficiently great that we have not pursued the characterization of these noncytotoxic antibodies.

Cells identified as positive for cytotoxic antibody were expanded into 2-ml wells (Linbro) seeded with 10^7 irradiated Lewis rat thymocyte feeder cells. The use of feeder cells at this stage improves the survival of the proliferating hybrid cells and effectively avoids the problem of decreased cell viability because of low cell density. Following this expansion, cells were cloned in semisoft agarose according to the method of Kennett *et al.* (1978; see Appendix). Alternatively, one can clone using limiting dilution techniques in fluid phase over feeder cells (see Appendix), but for high-volume work, the tube method of Kennett appears to be more advantageous.

Clones of cells are picked from the agarose and grown to large volume in Dulbecco's Modified Eagle's Medium (DMEM) with 20% serum supplement. We have recently converted from using fetal calf serum to agamma horse serum and find that selected lots of agamma horse serum are entirely satisfactory for selection, cloning, and growth of hybridomas in bulk culture. This may be of some practical importance given the decreasing availability of fetal calf serum in the United States.

Cloned lines were characterized with regard to antibody specificity and rat H and L chain class. Table III provides a summary of the cytotoxicity and hemagglutination patterns of 9 such Lewis anti-BN hybridoma antibodies. Of the 9 hybridoma antibodies 7 are IgM and 8 secrete a rat κ light chain as measured by inhibition of an anti-light-chain allotype passive hemagglutination reaction (Gutman and Weissman, 1971). The one rat hybridoma that does not react in the antiallotype reaction does, however, secrete a rat light chain as shown on sodium dodecyl sulfate–polyacrylamide gel electrophoresis (SDS-PAGE) (McKearn et al., 1979b). Therefore, this rat hybridoma may either be secreting a rat λ light chain or some variant of rat κ which does not display the κ allotype marker. Additional experiments have confirmed that most rat–mouse hybridomas secrete a rat κ allotype marker, and in one study, 127 of 131 consecutively tested hybridomas were positive for the rat κ allotype (T. McKearn, unpublished data).

All of these 9 hybridomas react in the cytotoxicity assay with determinants that are encoded by the MHC of BN. That is, the antibodies are cytotoxic for

TABLE III
Characteristics of Rat Anti-MHC Hybridomas[a]

Hybridoma	Heavy chain	Light chain	Cytotoxicity pattern			Hemagglutination pattern		
			BN	Lewis B3	BN.B1	BN	Lewis B3	BN.B1
D4,37	μ	Lacks κ allotype	+	+	−	+	+	−
D4,68	γ2b	κ	+	+	−	+	+	−
D4,69	γ2c	κ	+	+	−	+	+	−
K2.3.17	μ	κ	+	+	−	+	+	−
K2.13.2	μ	κ	+	+	−	+	+	−
N2.9.2	μ	κ	+	+	−	−	−	−
N2.11.6	μ	κ	+	+	−	+	+	−
N2.27.30	μ	κ	+	+	−	+	+	−
N2.54.3	μ	κ	+	+	−	+	+	−

[a]Summary of the characteristics of 9 hybridoma antibody culture supernatants. Rat heavy-chain isotype was determined using typing sera from Bazin et al. (1974). Rat κ light chain was assigned if the supernatants inhibited the agglutination of allotype-coated erythrocytes caused by limiting amounts of antiallotypic antisera (Gutman and Weissman, 1971). The cytotoxicity data were derived using ^{51}Cr-labeled Con A blast cells and rabbit complement. Hemagglutination was performed by a modification (McKearn et al., 1979a) of the method of Severson and Thompson (1966).

both BN and the congenic Lewis.B3 which contains the MHC of BN (Ag-B3) on a Lewis background. Moreover, these antibodies fail to lyse cells from BN.B1 animals that contain the MHC of Lewis (Ag-B1) on a BN genetic background. Since these hybridomas were derived from Lewis animals immunized with fully allogeneic BN spleen cells, one might not have expected that all of the Lewis anti-BN hybridomas tested would show such predilection for reactivity against the BN MHC antigens. In fact our overall experience to date suggests that the proportion of hybridomas that react with MHC determinants may largely be a function of the strain combinations used for immunization (T. McKearn, unpublished data).

Cytotoxicity titers of these hybridoma supernatants on BN targets vary from $1:64$ to $1:10^7$. The complement source used in the cytotoxicity assay has proven to be a critical factor in the magnitude of the cytotoxicity titer seen with a given monoclonal antibody. To optimize titers we have screened panels of rabbit sera to identify those relatively few individual rabbits whose sera will support lysis at high dilutions of hybridoma antibody without causing significant spontaneous lysis of the targets. It should be noted in passing that we have not observed the phenomena of "partial" or "synergistic" lysis as reported by Howard et al. (1978). Perhaps this is because we are primarily studying immunoglobulin M (IgM) antibodies and using rabbit complement, while Howard et al. use guinea pig complement with their IgG antibodies.

When tested on BN or Lewis.B3 target cells, these 9 hybridomas all gave 100% lysis of Con A blast target cells and, moreover, in every case tested, the cytotoxicity against the fully allogeneic BN targets could be completely absorbed on cells from Lewis.B3 congenic strain. The MHC determinants recognized by these hybridomas are therefore found on all lymphoid cells and would be considered the K/D equivalent or Class I MHC molecules in the terminology suggested by Klein (1977). If these antibodies are indeed reactive with Class I MHC determinants, one would predict that most of these hybridomas should also react with BN erythrocytes. Table III shows that 8 of 9 hybridomas do agglutinate BN and Lewis.B3 erythrocytes. With several of the antibodies (e.g., D4,68 and D4,69) hemagglutination is only seen after addition of a secondary anti-Ig antiserum.

The patterns of cross-reactivity on other inbred rat strains were then tested in the ^{51}Cr-release assay. Whenever possible, cells from MHC congenic animals were used in order to better define the genetic disparity between groups of animals. Table IV shows the cross-reactivity pattern of these antibodies on rats representing six MHC haplotypes. As noted earlier, with BN and Lewis.B3 target cells, the lysis appeared, with few exceptions, to be an all-or-none phenomenon. However, it is clear that the cytotoxicity titers against the cross-reactive targets often were considerably lower than the titers on the homologous BN or Lewis.B3 targets. These findings were further corroborated by cold-target inhibition studies in which, for example, the homologous BN target would cold-compete much more effectively for limiting amounts of D4,37 antibody than would DA target cells. We believe that such patterns of reactivity could reflect differences in relative avidity of binding of the various antibodies for different

Table IV
Summary of the Cytotoxic Cross-Reactivities of Hybridoma Antibodies[a]

	Rat AgB haplotype						Mouse H-2 haplotype					Human PBLs							
	1	2	3	4	5	6	d	k	b	q	s	a	b	c	d	e	f	g	RP
N2.9.2	−	−	+	−	⁓		−	−	−	−	−	−	−	−	−	−	−	−	1
N2.54.3	−	−	+	−	−	−	+	−	−	−	−	−	−	−	−	−	−	⁓	2
N2.27.30	−	−	+	−	−	−	+	−	−	−	−	−	−	−	−	−	+/−	−	3
N2.11.6	−	−	+	−	−	−	+	−	−	−	−	+/−	−	−	−	−	+	−	4
K2.3.17	−	−	+	−	−	−	+	+	−	−	−	+	+	+	−	+	+	+	5
D4,68	−	−	+	−	+	−	−	−	−	−	−	−	−	−	−	−	−	−	6
D4,69	−	−	+	−	+	−	−	−	−	−	−	−	−	−	−	−	−	−	6
K2.13.2	−	−	+	+	+	−	−	−	−	−	−	−	−	−	−	−	−	−	7
D4.37	−	+	+	+	−	+	+	+	+	+	+	+	+	+	+	+	+	+	8

[a]Summary of the cytotoxic cross-reactivities of hybridoma culture supernatants on rat, mouse, and human cells. The following rat strains were used: Ag-B1-Lewis, Fisher, A990, BH and BN.B1; Ag-B2-Wistar/Furth, BN.B2; Ag-B3-BN, LEW.B3; Ag-B4-DA,ACI, L.AVN; Ag-B5-August; Ag-B6-Buffalo. The mouse strains used included H-2^d-BALB/c, DBA/2, B10.D2; H-2^k-C3H, CBA, BALB.K; H-2^b C57BL/10, C57BL/6, BALB.B; H-2^q-DBA/1, B10.Q; H-2^s-SJL, B10.S. The human cells were peripheral blood lymphocytes derived from 7 randomly chosen volunteers. + Signifies greater than 60% lysis of target cells. +/− Signifies 20–60% lysis of target cells. Different reactivity patterns (RP) were assigned arbitrarily to those antibodies which gave differing patterns of lysis on this panel of cells.

targets, but we do not, as yet, have any direct measure of the relative avidities or affinities of these hybridoma antibodies.

The data on cross-reactive specificities was then pursued further by asking whether these hybridoma antibodies would lyse murine lymphoid cells. Table IV shows that 5 of 9 hybridomas do, indeed, lyse lymphoid cells from various mouse strains and that the pattern of lysis seen may either be nonpolymorphic (e.g., D4,37) or polymorphic (e.g., N2.11.6). The nonpolymorphic reactivity of D4,37 for murine lymphoid cells has now been verified on over 35 mouse strains, including several H-2 mutant mice and several wild mice. We therefore cannot assign by genetic analysis the determinant being recognized in the mouse by hybridoma D4,37.

The antibodies against polymorphic determinants, on the other hand, all can be assigned reactivity against H-2-encoded determinants by using the appropriate congenic partners. Thus, as shown in Table IV, hybridoma N2.11.6 fails to lyse C57BL/10 cells but does lyse cells from DBA/2 and the congenic strain B10.D2, implying reactivity against the MHC-encoded determinants of H-2^d. Additional data directed toward this same point were obtained, using MHC congenic mice on a BALB/c background where N2.11.6 showed lysis of BALB/c but not the MHC congenic strains BALB.B (H-2^b) or BALB.K (H-2^k).

A further evaluation of reactivity to subregions of the H-2 complex were then undertaken using H-2 recombinant mice (Table V). These studies showed that the determinants detected by K2.3.17 and N2.11.6 mapped to the left end of the H-2 complex. When positive these antibodies gave 100% lysis of either unstimulated murine lymph node cells or Con A blasts and, moreover, were

TABLE V
Cytotoxic Patterns on Selected Mouse Strains[a]

	H-2 subregions									Hybridoma			
	K	IA	IB	IJ	IE	IC	S	G	D	D4,37	K2.3.17	N2.11.6	P3/X63
DBA/2	d	d	d	d	d	d	d	d	d	+	+	+	−
B10.D2	d	d	d	d	d	d	d	d	d	+	+	+	−
C3H.0L	d	d	d	d	d	d	k	k	k	+	+	+	−
D2.GD	d	d	b	b	b	b	b	b	b	+	+	+	−
A/J	k	k	k	k	k	d	d	d	d	+	+	−	−
B10.A(4R)	k	k	b	b	b	b	b	b	b	+	+	−	−
A.TL	s	k	k	k	k	k	k	k	d	+	−	−	−
B10.A(5R)	b	b	b	k	k	d	d	d	d	+	−	−	−
C57BL/10	b	b	b	b	b	b	b	b	b	+	−	−	−

[a]Cytotoxic cross-reactivity patterns on selected mouse strains including H-2 congenic and H-2 recombinant mice. The *H-2* subregion assignments are according to Klein *et al.* (1978).

reactive with the appropriate erythrocytes in the PVP hemagglutination assay (D. Shreffler, personal communication). These antibodies therefore are probably cross-reactive with Class I molecules in the mouse and may well define some previously unrecognized patterns of cross-reactivity both between rat and mouse and between various mouse strains. The implication of such cross-reactivities will be discussed below.

Since several of these rat anti-MHC hybridomas were cross-reactive with *H-2*-encoded determinants, it seemed reasonable to ask whether such hybridoma antibodies might not also detect MHC determinants on cells from other species such as human. Table IV shows that 4 of 9 hybridomas are reactive with peripheral blood lymphocytes from randomly chosen humans in a complement-mediated cytotoxicity assay. As noted previously with murine cells, hybridoma D4,37 reacts in a nonpolymorphic fashion with all members of this small panel and, upon further testing, has lysed peripheral blood lymphocytes from over 100 consecutive humans (C. Zmijewski, personal communication). Hybridoma D4,37, however, fails to lyse both the Daudi cell line and human erythrocytes (data not shown), both of which are known to lack HLA-A, -B, and -C determinants.

The other positive hybridoma antibodies lyse cells from this panel in a polymorphic fashion and tend, as noted before, to give "all-or-none" lysis on the various target cells. Much larger panels of cells, including cells from selected family members, will be required in order to determine genetically whether the determinants detected by these hybridomas are linked to the *HLA* locus.

The combined cytotoxicity data from rats, mice, and humans (Table IV) portray better the overall reactivity patterns of these monoclonal antibodies. In fact, by using the strategy of reactivity pattern analysis as described by Cancro *et al.* (1978), one can argue that those monoclonal antibodies which differ in their reactivity on this panel of cells represent different antibody specificities. The reactivity pattern therefore becomes a rapid and powerful means for analyzing the fine specificity of these monoclonal antibodies. From the data shown here, one would conclude that these 9 hybridoma antibodies represent a minimum of 8 antibody specificities. Clearly therefore the B-cell response to MHC alloantigens as reflected in this small collection of hybridoma antibodies is not highly restricted, and in fact the overall anti-MHC B-cell repertoire may be quite diverse. The degree of that diversity and the manner in which it is generated are critical considerations for those models of the immune system which postulate sharing of B- and T-cell idiotypes specific for MHC alloantigens.

The biological properties of selected hybridoma antibodies have been studied both *in vitro* and *in vivo* and the results of these studies have been published (McKearn *et al.* 1978, 1979a,b). In brief, we have not succeeded in blocking the primary mixed lymphocyte reaction (MLR) with these hybridoma antibodies. This perhaps was to be expected, since these antibodies react with Class I MHC determinants, while Class II MHC determinants generally function as the major stimulus in the primary MLR (Bach *et al.*, 1977).

Certain of the hybridoma antibodies (e.g., D4,37) are capable of blocking the cytolytic activity of allogeneic killer T cells in a 6-hr cell-mediated lympholysis (CML) assay (McKearn *et al.*, 1979a). However, the degree of inhibition seen with D4,37 in this assay can vary remarkably from one experiment to another, which perhaps suggests that there may be substantial day-to-day variation in the number and/or proportion of killer T cells which are specific for the determinants recognized by D4,37. Further studies in this area are clearly needed before any firm conclusions are warranted.

More compelling evidence for biological effectiveness of these monoclonal antibodies has come from studies of primary antibody responses and suppression of renal allograft rejection. Table VI summarizes the findings in these two systems. Significant suppression of both primary antibody responses and renal allograft rejection were seen with hybridoma antibody D4,68. The specificity of such suppressed reactivity was ascertained by showing that Lewis animals injected with D4,68 mounted normal serum antibody responses following chal-

Table VI

Effect of Hybridoma Antibodies on Primary Antibody Responses and Renal Allograft Rejection[a]

	Suppression of primary anti-BN antibody responses	Suppression of L/BN renal allograft rejection
D4,37	−	−
D4,68	+	+
D4,69	−	−
K2.3.17	+	+ (2/3)
K2.13.2	+	+ (1/3)
N2.9.2	−	n.d.
N2.11.6	−	n.d.
N2.27.30	+	n.d.
N2.54.3	−	n.d.

[a]Effect of hybridoma antibodies on primary antibody responses and renal allograft rejection. Details of the experimental design and controls are found in references (McKearn *et al.*, 1978, 1979a,b).

lenge with ACI (AgB-4) cells. Moreover, animals pretreated with D4,68 and F_1 antigen in the manner which optimizes the suppression of HBN renal allograft rejection, rejected an L/ACI renal allograft in normal fashion.

Two additional antibodies (K2.3.17 and K2.13.2) caused suppression of the primary antibody response and induced some degree of suppression of renal allograft rejection. Likewise, antibody N2.27.30 suppressed serum antibody responses. However, the effect on renal allograft rejection is not yet known. The remaining antibodies were ineffective in suppressing primary antibody responses and, in those cases tested, were also unable to induce renal allograft enhancement.

Although more data are required to firmly establish the point, it appears that a correlation does exist between the ability of a given monoclonal antibody to suppress primary antibody responses and to induce renal allograft enhancement. It is worth noting that the "effective" antibodies (D4,68, K2.3.17, K2.13.2, and N2.27.30) differ from one another in both heavy-chain class and reactivity pattern (Tables I and IV). Moreover, preliminary data using rabbit antiidiotypic antibodies specific for D4,68 fail to detect any cross-reactive idiotypic determinants on these other hybridomas (T. McKearn, unpublished data).

It appears therefore that antibodies differing in heavy-chain class, antibody specificity, and (perhaps) idiotypic specificities are capable of inducing suppression. We are currently pursuing the question of determinant mapping as a final reasonable parameter, which could be an important indicator of the ability of antibody to induce suppression, i.e., it is possible that the most important factor in inducing suppression is the binding of a monoclonal antibody to a particular antigenic determinant on the allogeneic cell. If this is so, then it follows that there must be some hierarchy of allogeneic MHC determinants recognized by the responder animal and that only certain of these determinants will trigger an antibody response and/or allograft rejection.

C. Discussion

The application of hybridoma technology to studies of rat MHC have permitted significant new approaches toward understanding the structure and function of this important gene complex. The latter portion of this chapter has reviewed our findings with 9 monoclonal antibodies selected for their reactivity against MHC determinants of the BN (AgB-3) haplotype.

Such antibodies show various patterns of cross-reactivity with *H-2*-encoded determinants in the mouse and with certain cell-surface antigenic determinants in man. In the case of antibody D4,37, the reactivity on allogeneic rat cells is polymorphic (AgB-1 and AgB-5 are not detected). However, reactivity of D4,37 against murine and human cells is nonpolymorphic. If we may assume for the sake of argument that the determinant seen by D4,37 in mouse and man is in fact an MHC determinant, then these data imply that certain MHC determinants can be widely conserved in nature, suggesting, perhaps, that these determinants are involved in some important physiologic function served by the MHC. One cannot conclude that this particular determinant is required for survival, however, since Ag-B1 and Ag-B5 animals both lack this determinant. Such data suggest that after speciation the AgB-1 and AgB-5 rats developed a mutation of the determinant recognized by D4,37 and now either lack this particular region or perhaps more likely, have evolved an alternative (allelic?) determinant.

It is of some interest to note that Brodsky et al. (1979) have also found certain of their BALB/c anti-HLA hybridoma antibodies to cross-react with lymphoid cells from lower primates. Anti-MHC hybridoma antibodies prepared either by alloimmunization or xenoimmunization therefore may show a surprising degree of interspecies cross-reactivity.

The cross-reactivity patterns of the other hybridoma antibodies pose additional interesting problems. These patterns of cross-reactivity on allogeneic rat strains define two new MHC determinants (D4,37 and K2.13.2) and confirm one previously reported pattern of cross-reactivity between AgB-3 and AgB-5 (D4, 68 and D4,69) (29) (Gunther and Stark, 1977). It is perhaps more intriguing to note the cross-reactivity patterns on mouse cells where H-2^d is the most frequently cross-reactive murine haplotype. This is rather unexpected since the parental plasmacytoma cell lines (P3/X63-Ag8 or SP-2/0-Ag14) display H-2^d surface antigens. These hybridoma antibodies are indeed cytotoxic for both the parental mutant myeloma cell lines and BALB/c lymphoid cells which rules out the possibility that they are reactive with some previously undescribed H-2^d determinant which is lacking from BALB/c. Moreover, if one adds rabbit complement alone to several of these hybridoma cell lines that produce anti-H-2^d antibody, the hybridoma cells are lysed, thus establishing that the hybridoma cells are secreting a cytotoxic antibody that reacts with a "self" membrane component. Perhaps the most reasonable explanation for such antibody activity is to assume that Ag-B3 and H-2^d are cross-reactive in an immunized Lewis rat. Experiments designed to test this prediction are currently underway.

The use of reactivity pattern analysis to sort the antibody specificities of these monoclonal antibodies has permitted a rapid assessment of the degree of B-cell heterogeneity in this response to MHC alloantigens. Clearly, more data are needed in order to arrive at a reasonable estimate of the diversity of the antibody response to MHC alloantigens, but even these preliminary results suggest strongly that the response is not highly restricted. If this proves to be the case and B-cell responses to MHC antigens are quite diverse, how does one account for observed sharing of idiotypic specificities between B and T cells? Is it necessary to postulate the existence of a population of T-cell idiotypes equal in number to the B-cell repertoire or is the number of T-cell idiotypes much smaller? From a different perspective, can one identify "germline" vs "somatically generated" B-cell idiotypes, and is there an equivalent degree of representation of these two groups of idiotypes on T cells? Finally, if the generation of T-cell diversity is critically dependent on the interaction of MHC antigens within the thymus (von Boehmer et al., 1978), is B-cell reactivity to MHC alloantigens also affected by the thymus or by T cells which have matured in a particular thymic microenvironment?

The studies on enhancement of renal allografts with hybridoma antibodies provide the first demonstration *in vivo,* wherein a monoclonal alloantibody induced a state of life-long immunological suppression. They also provide compelling evidence that passively administered alloantibodies against Class I MHC determinants are fully capable of inducing a state of immunological enhancement. This does not rule out the possibility that monoclonal alloantibodies reactive with Class II MHC determinants might also be capable of inducing enhancement, and we are currently pursuing the derivation of such hybridomas in order to test this possibility.

The mechanisms whereby monoclonal alloantibodies induce immunological enhancement are currently obscure. As mentioned above, those three hybridoma antibodies which to date have shown some degree of suppression of renal allograft rejection differ from one another in terms of antibody specificities, heavy-chain isotypes, and idiotypic specificities. It is difficult to envision therefore, how any of these three factors could alone predominate as the single most important prognostic indicator of an "effective" enhancing antibody. Indeed, the observation that several of these hybridoma antibodies will induce some degree of enhancement and the apparent correlation of this enhancing property with the ability of these hybridomas to suppress primary antibody responses suggests that there may be multiple pathways by which one can arrive at the same immunological endpoint.

Acknowledgments

We are indebted to Drs. G. Köhler, C. Milstein, R. Kennett, and M. Scharff for providing us with cell lines for use in these studies. It is a pleasure to acknowledge the stimulating discussions and suggestions from our colleagues both in Chicago and Philadelphia, which have greatly benefited these studies. The excellent technical assistance of F. Buckingham, C. Buettger, L. Decker, Y. Hamada, M. Neu, and L. Ziegenfus is gratefully acknowledged.

This research was supported by U.S. Public Health Service grants AI-09268, AI-10961, CA-09140, CA-15822, and CA-20091; U.S. Public Health Service contract NCI-CB-74149-31; and a grant from the Leukemia Research Foundation.

References

Bach, F. H., Grillot-Courvalin, C., Kuperman, O. J., Sollinger, H. W., Hayes, C., Sondel, P. M., Alter, B. J., and Bach, M. L., 1977, Antigenic requirements for triggering of cytotoxic T lymphocytes, *Immunol. Rev.* **35**:76.

Bazin, H., Beckers, A., and Querinjean, P., 1974, Three classes and four (sub)classes of rat immunoglobulins: IgM, IgA, IgE and IgG1, IgG2a, IgG2b, IgG2c, *Eur. J. Immunol.* **4**:44.

Benacerraf, B., and Germain, R. N., 1978, The immune response genes of the major histocompatibility complex, *Immunol. Rev.* **38**:70.

Binz, H., and Wigzell, H., 1975, Shared idiotypic determinants on T and B cells reactive against the same antigenic determinants, *J. Exp. Med.* **142**:197.

von Boehmer, H., Hass, H., and Jerne, N. K., 1978, Major histocompatibility complex-linked immune-responsiveness is acquired by lymphocytes of low-responder mice differentiating in thymus of high-responder mice, *Proc. Natl. Acad. Sci. USA* **75**:2439.

Brodsky, F. M., Parham, P., Barnstable, C. J., Crumpton, M.J., and Bodmer, W. F., 1979, Monoclonal antibodies for analysis of the HLA system, *Immunol. Rev.* **47**:1.

Butcher, G. W., and Howard, J. C., 1977, A recombinant in the major histocompatibility complex of the rat, *Nature* **266**:362.

Cancro, M. P., Gerhard, W., and Klinman, N. K., 1978, The diversity of the influenza-specific B-cell repertoire in BALB/c mice, *J. Exp. Med.* **147**:776.

Davis, D. A. L., and Alkins, B. J., 1974, What abrogates heart transplant rejection in immunological enhancement? *Nature* **247**:294.

Doherty, P. C., Blanden, R. V., and Zinkernagel, R. M., 1976, Specificity of virus-immune effector T cells for H-2K compabtible interactions: Implications for H-antigen diversity, *Transplant. Rev.* **29**:89.

Gomez, C. M., Richman, D. P., Berman, P. W., Bemes, S. A., Arnason, B. G. W., and Fitch, F. W., 1979, Monoclonal antibodies against purified nicotinic acetylcholine receptor, *Biochem. Biophys. Res. Commun.* **88**:575.

Greene, L., Fitch, F. W., and Jensen, E. V., 1980, Monoclonal antibodies to estrophilin: A new approach to the study of estrogen receptors, *Proc. Natl. Acad. Sci. USA* **77**:157.

Gunther, E., and Stark, O., 1977, The major histocompatibility system of the rat (Ag-B or H-1 system), in: *The Major Histocompatibility System in Man and Animals* (D. Gotze, ed.), Springer-Verlag, New York, p. 207.

Gutman, G. A., and Weissman, I. L., 1977, Inheritance and strain distribution of a rat immunoglobulin allotype, *J. Immunol.* **107**:1390.

Howard, J. C., Butcher, G. W., Galfrè, G., and Milstein, G., 1978, Monoclonal anti-rat MHC (H-1) alloantibodies, *Curr. Top. Microbiol. Immunol.* **81**:54.

Hudson, L., and Sprent, J., 1976, Specific adsorption of IgM antibody onto H-2 activated mouse T lymphocytes, *J. Exp. Med.* **143**:44.

Jerne, N. K., 1974, Towards a network theory of the immune system, *Ann. Immunol. (Paris)* **125c**:373.

Jones, J. M., Peter, H. H., and Feldman, J. D., 1972, Binding *in vivo* of enhancing antibodies to skin allografts and specific allogeneic tissues, *J. Immunol.* **108**:301.

Kennett, R. H., Denis, K. A., Tung, A., and Klinman, N. R., 1978, Hybrid plasmacytoma production: Fusions with adult spleen cells, monoclonal spleen fragments, neonatal spleen cells and human spleen cells, *Curr. Top. Microbiol. Immunol.* **81**:77.

Klein, J., 1977, Evolution and function of the major histocompatibility system: Facts and speculations, in: *The Major Histocompatibility System in Man and Animals* (D. Gotze, ed.), Springer-Verlag, New York, p. 339.

Klein, J., and Park, J. M., 1973, Graft-vs-host reaction across different regions of the H-2 complex of the mouse, *J. Exp. Med.* **137**:1213.

Klein, J., Flaherty, L., Van de Berg, J. L., and Shreffler, D. C., 1978, H-2 haplotypes, genes, regions and antigens: First listing, *Immunogenetics* **6**:489.

McKearn, T. J., 1974, Antireceptor antiserum causes specific inhibition of reactivity to rat histocompatibility antigens, *Science* **183**:94.

McKearn, T. J., Sarmiento, M., Weiss, A., Stuart, F. P., and Fitch, F. W., 1978, Suppression of reactivity to rat histocompatibility antigens by monoclonal antibody, *Curr. Top. Microbiol. Immunol.* **81**:61.

McKearn, T. J., Fitch, F. W., Smilek, D. E., Sarmiento, M., and Stuart, F. P., 1979a, Properties of rat anti-MHC antibodies produced by cloned rat–mouse hybridomas, *Immunol. Rev.* **47**:91.

McKearn, T. J., Weiss, A., Stuart, F. P., and Fitch, F. W., 1979b, Selective suppression of humoral and cell-mediated immune responses to rat alloantigens by monoclonal antibodies produced by hybridoma cell lines, *Transplant. Proc.* **11**:932.

Nabholz, M., Vives, J., Young, H. M., Meo, T., Miggiano, V., Rijnbeek, A., and Shreffler, D. C., 1974,

Cell-mediated cell lysis *in vitro:* Genetic control of killer cell production and target specificities in the mouse, *Eur. J. Immunol.* **4:**378.

Niederhuber, J. E., 1978, The role of I region gene products in macrophage–T lymphocyte interaction, *Immunol. Rev.* **40:**28.

Ramseier, H., 1974, Spontaneous release of T-cell receptors for alloantigens. I. Reconition of alloantigens and receptor release dynamics, *J. Exp. Med.* **140:**603.

Rowley, D. A., 1950, The effect of splenectomy on the formation of circulating antibody in the adult male albino rat, *J. Immunol.* **64:**289.

Severson, C. D., and Thompson, J. S., 1966, Quantitative semi-micro hemagglutination, *J. Immunol.* **96:**785.

Soulillou, J.-P., Carpenter, C. B., d'Apice, A. J. F., and Strom, T. B., 1976, The role of nonclassical, Fc receptor-associated Ag-B antigens (Ia) in rat allograft enhancement, *J. Exp. Med.* **143:**405.

Stark, O., Gunther, E., Kohoutova, M., and Vojcik, L., 1977, Genetic recombination in the major histocompatibility complex (H-1, Ag-B) of the rat, *Immunogenetics* **5:**183.

Stuart, F. P., Saitoh, T., and Fitch, F. W., 1968, Rejection of renal allografts: Specific immunological suppression, *Science* **160:**1463.

Tada, T., Taniguchi, M., and David, C. S., 1977, Suppressive and enhancing T-cell factors as I-region gene products: Properties and the subregion assignment, *Cold Spring Harbor Symp. Quant. Biol.* **41:**119.

Taussig, M. J., Corvalan, J. R. F., Binns, R. M., and Holliman, A., 1979, Production of an H-2-related suppressor factor by a hybrid T-cell line, *Nature* **277:**305.

14
Murine T-Cell Differentiation Antigens Detected by Monoclonal Antibodies

JEFFREY A. LEDBETTER, JAMES W. GODING,
TAKESHI TOKUHISA, AND LEONARD A. HERZENBERG

I. Introduction

Monoclonal antibodies can now be produced in unlimited quantities by making "hybridomas" (Köhler and Milstein, 1975). These antibodies introduced a new era in serology, making it possible to distinguish single antigenic specificities among a complex array of antigens. Monoclonal antibodies have been used to discover new antigenic specificities on the surface of lymphoid cells of rats and mice (Williams *et al.*, 1977; Springer *et al.*, 1978a,b; Ledbetter and Herzenberg, 1979; Stern *et al.*, 1978; Trowbridge, 1978), and to characterize biochemically many of the molecules that express these antigens. In other cases monoclonal antibodies have made it possible to distinguish multiple antigenic sites on complex molecules. For example, using monoclonal antibodies, five allotypic sites have been defined and located on mouse IgG2a heavy chain (Oi and Herzenberg, 1979a,b). Similarly, two allotypic sites on mouse immunoglobulin D (IgD) have been located with monoclonal antibodies (Goding, 1980).

In this chapter, we describe a series of monoclonal antibodies that recognize T-lymphocyte surface antigens. These antibodies were produced by immunization of LOU/Ws1/M rats with mouse spleen or thymus cells, followed by fusion of the rat spleen with the myeloma parental line NS1. Xenogeneic immunizations were used because of the potential of detecting both polymorphic and

JEFFREY A. LEDBETTER, JAMES W. GODING, TAKESHI TOKUHISA, AND LEONARD A. HERZEN-
BERG • Department of Genetics, Stanford University School of Medicine, Stanford, California
94305.

nonpolymorphic antigens. We chose for detailed study those antibodies that react with differentiation antigens of T cells. Monoclonal antibodies that are described here recognize the previously known T-cell differentiation antigens Thy-1, Lyt-1, and Lyt-2 plus two previously undescribed T-cell differentiation antigens.

For all of the monoclonal antibodies in the series, we present fluorescence-activated cell sorter (FACS) analysis showing the distribution of the target antigens on lymphoid subpopulations. For those antibodies that precipitate detectable amounts of glycoproteins from NP-40 detergent extracts of surface-labeled cells, we show two-dimensional (2D) gel characterization of charge, size, and subunit structure of the target antigens. In addition, we present functional studies using fluorescence-activated cell sorting with one of our monoclonal antibodies, demonstrating the presence of Lyt-2 determinants on the T cells that exhibit allotype suppressive activity (Herzenberg et al., 1975).

II. Detection and Analysis of Monoclonal Antibodies Reactive with Cell-Surface Antigens

The initial fusions were performed according to the procedures of Oi et al. (1978) and Oi and Herzenberg (1979a) using 1:1 ratios of NS1 myeloma cells to spleen cells from rats that had been immunized i.p. with 10^7 mouse thymus or spleen cells and boosted with an equal number of cells 4 weeks later. Three days after the boost, cells were fused and plated into a 96-well plate (Costar # 3596, Division of Dynatech Laboratories, Alexandria, Virginia) at 10^6 cells/well. Growing hybrids were detected in every well within 15 days.

Our strategy for isolating hybrid clones depends on using the FACS both to identify wells containing hybrids that produce antibodies that bind to thymic or splenic subpopulations and to rapidly clone hybrids from positive initial wells (Parks et al., 1979) before the desired hybrids are overgrown by other cells in the well. Examples of FACS staining profiles of supernates from three positive wells of the initial culture dish are shown in Fig. 1. The bound monoclonal antibodies are revealed by "second-step" staining with a fluorescein-conjugated mouse (SJL/J) anti-rat IgG. We used this second-step reagent to avoid cross-reaction with mouse Ig. Antibodies that were obtained from the wells shown in Fig. 1 were later found to be detecting the lymphocyte differentiation antigens Lyt-1, Lyt-2, and Thy-1.2 (see Sections III and IV).

After the identification of positive initial wells, we used a new modification of the FACS to clone viable hybrids into microtiter plates containing mouse thymocytes as feeder cells (Parks et al., 1979). This allowed rapid cloning from each well and avoided overgrowth of the desired hybrid by other cells. The FACS with this cloning modification deposits one cell in each well of a cloning plate, thus avoiding the problems associated with limiting dilution or soft agar cloning of hybrids.

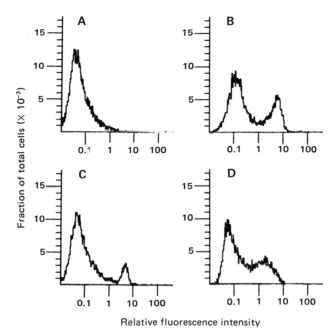

FIGURE 1. Immunofluorescent staining of C3H/HeJ spleen cells with supernates from initial hybrid wells. After reaction with hybrid supernates, bound antibody was detected by reaction with FITC-conjugated second-step antibody (SJL/J anti-Rat Ig). (A) Background staining with second step only. (B) Monoclonal antibody 30-H12 (anti-Thy-1.2). (C) Monoclonal antibody 53-6.7 (anti-Lyt-2). (D) Monoclonal antibody 53-7.3 (anti-Lyt-1). Stained cells were analyzed using the FACS-II with a logarithmic amplifier.

Screening for antibody in supernatants from hybrid cells with fluorescence staining provided the major assay system for detection of antibody activity. Positive supernatants were also tested by radioimmune binding, cytotoxicity, and immunoprecipitation; however, these assays were less reliable for detection of antibodies reactive with subpopulations of lymphocytes. The reactivities of the antibodies in these assays are summarized in Table I.

Immunoprecipitation and 2D gel analysis provided a second major assay system for characterizing target determinants. All but one of the monoclonal antibodies described here reacted with cell-surface glycoproteins that were detected by immunoprecipitations from NP40 extracts of cells that were surface-labeled with ^{125}I using the lactoperoxidase technique. Immunoprecipitated proteins were characterized by 2D gel electrophoresis, a system that separates proteins based upon charge-dependent migration properties in the first dimension and size-dependent migration in the second dimension. We used nonequilibrium pH gradient electrophoresis (NEPHGE) in the first dimension to resolve basic as well as acidic proteins and 10% SDS gels in the second dimension (O'Farrell, 1975; O'Farrell et al., 1977).

TABLE I

Rat Monoclonal Antibodies to Mouse Cell-Surface Antigens

Antibody	Target antigen	H-chain isotype[a]	Cyto-toxicity	RIA[b]	Protein A binding[c]	FACS analysis[d]				
						Spleen (%)	T	B	Thymus (%)	Bone marrow (%)
30-H12	Thy-1.2	IgG2b	+	29	−	37	+	−	>97	<1
53-2.1	Thy-1.2	IgG2a	+	34	+/−	39	+	−	>98	<1
53-3.1	Thy-1	IgM	+	18	−	37	+	−	>98	<1
53-8.1	T-30[e]	IgG2c	+	6.9	+	30	+	−	>97	<1
53-7.3	Lyt-1	IgG2a	+/−	6.2	−	35	+	−	>98	<1
53-6.7	Lyt-2	IgG2a	+/−	9.0	+/−	11	+	−	90	<1
53-5.8	Lyt-2	IgG1	−	8.4	−	10	+	−	89	<1
30-H11[e]	—	IgG2b	+	3.7	−	43	+	−	>96	49

[a]Determined by double diffusion with class-specific antisera (Miles).
[b]Radioimmune binding is expressed as specific binding/background assayed on thymocyte membranes.
[c]Determined by reactivity of the antibodies with [^{125}I]Protein A in radioimmune assays.
[d]Determined by fluorescence staining and analysis using the FACS II.
[e]Previously undescribed (see text).

Figure 2 shows the 2D gel pattern of total thymocyte-surface proteins and surface glycoproteins that were specifically precipitated by one of the monoclonal antibodies (30-H12) that recognizes Thy-1.2. In the sections that follow we present some detailed studies using individual monoclonal antibodies to investigate the expression and biochemical properties of target antigens. The first sections describe characteristics of Thy-1, Lyt-1, and Lyt-2. The last section is concerned with two previously unknown T-cell-differentiation antigens.

III. Two Antigenic Specificities of Mouse Thy-1 Recognized by Monoclonal Antibodies

The Thy-1 antigen, discovered by Reif and Allen (1964), is expressed on thymocytes and thymus-dependent cells in the spleen but is absent on bone marrow cells. It also is expressed on brain cells, epithelial cells, and fibroblasts (Barclay *et al.*, 1976; Hilgers *et al.*, 1975; Scheid *et al.*, 1972; Stern, 1973). Two Thy-1 alloantigenic determinants, Thy-1.1 and Thy-1.2 are known in mice. These are coded for by alleles of the *Thy-1* locus on chromosome 9 (Itakura *et al.*, 1972, 1974; Blankenhorn and Douglas, 1972). Thy-1.1 antigenic determinants have also been detected on rat thymocytes with mouse alloantisera, but Thy-1.2 antigenic determinants have not been seen in any rat strains (Douglas, 1972; Williams, 1977).

Thy-1 has been purified from both rat brain and rat thymus and character-

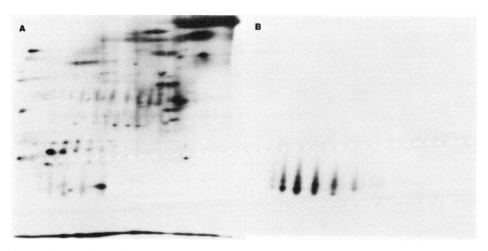

Figure 2. Two-dimensional gel electrophoresis of cell-surface glycoproteins immunoprecipitated with a monoclonal rat antibody from NP40 extracts of [125I]lactoperoxidase-labeled BALB/c thymocytes. (A) Total 125I-labeled thymocyte proteins; (B) Immunoprecipitate using antibody 30-H12 (anti-Thy-1.2). The first dimension separations were by NEPHGE (acidic proteins are on the right and basic proteins are on the left). The second-dimension separations were by SDS-PAGE on 10% gels (from top to bottom).

ized biochemically (Letarte-Muirhead et al., 1974; Barclay et al., 1975). Two forms of rat thymocyte Thy-1 were identified on the basis of ability to bind to lentil lectin affinity columns. The lentil lectin binding form was a glycoprotein of 25,000 daltons. Rat brain Thy-1 was found to differ from both of these forms in molecular weight and was a glycoprotein of 24,000 daltons.

Amino acid and carbohydrate composition studies of the three forms of rat Thy-1 have been reported (Barclay et al., 1976). These studies indicated that the amino acid compositions are very similar for all three; however, the carbohydrate compositions were markedly different for brain Thy-1 as opposed to either form of thymocyte Thy-1. Smaller carbohydrate differences between thymocyte lentil lectin binding and nonbinding Thy-1 also were apparent. Thus in the rat, the brain and thymus forms of Thy-1 appear to have the same polypeptide chain associated with different carbohydrate structures.

Mouse Thy-1 antigenic determinants are on a 25,000-dalton glycoprotein similar to the rat molecule. Trowbridge et al. (1975) used antiserum against rat brain that cross-reacts with mouse Thy-1.1 to immunoprecipitate a 25,000-dalton species from mouse thymocytes that were labeled metabolically with radioactive sugars or by 125I with the lactoperoxidase technique. Several reports have suggested that Thy-1 determinants are expressed on glycolipids (Miller and Esselman, 1975; Wang et al., 1978). The monoclonal antibodies we produced, which have staining and cytotoxic properties indistinguishable from conventional anti-Thy-1, precipitate a family of thymocyte glycoproteins with molecular weights of 25,000–30,000 that have biochemical properties very similar to rat

Thy-1. We have not yet examined glycolipids for reactivity with our monoclonal Thy-1 antibodies.

Our monoclonal Thy-1 antibodies identify at least two antigenic determinants on mouse Thy-1. One antibody (30-H12) is specific for a Thy-1.2 antigenic determinant. It stains AKR/Cu (Thy-1.2) thymocytes and immunoprecipitates a glycoprotein from these thymocytes, but it is unreactive with thymocytes from a congenic strain (AKR/J) carrying the Thy-1.1 allele. A second antibody (53-3.1) identifies a framework (nonpolymorphic) determinant on both Thy-1.1 and Thy-1.2 but not on rat Thy-1. This distinction between rat and mouse Thy-1 confirms previous data from absorption studies with conventional xenogencic antisera showing that mouse and rat Thy-1 each have distinct antigenic determinants (Clagett et al., 1973; Thiele et al., 1972; Morris and Williams, 1975).

The 2D gel pattern of Thy-1 immunoprecipitated from thymocytes (Fig. 2) was obtained with the 30-H12 monoclonal antibody and is identical to patterns obtained with all other anti-Thy-1 antibodies in the series. It shows a family of proteins of 25,000–30,000 daltons with extensive charge and size heterogeneity. Neuraminidase digestions of whole thymocyte extracts (Fig. 3) show that the charge heterogeneity of Thy-1 is caused by variable amounts of terminal sialic acid on the glycoprotein. The size heterogeneity of Thy-1 is most likely due to variable amounts of neutral sugars, since the series of Thy-1 glycoproteins are divided based on size into a lentil lectin binding fraction (25,000 daltons) and a

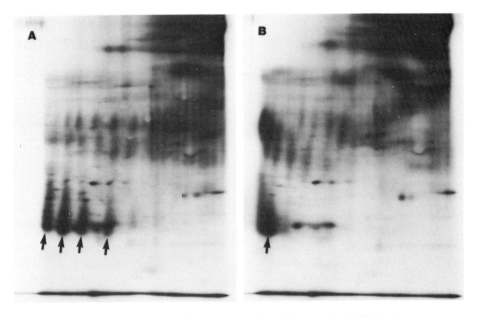

FIGURE 3. Neuraminidase digestion of thymocyte-surface glycoproteins. BALB/c thymocytes were labeled with ^{125}I using the lactoperoxidase technique and then extracted with 0.5% NP40. (A) ^{125}I-labeled thymocyte glycoproteins before neuraminidase digestion; (B) ^{125}I-labeled thymocyte glycoproteins after neuraminidase digestion. The arrows in each panel point to the Thy-1 glycoprotein. Autoradiographs of the 2D gels are positioned as described in the legend to Fig. 2.

lentil lectin nonbinding fraction (26,000–30,000 daltons; see Fig. 4). These data demonstrate that mouse Thy-1, like rat (Williams, 1977), most likely consists of a single polypeptide chain with heterogeneity in its glycosylation. Note that the lentil lectin binding forms of mouse thymocyte Thy-1 migrate with an apparently smaller molecular weight on sodium dodecyl sulfate (SDS) gels compared to the lentil lectin nonbinding forms (Fig. 4). Therefore the ability of Thy-1 to bind to lentil lectin does not appear to be directly related to its degree of glycosylation.

IV. Characterization of Lyt-1 and Lyt-2 Glycoproteins with Monoclonal Antibodies

Three T-lymphocyte differentiation antigens, Lyt-1, Lyt-2, and Lyt-3, have been described using conventional cytotoxic alloantisera (Boyse et al., 1968; 1971). Genetic mapping studies indicated that the *Lyt-1* locus is on mouse chromosome 19 (Itakura et al., 1974) and that the *Lyt-2* and *Lyt-3* loci are closely linked to each other on mouse chromosome 6 (Itakura et al., 1972). Two alleles are known at each locus, e.g., *Lyt-1.1*, *Lyt-1.2*. The identification of the Lyt-1, Lyt-2 and Lyt-3 alloantigens is currently based upon the presence of cell-surface determinants of Lyt congenic pairs of the C57BL/6 background (Shen et al., 1976).

Functional subclasses of T lymphocytes have been identified based on their differential expression of Lyt antigens (Cantor and Boyse, 1975a,b). T cells that

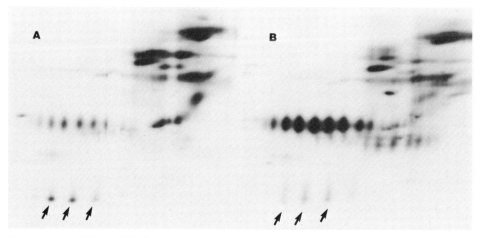

FIGURE 4. Lentil lectin binding and nonbinding surface glycoproteins. C57BL/6 EL4 cells were surface ^{125}I-labeled with the lactoperoxidase technique and extracted with 0.5% NP40. The cell lysate was then separated into binding and nonbinding fractions using lentil lectin–Sepharose. (A) Lentil lectin bound glycoproteins. (B) Lentil lectin nonbound glycoproteins. The arrows in each panel point to the Thy-1 glycoprotein. Autoradiographs of the 2D gels are positioned as described in the legend to Fig. 2.

demonstrate suppressor activity and T cells with cytotoxic killer activity (Cantor and Boyse, 1975a; Cantor *et al.*, 1976; Beverley *et al.*, 1976; Herzenberg *et al.*, 1976) are killed by anti-Lyt-2 serum but not by anti-Lyt-1 serum. Cells with phenotype Lyt-1$^+$2$^+$3$^+$ appear to be mainly precursors of the above subsets (Huber *et al.*, 1976) although there are several examples where cytotoxic killer T cells have been removed by cytotoxic treatment with either anti-Lyt-1 or anti-Lyt-2,3 (Beverley *et al.*, 1976; Shiku *et al.*, 1975).

The target antigens of the conventional anti-Lyt antisera have been biochemically characterized by immunoprecipitation from detergent extracts of thymocytes that were ^{125}I-labeled by the lactoperoxidase technique. Anti-Lyt-1 antisera precipitated a 67,000-dalton glycoprotein and a glycoprotein of 87,000 daltons that could be labeled with [^{3}H$_4$]NaB and galactose oxidase but not with the [^{125}I]lactoperoxidase method (Durda *et al.*, 1978). The Lyt-2 and Lyt-3 antigens were found on cell-surface glycoproteins labeled with the [^{125}I]lactoperoxidase method (Durda and Gottleib, 1976). Immune precipitations with anti-Lyt-3 serum showed a 35,000-dalton protein on SDS gels. Anti-Lyt-2 serum also immunoprecipitated a 35,000-dalton protein. It is not yet clear whether Lyt-2 and Lyt-3 antigens are expressed on the same or different proteins.

The data presented here using monoclonal antibodies confirm and extend the findings with conventional sera. The 2D gel analysis of immunoprecipitates with antibodies to Lyt-1 and Lyt-2 shows the charge, molecular weight, and subunit structure of the lymphocyte-surface molecule carrying these determinants. Comparative 2D gel immunoprecipitation studies with C57BL/6 Ly congenic strains show that our monoclonal Lyt-1 and Lyt-2 antibodies precipitate the same molecular species as conventional Ly alloantisera (Ledbetter and Herzenberg, 1979). Our rat antibodies differ from the conventional (allogenic) sera in that ours precipitate both allelic forms of Lyt-1 or Lyt-2 and therefore must recognize framework or species (nonpolymorphic) determinants on the Lyt-1 and Lyt-2 proteins.

The anti-Lyt-1 monoclonal (53-7.3) precipitated a protein of approximately 70,000 daltons that exhibited extensive charge heterogeneity on 2D gel (Fig. 5).

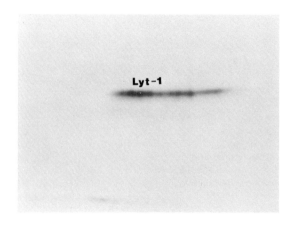

FIGURE 5. 2D gel electrophoresis of Lyt-1 glycoprotein immunoprecipitated with a monoclonal antibody (53-7.3) from an NP40 extract of [^{125}I]lactoperoxidase-labeled BALB/c thymocytes. The 2D gel autoradiograph is positioned as described in the legend to Fig. 2.

This molecule ran identically in gels under both reducing and nonreducing conditions; thus it appears to be composed of a single polypeptide chain rather than sulfhydryl-linked subunits.

In contrast, Lyt-2 appears to consist of two subunits of approximately 30,000 and 35,000 daltons that resolved on 2D gels under reducing conditions. Under nonreducing conditions, the 30,000- and 35,000-dalton proteins are not present; instead a 65,000-dalton glycoprotein appears which runs with the same charge characteristics (extremely basic) as the two small subunits found under reducing conditions (Fig. 6). Therefore the 30,000- and 35,000-dalton proteins most likely constitute a disulfide-bonded cell-surface molecule.

The identification of Lyt-1 and Lyt-2 as the target antigens of several of our monoclonal antibodies relied upon the immunoprecipitation of glycoproteins from thymocytes of the C57BL/6 Ly congenic strains. However, in view of the expression of Lyt-1 and Lyt-2 alloantigens on functional subsets of T cells, we felt it necessary to demonstrate the presence of the immunoprecipitated glycoproteins on functional T-cell populations.

For Lyt-1, FACS analysis (see Table II) indicates that this antigen is present on essentially all thymocytes and peripheral T cells. Our 53-7.3 antibody that recognizes the same 70,000-dalton glycoprotein recognized by a conventional anti-Lyt-1.1 serum shows a 14-fold variation in the brightness of staining among splenic T cells (Fig. 1), indicating that Lyt-1 is expressed in different quantities on different T cells. If functionally distinct T cells express different amounts of Lyt-1 antigen, then the cells with low Lyt-1 expression may be difficult to kill with antibody and complement. This may explain discrepancies among different lab-

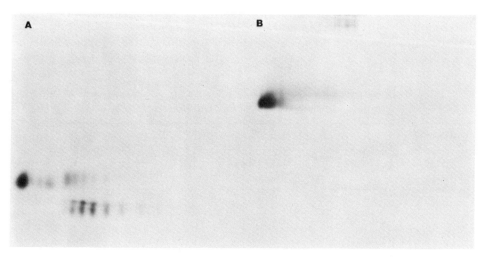

FIGURE 6. Reduced vs. nonreduced forms of the Lyt-2 glycoprotein. Thymocytes from BALB/c mice were labeled with ^{125}I using the lactoperoxidase technique and extracted with 0.5% NP40. Lyt-2 was immunoprecipitated from the cell lysate with monoclonal rat antibody 53-6.7 and divided into two aliquots for (A) electrophoresis under reducing conditions, and (B) electrophoresis under nonreducing conditions. Autoradiograms of the 2D gels are positioned as described in the legend to Fig. 2.

TABLE II

Expression of T-Cell Differentiation Markers Among Lymphoid Cells[a]

BALB/c lymphoid cell suspension	Monoclonal antibody				
	Anti-Thy-1.2 (30-H12)	Anti-Lyt-1 (53-7.3)	Anti-Lyt-2 (53-6.7)	Anti-T30 (53-8.1)	(30-H11)
Thymus					
All cells	>99	>99	91	>95	>95
Cortisone-resistant[b]	>99	>99	50	n.d.	>95
Spleen					
All cells	34	30	11	25	40
Nylon-passed[c]	87	84	28	65	92
Lymph node	78	80	25	40	75
Bone marrow	<1	<1	<1	<1	50
Peripheral blood lymphocytes[d]	61	63	12	37	60

[a]Expressed as percentage of cells under the positive peak determined by quantitative fluorescence staining using the FACS-II.
[b]Cortisone-resistant thymocytes were produced by intraperitoneal injection of 2.5 mg of hydrocortisone acetate per animal 48 hr prior to assay.
[c]Splenic T cells were enriched using nylon columns as described by Julius et al. (1973).
[d]Peripheral blood lymphocytes were purified on Ficoll–Hypaque (Pharmacia).

oratories in the ability to remove cytotoxic killer T cells with anti-Lyt-1 and complement (Shiku et al., 1975; Beverley et al., 1976; Nakayama et al., 1979).

For Lyt-2, where a subpopulation of peripheral T cells carries the antigen, FACS staining and separation could be performed. We used our 53-6.7 monoclonal antibody to show that the glycoprotein it detects (Fig. 6) is expressed on allotype suppressor T cells (Table III). The use of a monoclonal antibody is the key factor in allowing the demonstration of the relationship of a surface molecu-

TABLE III

Ig1b Allotype Suppressor T Cells Express Lyt-2 Determinants Detected
by A Monoclonal Rat Antibody

(SJL × BALB/c)F$_1$ spleen cells transferred (× 10^6)		Anti-DNP response (RIA)[a]	
DNP-KLH primed normal	Unprimed suppressed[b]	Ig1a	Ig1b
10	—	122	120
10	5 (Stained, unseparated)[c]	120	36
10	0.5 (Lyt-2 positive)	112	36
10	5 (Lyt-2 negative)	104	84

[a]Units of a standard anti-DNP serum. One unit = 1% of the binding activity of the standard, measured on DNP$_{42}$-BSA. Response measured 14 days after transfer.
[b]Suppressed by exposure to maternal anti-Ig1b (Herzenberg et al., 1975).
[c]Stained with monoclonal rat antibody 53-6.7 (anti-Lyt-2). See Fig. 1 for staining pattern of spleen cells with this antibody.

lar structure (the Lyt-2 glycoprotein) to a functional T-cell subpopulation (suppressor T cells). In several cases conventionally prepared anti-Ly sera were shown to contain antibodies to other, non-Ly determinants (Glimcher et al., 1977; Durda et al., 1979) and thus Shen et al. (1976) have advised caution in the use of the standard, noncongenic anti-Ly alloantisera.

Since the Lyt-2 glycoprotein is expressed on only 30% of splenic T cells (Table II) it is possible that the Lyt-2 glycoprotein plays a role in the functions of the cells that express it (suppressor and cytotoxic T cells). Recent experiments show that conventional or monoclonal Lyt-2 antisera specifically block the killing ability of cytotoxic T cells (Nakayama et al., 1979; Shinohara and Sachs, 1979). However, it is not yet known whether Lyt-2 is involved in the recognition stages or in the effector stages of T-cell killing.

V. Identification of Two Previously Unknown T-Cell Differentiation Antigens

In the sections above we described monoclonal antibodies that detect determinants on the Thy-1, Lyt-1, and Lyt-2 glycoproteins. In this section we describe two monoclonal antibodies (30-H11 and 53-8.1) derived from xenogeneic immunizations that recognize nonpolymorphic (species) determinants expressed on T cells. To our knowledge, these two antigens have not previously been described with conventional antisera.

FACS analysis showed that the 53-8.1 monoclonal antibody reacts with thymocytes (Fig. 7). Fluorescence staining in the spleen showed that 53-8.1 reacts with a splenic subpopulation (Fig. 7). There was no apparent staining with 53-8.1 in the bone marrow. Thymocytes stained much brighter than peripheral T cells with this antibody, indicating that the antigen it detects is expressed in greater amounts on thymocytes than on splenic or lymph node T cells (Fig. 7). Although the staining in the peripheral lymphoid tissues with 53-8.1 was quite dull, it was apparent that the antigen it detects may be expressed on a subpopulation of peripheral T cells. For example, fluorescence analysis indicated that a nylon passed population from spleen consisted of 87% Thy-1 positive cells. However, only 65% of these cells were stained with 53-8.1 (Table II and Fig. 7).

Immunoprecipitations with the 53-8.1 monoclonal antibody demonstrated that it specifically recognizes a 30,000-dalton thymocyte protein (Fig. 8). Since this species appears to be selectively expressed on thymocytes and peripheral T cells, we named it T30.

The 30-H11 antibody recognizes an antigen that is present on thymocytes and peripheral T cells (Fig. 9). We used two-color immunofluorescence to show that splenic IgM bearing cells do not express this antigen (not shown). The antigen is not restricted to T cells, however, since the large bone marrow cells of the granulocyte–macrophage lineage are stained positively by the 30-H11 antibody.

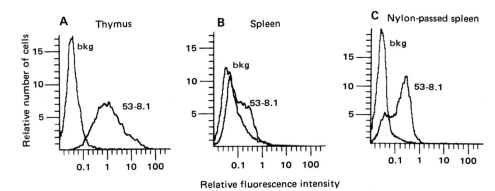

FIGURE 7. Immunofluorescent staining of BALB/c thymocytes (A), spleen cells (B), and nylon-enriched splenic T cells (C) with monoclonal antibody 53-8.1 (anti-T30). After reaction with hybrid supernates, bound antibody was detected by reaction with FITC-conjugated second-step antibody (SJL/J anti-Rat Ig). Stained cells were analyzed using the FACS II with a logarithmic amplifier. Background staining (second step alone) is shown in each panel.

The pattern of 30-H11 reactivity with lymphoid tumors mirrors its reactivity with normal lymphoid cells (N. Warner, personal communication). The 30-H11 antibody does not react with B lymphomas, although thymic and peripheral T lymphomas stain positively with 30-H11, reflecting the reactivity of this antibody with T cells plus some other non-B cells in normal animals.

The 30-H11 antibody does not immunoprecipitate detectable amounts of any glycoprotein from NP40 extracts of thymocytes labeled with ^{125}I by the lactoperoxidase method. The target antigen of this antibody may be a glycoprotein that either (1) does not contain exposed tyrosines and thus is not labeled by the lactoperoxidase technique; (2) is not solubilized by 0.5% NP40; or (3) is extracted into but not immunoprecipitable from 0.5% NP40. Alternatively, 30-H11 may recognize carbohydrate determinants on a membrane glycolipid that is not detectable on SDS gels.

Table II shows the expression of the antigens detected by antibodies

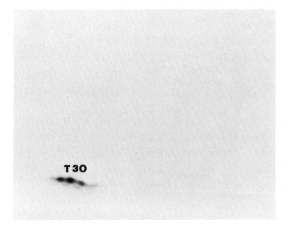

FIGURE 8. Immunoprecipitation of a thymocyte-surface protein T30 with a monoclonal antibody (53-8.1). BALB/c thymocytes were surface-labeled with ^{125}I using the lactoperoxidase technique and extracted with 0.5% NP40. Immunoprecipitated proteins were separated on 2D gels. The autoradiograph is positioned as described in the legend to Fig. 2.

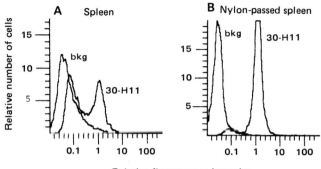

FIGURE 9. Immunofluorescent staining of BALB/c spleen cells (A) and nylon-enriched splenic T cells (B) with monoclonal antibody 30-H11. After reaction with hybrid supernatants, bound antibody was detected by reaction with FITC-conjugated second-step antibody (SJL/J anti-rat Ig). Stained cells were analyzed using the FACS II with a logarithmic amplifier. Background staining (second step alone) is shown in each panel.

30-H11 and 53-8.1 on cells from various lymphoid organs. The 30-H11 antibody consistently reacted with 5–10% more cells in the spleen and lymph nodes than an anti-Thy-1.2 monoclonal (30-H12), further indicating that 30-H11 reacts with some non-T cells. For 53-8.1, the fluorescence staining in peripheral lymphoid tissues indicates that T30 may be expressed on a T-cell subpopulation.

ACKNOWLEDGMENTS

This work was supported in part by grants from the National Institutes of Health (GM-17367 and CA-04681).

The authors wish to thank Mr. Theta Tsu for his excellent technical assistance and Miss Leslie Brenner for her help in preparing this manuscript.

J. A. Ledbetter is a Research Fellow of the National Cancer Institute (CA-06207). J. W. Goding is C. J. Martin Fellow of the National Health and Medical Research Council of Australia.

References

Barclay, A. N., Letarte-Muirhead, M., and Williams, A. F., 1975, Purification of the Thy-1 molecule from rat brain, *Biochem. J.* **151**:699.

Barclay, A. N., Letarte-Muirhead, M., Williams, A. F., and Faulkes, R. A., 1976, Chemical characterization of the Thy-1 glycoproteins from the membranes of rat thymocytes and brain, *Nature* **263**:563.

Beverley, P. C. L., Woody, J., Dunkley, M., Feldmann, M., and McKenzie, I., 1976, Separation of suppressor and killer T cells by surface phenotype, *Nature* **262**:495.

Blankenhorn, E. P., and Douglas, T. C., 1972, Location of the gene for theta antigen in the mouse, *J. Hered.* **63**:259.

Boyse, E. Z., Miyazawa, M., Aoki, T., and Old, L. J., 1968, Ly-A and Ly-B: Two systems of lymphocyte isoantigens in the mouse, *Proc. R. Soc. Lond. [Biol.]* **170:**175.

Boyse, E. A., Itakura, K., Stockert, E., Iritani, C. A., and Miura, M., 1971, Lyc: A third locus specifying alloantigens expressed only on thymocytes and lymphocytes, *Transplantation* **11:**351.

Cantor, H., and Boyse, E. A., 1975a, Functional subclasses of T lymphocytes bearing different Ly antigens. I. The generation of functionally distinct T-cell subclasses in a differentiative process independent of antigen, *J. Exp. Med.* **141:**1376.

Cantor, H., and Boyse, E. A., 1975b, Functional subclasses of T lymphocytes bearing different Ly antigens. II. Cooperation between subclasses of Lyt cells in the generation of killer activity, *J. Exp. Med.* **141:**1390.

Cantor, H., Shen, F. W., and Boyse, E. A., 1976, Separation of helper from suppressor T cells expressing Ly components. II. Activation by antigen: After immunization, antigen specific suppressor and helper activities are mediated by distinct T-cell subclasses, *J. Exp. Med.* **143:**1391.

Clagett, J., Peter, H. H., Feldman, J. D., and Weigle, W. O., 1973, Rabbit antiserum to brain-associated thymus antigens of mouse and rat. II. Analysis of species-specific and cross-reacting antibodies, *J. Immunol.* **110:**1085.

Douglas, T. C., 1972, Occurrence of a theta-like antigen in rats, *J. Exp. Med.* **136:**1054.

Durda, P. J., and Gottlieb, P. D., 1976, The Ly-3 antigens on mouse thymocytes: Immune precipitation and molecular weight characterization, *J. Exp. Med.* **144:**476.

Durda, P. J., Shapireo, C., and Gottlieb, P. D., 1978, Partial molecular characterization of the Ly-1 alloantigen on mouse thymocytes, *J. Immunol.* **120:**53.

Durda, P. J., Boos, B. C., and Gottlieb, P. D., 1979, T100: A new murine cell surface glycoprotein detected by anti-Ly 2.1 serum, *J. Immunol.* **122:**1407.

Glimcher, L., Shen, F. W., and Cantor, H., 1977, Identification of a cell surface antigen expressed on the natural killer cell, *J. Exp. Med.* **145:**1.

Goding, J. W., 1980, Structural studies of murine lymphocyte surface IgD, *J. Immunol.* (in press).

Herzenberg, L. A., Okumura, K., and Metzler, C. M., 1975, Regulation of immunoglobulin and antibody production by allotype suppressor T cells in mice, *Transplant. Rev.* **27:**56.

Herzenberg, L. A., Okumura, K., Cantor, H., Sato, V. L., Shen, F. W., Boyse, E. A., and Herzenberg, L. A., 1976, T cell regulation of antibody responses: Demonstration of allotype-specific helper T cells and their specific removal by suppressor T cells, *J. Exp. Med.* **144:**330.

Hilger, J., Haverman, J., Nusse, R., Van Blitterwijk, W. J., Cleton, F. J., Hegeman, P. C., van Nie, R., and Calafat, J., 1975, Immunologic, virologic, and genetic aspects of mammary tumor virus-induced cell surface antigens: Presence of these antigens and the Thy-1.2 antigen on murine mammary gland and tumor cells, *J. Natl. Cancer Inst.* **54:**1323.

Huber, B., Devinsky, O., Gershon, R. K., and Cantor, H., 1976, Cell-mediated immunity: Delayed-type hypersensitivity and cytotoxic responses are mediated by different T-cell subclasses, *J. Exp. Med.* **143:**1534.

Itakura, K., Hutton, J. J., Boyse, E. A., and Old, L. J., 1972, Genetic linkage relationships of loci specifying differentiation alloantigens in the mouse, *Transplantation* **13:**239.

Itakura, K., Hutton, J. J., Boyse, E. A., and Old, L. J., 1974, Linkage groups of the Θ and Ly-A loci, *Nature [New Biol.]* **230:**126.

Julius, M. H., Simpson, E., and Herzenberg, L. A., 1973, A rapid method for isolation of functional thymus derived murine lymphocytes, *Eur. J. Immunol.* **3:**645.

Köhler, G., and Milstein, C., 1975, Continuous cultures of fused cells secreting antibody of predefined specificity, *Nature* **256:**495.

Ledbetter, J. A., and Herzenberg, L. A., 1979, Xenogeneic monoclonal antibodies to mouse lymphoid differentiation antigens, *Immunol. Rev.* **47:**63.

Letarte-Muirhead, M., Barclay, A. N., and Williams, A. F., 1974, Purification of the Thy-1 molecule, a major cell surface glycoprotein of rat thymocytes, *Biochem. J.* **151:**685.

Loken, M. R., and Herzenberg, L. A., 1975, Analysis of cell populations using a fluorescence-activated cell sorter, *Ann. NY Acad. Sci.* **254:**163.

Miller, H. C., and Esselman, W. J., 1975, Modulation of the immune response by antigen-reactive lymphocytes after cultivation with gangliosides, *J. Immunol.* **115:**839.

Morris, R. J., and Williams, A. F., 1975, Antigens on mouse and rat lymphocytes recognized by rabbit antiserum against rat brain: The quantitative analysis of a xenogeneic antiserum. *Eur. J. Immunol.* **5:**274.

Nakayama, E., Shiku, H., Stockert, E., Oettgen, H. F., and Old, L. J., 1979, Cytotoxic T cells: Lyt phenotype and blocking of killing activity by Lyt antisera, *Proc. Natl. Acad. Sci. USA* **76:**1977.

O'Farrell, P. H., 1975, High resolution two-dimensional electrophoresis of proteins, *J. Biol. Chem.* **250:**4007.

O'Farrell, P. Z., Goodman, H. M., and O'Farrell, P. H., 1977, High resolution two-dimensional electrophoresis of basic as well as acidic proteins, *Cell* **12:**1133.

Oi, V. T., and Herzenberg, L. A., 1979a, Immunoglobulin-producing hybrid cell lines, in: *Selected Methods in Cellular Immunology* (B. B. Mishell and S. M. Shiji, eds.), W. H. Freeman, San Francisco, Chapter 17.

Oi, V. T., and Herzenberg, L. A., 1979b, Localization of murine Ig-1b and Ig-1a (IgG2a): Allotypic determinants defined with monoclonal antibodies, *Mol. Immunol.* **16:**1005.

Oi, V. T., Jones, P. P., Goding, J. W., Herzenberg, L. A., and Herzenberg, L. A., 1978, Properties of monoclonal antibodies to mouse Ig allotypes, H-2, and Ia antigens, *Curr. Top. Microbiol. Immunol.* **81:** 115.

Parks, D. R., Bryan, V. M., Oi, V. T., and Herzenberg, L. A., 1979, Antigen specific identification and cloning of hybridomas with a fluorescence-activated cell sorter (FACS), *Proc. Natl. Acad. Sci. USA* **76:**1962.

Pickel, K., Hammerling, U., and Hoffman, M. K., 1976, Ly phenotype of T-cells releasing T-cell replacing factor, *Nature* **264:**72.

Reif, A. E., and Allen, J. M. V., 1964, The AKR thymic antigen and its distribution in leukemias and nervous tissues, *J. Exp. Med.* **120:**413.

Scheid, M., Boyse, E. A., Carswell, E. A., and Old, L. J., 1972, Serologically demonstrable alloantigens of mouse epidermal cells, *J. Exp. Med.* **135:**938.

Shen, F. W., Boyse, E. A., and Cantor, H., 1976, Preparation and use of Ly antiserum, *Immunogenetics* **2:**591.

Shiku, H., Kisielow, P., Bean, M. A., Takahashi, T., Boyse, E. A., Oettgen, H. F., and Old, L. J., 1975, Expression of T cell differentiation antigens on effector cells in cell-mediated cytotoxicity in vitro, *J. Exp. Med.* **141:**227.

Shinohara, N., and Sachs, D. H., 1979, Mouse alloantibodies capable of blocking cytotoxic T-cell function. I. Relationship between the antigen reactive with blocking antibodies and the *Lyt-2* locus, *J. Exp. Med.* **150:**432.

Springer, T., Galfrè, G., Secher, D. S., and Milstein, C., 1978a, Monoclonal xenogenic antibodies to murine cell surface antigens: Identification of novel leukocyte differentiation antigens, *Eur. J. Immunol.* **8:**539.

Springer, T., Galfrè, G., Secher, D., and Milstein, C., 1978b, Monoclonal xenogenic antibodies to mouse leukocyte antigens: Identification of macrophage-specific and other differentiation antigens, *Curr. Top. Microbiol. Immunol.* **81:**45.

Stern, P. L., 1973, Θ alloantigens on mouse and rat fibroblasts, *Nature [New Biol.]* **246:**76.

Stern, P. L., Willison, K. R., Lennox, E., Galfrè, G., Milstein, C., Secher, D., and Ziegler, A., 1978, Monoclonal antibodies as probes for differentiation and tumor-associated antigens: A Forssman specificity on teratocarcinoma stem cells, *Cell* **14:**775.

Thiele, H.-G., Stark, R., and D. Keeser, 1972, Antigenic correlations between brain and thymus. I. Common antigenic structures in rat and mouse brain tissue and thymocytes, *Eur. J. Immunol.* **2:**424.

Trowbridge, I. S., 1978, Interspecies spleen-myeloma hybrid producing monoclonal antibodies against the mouse lymphocyte surface glycoprotein T200, *J. Exp. Med.* **148:**313.

Trowbridge, I. S., Weissman, I., and Bevan, M. J., 1975, Mouse T-cell surface glycoprotein recognized by heterologous anti-thymocyte sera and its relationship to Thy-1 antigen, *Nature* **256:**652.

Wang, T. J., Freimuth, W. W., Miller, H. C., and Esselman, W. J., 1978, Thy-1 antigenicity is associated with glycolipids of brain and thymocytes, *J. Immunol.* **121:**1361.

Williams, A. F., 1977, Differentiation antigens of the lymphocyte cell surface, *Contemp. Top. Mol. Immunol.* **6:**83.

Williams, A. F., Giovanni, G., and Milstein, C., 1977, Analysis of cell surface by xenogenic myeloma hybrid antibodies: Differentiation antigens of rat lymphocytes, *Cell* **12:**663.

15
Monoclonal Antibodies That Define T-Lymphocyte Subsets in the Rat

DONALD W. MASON, ROGER J. BRIDEAU,
W. ROBERT McMASTER, MICHAEL WEBB,
ROBERT A. H. WHITE, AND ALAN F. WILLIAMS

I. Introduction

All lymphocytes have the same morphological appearance, but they can be functionally split into two main categories. B lymphocytes differentiate in the bursa (avia) or bone marrow (mammalia) and give rise to antibody-secreting cells, while T lymphocytes differentiate in the thymus and are responsible for cell-mediated immunity (Möller, 1969). These differences in function and ontogeny correlate with the expression of different cell-surface molecules (antigens) on B and T lymphocytes and antibodies to these molecules have been important as markers for identifying and separating different cell types (Raff, 1971). The possibility that marker antigens have important functional roles is illustrated by the fact that cell-surface immunoglobulin (sIg) is a standard marker for B lymphocytes and is also the receptor for antigen on these cells.

T lymphocytes mediate a variety of functions, including allogeneic immunity as measured by graft-vs.-host (GVH) and mixed lymphocyte responses

DONALD W. MASON, ROGER J. BRIDEAU, W. ROBERT McMASTER, MICHAEL WEBB, ROBERT A. H. WHITE, AND ALAN F. WILLIAMS • MRC Cellular Immunology Unit, Sir William Dunn School of Pathology, University of Oxford, Oxford OX1 3RE, England.

(MLR), cell-mediated cytotoxicity, and control of antibody responses via helper or suppressor activity. In the mouse it has been shown that the cells responsible for these functions can be divided into subsets on the basis of their expression of the Lyt-1,2,3 alloantigens. Helper cells have been shown to be Lyt-$1^+2^-3^-$, while cells with cytotoxicity and suppressor functions have been classified as Lyt-$1^-2^+3^+$ (Cantor and Boyse, 1976). More recent data suggests that Lyt-1 antigen is present on all T cells and that Lyt-2,3 antigens may be the only true T subset markers defined in the mouse (Scollay *et al.*, 1978; Nakayama *et al.*, 1979).

The use of antibodies as markers for lymphocyte subsets has been limited by problems of specificity. One needs specific antibodies to cell-surface molecules that are uncharacterized. In the past antisera have mainly been raised against polymorphic determinants within the species (alloantisera), since in this case there is a genetic criterion for specificity, namely, the production of congenic strains of animals. The disadvantage of alloantisera is that the antibody concentration is often low and only those cell-surface molecules that are polymorphic can be detected. Furthermore, in labeling studies there are difficulties if the binding of alloantibodies is detected with anti-Ig reagents, since these will also bind to endogenous-cell-membrane Ig.

If antibodies are raised between species (xenoantisera), then potentially all protein molecules will be antigenic due to evolutionary divergence between species. The difficulty here is that unless pure antigen is available specific antisera cannot be raised, and there is no satisfactory criterion for specificity. Xenoantibodies are preferable in labeling studies, since an anti-Ig used as a second reagent to detect binding can be made specific for the xenoantibodies and thus will not bind to endogenous Ig.

The problems of obtaining specific antibodies after xenoimmunizations are solved by producing monoclonal antibodies (Köhler and Milstein, 1976; Williams *et al.*, 1977). The procedures are illustrated in Fig. 1 with reference to the production of mouse anti-rat antibodies as used in the experiments to be described. Mice were hyperimmunized with membranes or glycoproteins from rat thymocytes. Immune spleen cells were then fused with the mouse myeloma cell line NS1 and hybrid cells were selected for with hypoxanthine–aminopterin–thymidine (HAT) medium. Hybrids secreting antibody were detected by assaying supernatants for antithymocyte antibody with an indirect radioactive binding assay and antibodies specific for lymphocyte subsets were detected by analysis of labeled cells with a fluorescence-activated cell sorter (FACS). Hybridoma production provides the advantage that the antibodies produced are monospecific, since they derive from a single antibody-forming cell, and it does not matter that the starting immunogen was a complex mixture of molecules. Monoclonal antibodies can be produced in large amounts by collecting ascitic fluid or blood from mice growing the antibody-secreting hybridomas as tumors.

In this chapter monoclonal antibodies that mark rat T-lymphocyte subsets will be described. Two clear sets of mature T cells are identified, and they have different functional capabilities. One of the subset specific antigens may play an important role in immune functions, since the monoclonal antibody against it inhibits mixed lymphocyte reactions.

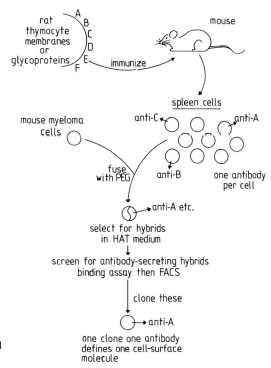

FIGURE 1. The production of monoclonal antibodies against cell-surface antigens.

II. Production and Detection of Antibodies

A. Monoclonal and Other Antibodies

The antibodies used were as follows (all were against determinants present on all rat strains tested):

W3/13 and W3/25 antibodies (Williams *et al.*, 1977). These were derived from a fusion using spleen cells from mice immunized with rat thymocyte membrane. Both are IgG antibodies with high affinities (Mason and Williams, 1980).

MRC OX 8 antibody (Brideau *et al.*, 1980). The spleen cells fused were from a mouse immunized with large glycoproteins from rat thymocyte membrane prepared using lentil lectin affinity chromatography and gel filtration (Letarte-Muirhead *et al.*, 1975) and depleted of the L-C antigen with an MRC OX 1 antibody column (Sunderland *et al.*, 1979).

Rabbit F(ab')2 antibodies against mouse and rat Fab or IgG. Prepared by affinity chromatography (Jensenius and Williams, 1974).

B. Serology

For all experiments binding techniques were used as shown in Fig. 2. Cells were incubated with the test antibody, washed, and then incubated again with the appropriate purified F(ab')₂ anti-Ig antibody to detect the binding of the first antibody, and washed again. The anti-Ig antibody was labeled with ^{125}I or fluorescein isothyocyanate (FITC) or coupled to sheep erythrocytes depending on the aim of the experiment. Radioactive binding assays were used to assay antibodies in the preparation of monoclonal antibodies and for setting up quantitative radioimmunoassays to detect antigen by absorption of a limiting amount of antibody (Williams, 1977). Fluorescein-labeled antibody was used when cells were to be analyzed or separated on the FACS (Loken and Herzenberg, 1975). Erythrocytes coated with antibody were used to form rosettes with antigen-positive cells to allow depletion of these cells by density gradient centrifugation (Parish and Hayward, 1974a).

The kinetic properties of antibodies are important in the interpretation of binding data and apparently confusing results can be obtained if antibodies show slow association and/or rapid dissociation kinetics. This is particularly seen with monoclonal antibodies which are homogeneous, in comparison with conventional xenoantibodies containing a mixture, of which the fast-reacting and slowly dissociating antibodies predominate in binding assays (Mason and Williams, 1980).

The effects of different kinetic parameters are particularly evident in absorption analysis, where a limiting amount of antibody is reacted with antigen and subsequently free antibody is assayed using the indirect binding assay. The

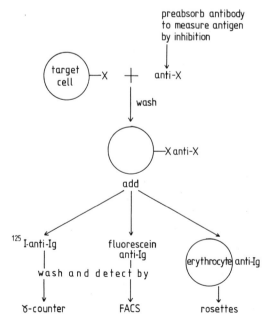

FIGURE 2. Binding assays for analysis of antibodies against cell-surface antigens.

association kinetics matter, since with slow-reacting antibodies the reaction with antigen may be far from complete in the 1- to 2-hr preincubation period that is normally used. For example, at saturation W3/13 antibody gave binding of about 35,000 molecules per thymocyte compared with 15,000 for W3/25 antibody. But in absorption analysis more thymocytes were needed to inhibit the binding of W3/13 antibody than W3/25 antibody (Williams *et al.*, 1977). However, the association constants for W3/13 and W3/25 antibody were found to be 0.8×10^5 and $11 \times 10^5 \, M^{-1} \, sec^{-1}$, respectively, and this 14-fold difference in reaction rate was responsible for the apparently anomalous results in absorption (Mason and Williams, 1980).

Dissociation rates become particularly important when absorption by monomeric antigen is compared with multimeric antigen, as is the case in a purification series going from membrane to detergent-solubilized extracts. The dissociation of antibody from multimeric antigen will be much slower then from monomeric antigen, since in the former case the antibody can bind bivalently. After preincubation of antigen with antibody, free antibody is assayed by addition of glutaraldehyde-fixed target cells that display multimeric antigen. If the monomeric interaction is rapidly dissociating, then antibody will accumulate on the target cells, and the amount of free antibody will be overestimated. However, if the dissociation for the monomeric interaction is of the same order or longer than the time for incubation with target cells, then the amount of free antibody is accurately assayed and the form of the antigen is unimportant. A simple experiment to test for rapid dissociation is to see whether addition of detergent in an absorption with membrane leads to an apparent reduction of inhibition (Mason and Williams, 1980).

III. Labeling of Rat Lymphoid Cells with the Monoclonal Antibodies

The most important monoclonal antibodies in the study of rat T lymphocytes are W3/25 and MRC OX 8. Both these antibodies give clear labeling of a subset of mature rat lymphoid cells, and this is shown in Fig. 3 for lymph node cells with binding analyzed by a FACS. MRC OX 8 antibody labeled 19% of the cells while W3/25 antibody labeled 31%. Also shown in Fig. 3 is labeling by W3/13 antibody and anti-Ig antibody, which label mature T and B lymphocytes, respectively (Williams *et al.*, 1977). It should be noted that W3/13 antibody is not a general marker for rat T lymphocytes because it is found on polymorphs (Williams *et al.*, 1977, and later in this section) and also on plasma cells (D. Secher, personal communication) despite its total absence from B lymphocytes. In lymphoid populations where polymorphs or plasma cells are present at only low frequency, W3/13 antibody can be useful to mark or separate T lymphocytes.

The relationship between the cell populations labeled by the various anti-

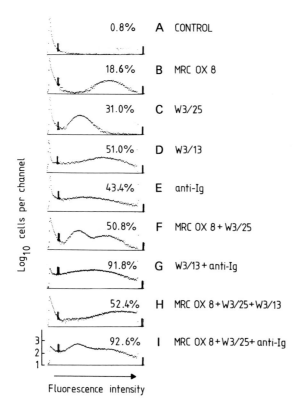

FIGURE 3. Labeling of rat lymphoid cells with monoclonal antibodies. Cells from the cervical lymph nodes of AO rats were incubated with the monoclonal antibodies shown on the figure, including a mouse anti-rat Ig monoclonal antibody provided by Dr. S. V. Hunt (called anti-Ig). Control labeling was with an anti-HLA-A, -B, -C antibody called W6/32. After washing, the cells were then incubated with fluorescein anti-mouse IgG antibody, washed again and analyzed with the FACS. The percentage of cells labeled above the marker is given on each profile.

bodies was examined by experiments in which the fluorescent profiles were measured after labeling with antibodies added alone or in mixtures. Some typical data are shown in Fig. 3. If cells are incubated with MRC OX 8 and W3/25 antibodies, then the percentage of cells labeled equals the sum of the individual labeling indices, and the individual modes of fluorescent labeling can be clearly detected in profiles where cells were labeled with both antibodies (Fig. 3B and C compared with F). A similar result is found if anti-Ig is added in addition to W3/25 and MRC OX 8 (Fig. 3I). This shows that MRC OX 8, W3/25 and anti-Ig antibodies label different cell populations, and a similar experiment establishes that W3/13 and anti-Ig antibodies label different sets of cells (Fig. 3G). In contrast to this, when cells are labeled with MRC OX 8, W3/13 and W3/25 antibodies mixed together the percentage of cells labeled equals that found with W3/13 antibody alone and the fluorescence profile has a mode of intensity higher than any of the individual patterns (Fig. 3H compared with B, C, and D). This shows that the MRC OX 8 and W3/25 positive cells also carry W3/13 antigen.

Labeling studies of the type shown in Fig. 3 have been carried out for thoracic duct lymphocytes (TDL), lymph node, spleen, thymus, and bone marrow of normal rats and for TDL, spleen, and bone marrow of congenitally athymic *rnu/rnu* rats. The results are summarized in bar charts shown in Figs. 4 and 5. Data for normal TDL are not shown, but this was very similar to lymph node except that the proportion of T cells which are MRC OX 8-positive is smaller (about 20%) (Brideau *et al.*, 1980).

In normal lymphoid tissues the situation can be summarized as follows. Among lymph node cells, surface Ig marks B lymphocytes, and these cells do not carry W3/13, W3/25, or MRC OX 8 antigen. The W3/13 antibody appears to label all T lymphocytes and the W/25 and MRC OX 8 antibodies split these into two populations constituting, respectively, about ²/₃ and ¹/₃ of the T lymphocytes. The pattern in spleen is similar except that the T lymphocyte population is equally divided among W3/25 positive and MRC OX 8-positive cells. No cells with both these markers have been detected. In contrast to this most but not all thymocytes carry both W3/25 and MRC OX 8 antigen, and virtually all are W3/13 antigen-positive. In bone marrow very few cells are labeled with W3/25 and MRC OX 8 antibody, while a clear subset, the polymorphs, are labeled by W3/13 antibody.

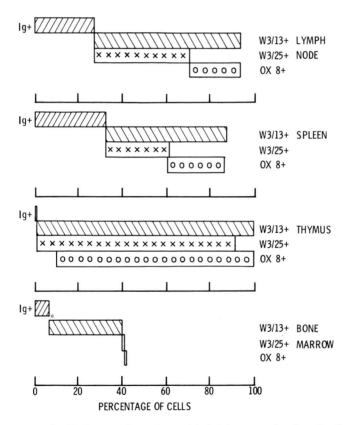

FIGURE 4. Percentage of cells from various tissues labeled by monoclonal antibodies. Different lymphoid cell populations from normal AO rats were analyzed for binding of antibodies and for overlap between different antibodies as in Fig. 3. The results are shown in the bar charts. *, Overlaps between Ig- and W3/13-positive cells in bone marrow were not tested but are likely to be distinct (Williams *et al.*, 1977). Also overlaps have not been tested in any case where only a few percent of cells were labeled.

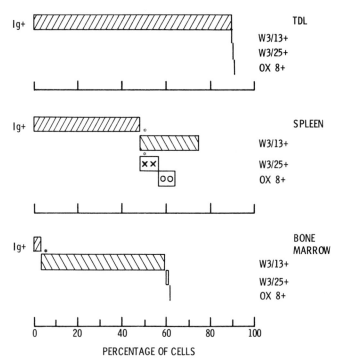

FIGURE 5. Labeling with monoclonal antibodies of lymphoid cells from rnu/rnu rats. Different lymphoid cell populations from rnu/rnu rats were analyzed for binding of antibodies as in Fig. 3. The results are shown on the bar charts. *, The only overlaps investigated were between W3/25- and MRC OX 8-positive cells for spleen.

In rnu/rnu rats the situation is very different (Fig. 5). Most TDL are sIg-positive and the proportion of cells labeled with W3/13, W3/25 or MRC OX 8 antibody was only 0.6% above background. In spleen 45% of cells were Ig-positive, 24% W3/13-positive and 8 and 7%, respectively, were positive for W3/25 and MRC OX 8 antigen. None of these latter cells appeared to carry both W3/25 and MRC OX 8 antigens, since when the antibodies were added together 17% of the cells were labeled, above the control (1.8% labeled). The nature of the W3/13 positive cells is open to question, particularly since the antigen is found on polymorphs and plasma cells. However, W3/25 and MRC OX 8 antigens have not been detected on cell types other than T lymphocytes. The spleen cells positive for these antigens do not seem to be thymocytelike in that they do not carry both antigens. In bone marrow of rnu/rnu rats, cells positive for W3/25 or MRC OX 8 antigen are rare (1.6 and 0.6%, respectively), while there is a large population of W3/13 positive cells, presumably polymorphs.

Two other antigens have been studied in the lymphoid populations shown in Figs. 4 and 5, namely, Ia antigen (Mason and Gallico, 1978; McMaster and Williams, 1979) and Thy-1 antigen (Williams et al., 1976; Hunt et al., 1977; Ritter et al., 1978). In brief the distribution of Ia-positive cells largely coincides with that of Ig-positive cells except that approximately 20% of thymocytes are Ia-positive. Rat Thy-1 antigen is found on all thymocytes and probably on all immature B lymphocytes, including stem cells. In spleen and lymph nodes it is found on a minor fraction of B and T lymphocytes.

In summary, the labeling studies showed that W3/25 and MRC OX 8 antigens seemed exclusive to thymocytes and T lymphocytes among lymphoid cell populations. In peripheral lymphoid organs they distinguish two subsets that display one antigen or the other but not both. In the nude rat the labeling patterns were consistent with the possibility that these animals lack T lymphocytes, with the exception that small fractions of W3/25-positive and MRC OX 8-positive cells were found in the spleen, and these might be related to T lymphocytes. The cells were not thymocytelike, since they did not display both antigens.

IV. Amount of Antigen per Cell and Expression on Other Tissues

The data in Table I summarize the number of molecules of monoclonal antibody that bind at saturation to thymocytes or antigen-positive T lympho-

TABLE I

Amounts of Antigens Assessed by Antibody Binding at Saturation and Absorption Analysis[a]

| Cell type | Molecules of monoclonal IgG or F(ab′)$_2$ antibody bound per cell at saturation $\times 10^{-3}$ | | | | |
	W3/13	W3/25	MRC OX 8	Thy-1 MRC OX 7	L-C MRC OX 1
Thymocytes	38	15	33	700	50
T cells from lymph node	34	22	65		

Tissue type	Absorptive capacity of tissue homogenates relative to thymocytes put at 100%				
Brain	100	<1	<1	80	<1
Kidney, liver	<1	<1	<1	<1	<1
Heart	—	<1	<1	<1	<1
Lung	—	<1	<1	<1	2
Testis, muscle	—	<1	<1	—	—

[a]The number of molecules bound at saturation was determined by standard techniques as used in Williams *et al.* (1977) (W3/13, W3/25), Sunderland *et al.* (1979) (L-C), Brideau *et al.* (1980) (MRC OX 8), and Mason and Williams (1980) (Thy-1). The percent absorptive capacity of a tissue homogenate relative to thymocytes is equal to 100 times the amount of thymocyte protein needed to absorb 50% of a limiting amount of antibody divided by the amount of tissue homogenate protein needed. The data are from experiments as in Williams *et al.* (1976) (Thy-1), Williams *et al.* (1977) (W3/13, W3/25), and Brideau *et al.* (1980) (MRC OX 8). However, in some cases the experiments have been repeated with tissues from animals given 1000-rad irradiation 3 days previously. This includes data for L-C antigen (Sunderland, unpublished) and for W3/25 antigen assayed on kidney, liver, heart, and lung (Williams, unpublished).

cytes. These are compared with data for Thy-1 and L-C antigens which are predominant cell-surface molecules of thymocytes. There is a large number of molecules of Thy-1 per thymocyte, but this molecule has a molecular weight of only 18,500. By contrast there are 14 times fewer L-C molecules per cell, but the molecular weight is about 150,000 and thus both Thy-1 and L-C antigen constitute roughly the same proportion of the membrane by weight (Sunderland et al., 1979).

The T-cell antigens are present in smaller amounts than either L-C or Thy-1 glycoproteins, although the number of molecules of W3/13 and MRC OX 8 antibody bound is not markedly less than that for L-C antigen. Binding of W3/25 antibody is markedly lower than the other antibodies. On peripheral T lymphocytes the labeled cells bound similar amounts of W3/13 and W3/25 antibodies as did thymocytes, but lymph node cells positive for MRC OX 8 bound about twice as much antibody as thymocytes. W3/13 antigen is known to be a glycoprotein of approximate molecular weight 95,000 (Standring et al., 1978), but the nature of W3/25 and MRC OX 8 antigens is at present unknown.

The presence of the antigens on other tissues was assessed by absorption analysis. W3/25 and MRC OX 8 antigens were not detectable on homogenates of nonlymphoid tissue assayed in comparison with thymocytes. Previously small amounts of W3/25 antigen were detected in normal kidney and liver homogenates (about 3% compared with thymocytes) and this was thought to be significant, since W3/13 antigen was detected in smaller amounts (Williams et al., 1977). It was considered that W3/13 absorption was a good control for contaminating lymphocytes, but with very small amounts of antigen the large amount of irrelevant protein could have a different effect in different assays. If the rate of reaction were slowed by irrelevant protein, then the absorptive capacity measured would be underestimated to a greater extent for antibodies with a low association constant (W3/13 antibody) compared with those with high intrinsic reaction rates (W3/25). In more recent experiments tissues were obtained from rats that had been irradiated 3 days before with 1000 rad to remove lymphocytes, and W3/25 antigen was not routinely detected in kidney and liver homogenates from these animals (Table I).

Given the data in Table I it seems reasonable to regard MRC OX 8 and W3/25 antigens as being substantially, if not totally, restricted to the T-lymphoid-cell lineage. In contrast to this, W3/13 antigen is found on brain as well as hemopoietic tissues, and this antigen is thus comparable to Thy-1, which is also found on a variety of tissues. The reason for the expression of the same molecule on apparently unrelated tissues, together with its total absence from many others, is at present not understood. However, the phenomenon is not uncommon, and the MRC OX 2 antigen shows this type of distribution as well as Thy-1 and W3/13 antigens (McMaster and Williams, 1979). Given these results it is clear that no antigen can be taken to define a cell type unless the function of the molecule is known, as is the case for cell-surface Ig. This does not detract from the value of marker antigens in allowing identification of different functions with subsets of cells.

V. Functional Studies

The observation that two subpopulations of peripheral T cells could be defined by the monoclonal antibodies W3/25 and MRC OX 8 prompted the question as to whether or not these subpopulations mediate different T-cell functions. Although on the basis of FACS analysis W3/25-positive and MRC OX 8-positive peripheral lymphocytes were completely mutually exclusive and the two subpopulations together appeared to account for all the peripheral T cells, it was important to show that functionally there were only two T-cell subpopulations. Labeling studies alone could not exclude the possible existence of a numerically small but functionally important population of T cells that carried both markers or neither of them. Accordingly T-cell subpopulations were isolated using the FACS to separate W3/25-positive or MRC OX 8-positive lymphocytes from complementary unlabeled populations and both positive and negative fractions were assayed for a number of T-cell functions.

A. Helper-Cell Function

The capacity of the T-cell subpopulations defined by W3/25 or MRC OX 8 to provide help for a B-cell antihapten response was determined by a classical adoptive transfer assay (White *et al.*, 1978; Brideau *et al.*, 1980). TDL from donors primed to dinitrophenyl bovine gamma globulin (DNPBGG) were labeled with the appropriate antibodies, fractionated on the FACS and transferred to irradiated syngeneic recipients that were simultaneously challenged with DNPBGG. Anti-DNP plaque-forming cell (PFC) assays were carried out on spleen cells of the recipients 7 days later. The donor TDL provided the source of primed B cells as well as primed T cells. When B cells were to be isolated together with the positively labeled T-cell subpopulation, the TDL were incubated with a mixture of rabbit anti-rat $F(ab')_2$-FITC and rabbit $F(ab')_2$ anti-mouse Ig-FITC in the second step. When it was required to isolate the B cells along with the unlabeled T cell subpopulation, the rabbit anti-rat $F(ab')_2$-FITC reagent was omitted.

In the first experiment (Fig. 6A) the helper activity of W3/25-positive T cells was examined. When unfractionated TDL were transferred the PFC response obtained in the sublethally irradiated host was in excess of 2×10^5 PFC/spleen (column 4). However, transfer of an equal number of antigen-primed B cells, together with W3/25-negative cells, yielded no response (Column 3). In contrast, when primed B cells were transferred with W3/25-positive cells (column 5), a response was obtained that equalled in magnitude that from unfractionated TDL. Finally, when the capacity of the two T-cell subpopulations to collaborate with radioresistant B cells in the host (Parish and Hayward, 1974b) was examined, only the W3/25-positive population did so (cf. columns 2 and 6).

These assays were repeated but using MRC OX 8 monoclonal antibody

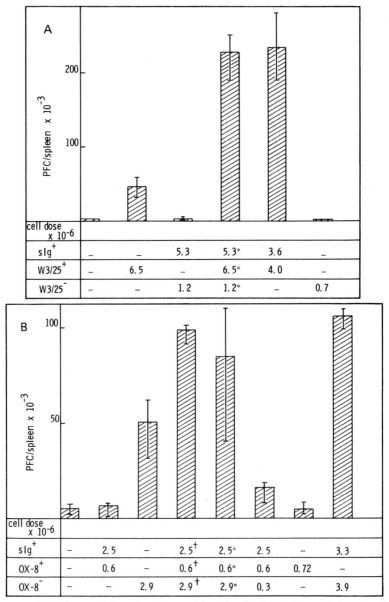

FIGURE 6. (A) The helper activity of W3/25-positive T cells. TDL from PVG rats primed to DNPBGG were labeled according to the procedures described in the text and separated on the FACS. The various cell combinations shown in the table were then transferred, together with 1 mg of DNPBGG into irradiated syngeneic recipients. Autoradiographic PFC assays (Mason, 1976) were carried out 7 days later. The vertical columns represent the average number of PFC/spleen and the bars indicate the range. Two to three recipients were used in each group. *, Unseparated TDL.

(B) The lack of helper activity in MRC OX 8-positive T cells. See legend to Fig. 6A and the main text. The reconstituted mixture of column 4 was obtained by combining, after FACS separation, MRC OX 8-negative cells with cells positive for surface Ig or MRC OX 8 antigen. It is evident, by comparing columns 4 and 5, that the fractionation procedure had no adverse effect on cell function. † Reconstituted mixture; *, unseparated TDL.

rather than W3/25 antibody to label the TDL. It was evident that only when MRC OX 8-negative cells were combined with primed B cells (Fig. 6B, column 8) did the response reach the control value obtained from unfractionated TDL (column 5).

In these experiments the various subpopulations were used in their physiological ratios. It could be argued that the failure to detect helper activity from W3/25-negative, MRC OX 8-positive cells was a consequence of the small numbers of these cells transferred. However, the helper activity of only 3×10^5 MRC OX 8-negative cells was readily detected in the assay system used (column 6) whereas twice this number of MRC OX 8-positive cells were without effect (column 2).

Taken together these data define the phenotype of the helper T cell for antihapten antibody responses as W3/25-positive, MRC OX 8-negative.

B. Graft-vs.-Host Reactivity

The popliteal lymph node assay of Ford et al. (1970) was used to assay the GVH reactivity of the various T-cell subpopulations (White et al., 1978; Brideau et al., 1980). Parental TDL were labeled with either W3/25 or MRC OX 8 and after separation of labeled and unlabeled cells in the FACS aliquots of separated cells were injected into the footpads of 6- to 7-week-old F_1 rats. The popliteal lymph nodes were removed and weighed 7 days later.

When the GVH activity of TDL subpopulations, defined by W3/25 monoclonal antibody, were assayed (Fig. 7A), it was apparent that virtually all the lymph node enlargement was mediated by W3/25-positive cells. Even when W3/25-negative cells were used in numbers 8 times greater than those present in unfractionated TDL (column 4), only a modest enlargement was obtained. This lymph node enlargement is of doubtful significance since apparently similar low levels of enlargement may be obtained with syngeneic cell transfer (Ford et al., 1970). Very similar results were obtained when the assays were repeated with the sIg-positive cells transferred together with the W3/25-positive T cells (data not shown) indicating that the donor B cells played no role in the assay.

Figure 7B shows the GVH assay results obtained when donor TDL were fractionated on the FACS using MRC OX 8 antibody to label the cells. Data obtained from two separate experiments are presented, one in which the B cells were transferred with the labeled T-cell subpopulation and one where the B cells accompanied the unlabeled cells. It is evident that MRC OX 8-positive cells are inactive in this assay, even when used in a large dose (column 5) and that virtually all the GVH reactivity is found in the MRC OX 8-negative cells. As with the previous experiment the donor B cells were incapable of mediating any host lymph node enlargement.

These two groups of experiments identify the donor T cell responsible for GVH reactivity as being W3/25-positive, MRC OX 8-negative, and it is thus phenotypically the same as the helper T cell.

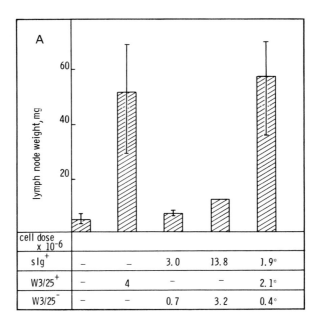

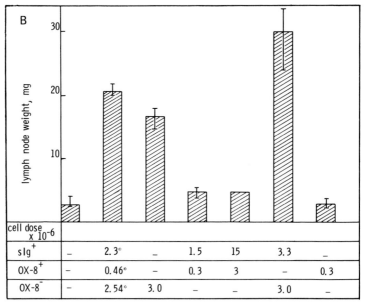

FIGURE 7. The GVH reactivity of W3/25-positive cells and MRC OX 8-positive cells. (PVG × DA)F₁ rats were injected in the footpads with PVG TDL subpopulations defined by W3/25 antibody (A) or MRC OX 8 antibody (B). Control rats received injections of medium only. Popliteal lymph nodes of the recipient rats were removed and weighed 7 days later. *, Unseparated TDL.

C. Mixed Lymphocyte Reactions

The mixed lymphocyte reaction (MLR) is generally considered to be the *in vitro* analogue of the GVH reaction, despite some differences (Cantor and Weissman, 1976). Accordingly it was anticipated that the responder cell in the MLR would be W3/25-positive, MRC OX 8-negative. This expectation was confirmed with regard to the W3/25 marker by using the FACS to separate TDL into positive and negative fractions and assaying the fractions independently for MLR reactivity (Webb *et al.*, 1979). A typical result is shown in Fig. 8. It is evident that W3/25-positive cells in this experiment were about 5 times more potent in terms of thymidine incorporation per responding cell as compared to the unlabeled cells. Several identical experiments have yielded a mean value of 8 for this ratio. The modest response from W3/25 negative cells is discussed below.

D. Proliferation of W3/25 Negative Cells in the MLR

Studies on the proliferation of W3/25 negative responders in the MLR have revealed a complex situation (D. W. Mason and M. Webb, unpublished observations). Both surface Ig-negative and MRC OX 8-negative fractions are capable of proliferation when allogeneic TDL are used as stimulators. This proliferation is inhibitable by W3/25 antibody and is dependent on the presence of W3/25-positive stimulator cells. This response thus appears to be the result of back

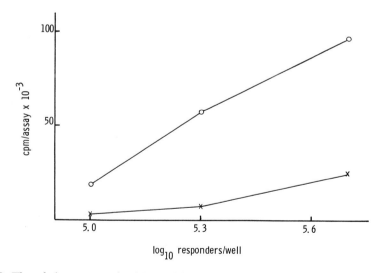

FIGURE 8. The relative potency of W3/25-positive and W3/25-negative responder cells in the mixed lymphocyte reaction. TDL from PVG (RT1c) rats were labeled with W3/25 antibody followed by fluorescein-conjugated anti-mouse Ig. Labeled and unlabeled cells were fractionated on the FACS and assayed for MLR at the doses indicated using 900-rad irradiated HO.B2 (RT1y) spleen cells as stimulators. Note that the unlabeled fraction contained surface-Ig-positive cells as well as W3/25-negative T cells. Assays were in triplicate. W3/25-positive (–o–); W3/25-negative (–×–).

stimulation; a similar phenomenon has been reported in the mouse MLR (Piguet *et al.*, 1975). Back stimulation should not occur if F_1 stimulators are used and W3/25-negative cells do not respond to F_1 TDL. However, F_1 spleen cells do stimulate W3/25-negative cells, despite the absence of back stimulation. Thus we conclude that W3/25-negative T cells can proliferate in an MLR under certain conditions.

E. Allogeneic Suppression

Sublethal irradiation of rats leaves a surviving population of radioresistant B cells that are capable of differentiating into antibody-forming cells. This differentiation is dependent on the provision of T cells from a nonirradiated donor so that such rats provide a convenient assay system for helper T cells. It has been observed that if an irradiated F_1 animal is reconstituted with parental T cells and the recipient rat challenged with antigen, the host PFC response is much less than that obtained by transferring the parental T cells into a fully syngeneic host (Parish and Hayward, 1974b; White *et al.*, 1978). Experiments were carried out to determine which T-cell subpopulation was responsible for the suppression of the PFC response in the transfer of parental cells into F_1 hosts. The results are illustrated in Fig. 9A,B (White *et al.*, 1978; Brideau *et al.*, 1980).

It is evident from Fig. 9A that when the W3/25-negative T-cell subpopulation was removed from the parental donor TDL, the F_1 host B cells were capable of making an antihapten response comparable in magnitude to that obtained in the parent to parent transfer. Similarly, as shown in Fig. 9B, the removal of the MRC OX 8-positive T-cell subpopulation from the parental cells also alleviated the suppression of the B-cell response in the F_1 host. In this experiment the suppression of the host response by unfractionated TDL was less profound than that obtained in the experiment using W3/25 antibody (contrast Fig. 9A column 3 with Fig. 9B column 1). The reasons for this remain to be established.

Taken together the data in Fig. 9A,B show that allogeneic suppressor cells are MRC OX 8-positive, W3/25-negative. Because W3/25-positive cells are required to provide T-cell help in these experiments it is not possible to ask whether T cell–T cell collaboration between MRC OX 8-positive and W3/25-positive cells is needed for the allogeneic suppression effect.

F. Summary of Functional Studies

The series of experiments described in the preceding sections amply confirm that the antigens recognized by the monoclonal antibodies W3/25 and MRC OX 8 serve as markers for functionally different T-cell subpopulations. The three assays of T-cell function are in accord with the labeling studies in defining two T-cell subpopulations. Thus on a functional basis T cells were either W3/25-positive, MRC OX 8-negative or W3/25-negative, MRC OX 8-positive. Table II summarizes the established roles of these T-cell subpopulations.

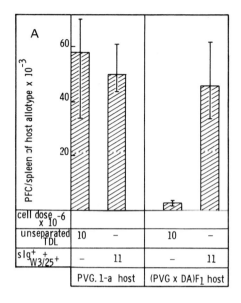
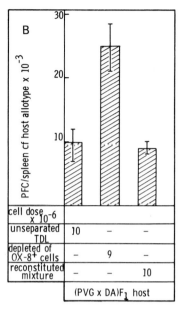

FIGURE 9. The ability of W3/25-negative, MRC OX 8-positive parental cells to suppress the antibody response of sublethally irradiated F_1 recipients. (A) TDL from PVG donors, primed to DNPBGG, were transferred, either unfractionated or depleted of W3/25-negative T cells, into 660-rad irradiated rats. These recipients were either PVG.1-a, congeneic with PVG but with the 1-a light-chain allotype of DA, or (PVG × DA)F_1. The anti-DNP response was assayed autoradiographically (Mason, 1976) using ^{125}I-labeled anti-1-a allotype to detect the plaques derived from host B cells. (B) The procedure was similar to that of Fig. 9A, except that MRC OX 8 monoclonal antibody was used to label the parental TDL. Recipients were all (PVG × DA)F_1.

VI. Inhibition of the Mixed Lymphocyte Reactions by W3/25 Antibody

Various monoclonal antibodies were added to the tissue culture medium in rat MLR to see if any of them influenced the proliferative response (Webb *et al.*, 1979). The antibodies used were W3/13, MRC OX 1, which labels all leukocytes (Sunderland *et al.*, 1979), MRC OX 7, a monoclonal anti-Thy-1.1 and W3/25. Of these antibodies only two had any effect. W3/25 antibody produced a profound suppression of the MLR that was fully developed at an initial antibody concentration of 25 ng/ml. In contrast W3/13 antibody produced a moderate but consistent increase in tritiated thymidine ([^{3}H]-Tdr) incorporation (Fig. 10). The suppression mediated by W3/25 antibody was also observed when the F(ab')$_2$ fragment of the antibody was used, indicating that the Fc fragment of the molecule was not involved in the inhibition (Fig. 10). That this suppression was dependent on the W3/25 antibody specificity was established by absorbing the antibody with equal numbers of rat or rabbit thymocytes. Absorption with rat

TABLE II

Functions of Rat T-Cell Subpopulations Defined by W3/25 and MRC OX 8 Monoclonal Antibodies

	T-cell function			
T-cell subset	Helper activity	GVH reactivity	Allogeneic suppression	MLR activity
W3/25+, OX 8−	+++	+++	−[a]	+++
W3/25−, OX 8+	−	±	+++	+

[a]Allogeneic suppression may require collaboration between W3/25-positive and W3/25-negative cells for its full expression (R. White, unpublished).

thymocytes completely removed suppressive activity whilst absorption with rabbit thymocytes left it intact (Fig. 11).

In order to exclude the possibility that W3/25 antibody was simply killing the responding cells in the MLR a preincubation in the presence or absence of W3/25 antibody was carried out. It was found that cells could be incubated for up to 24 hr in the presence of antibody without a decline in their ability to

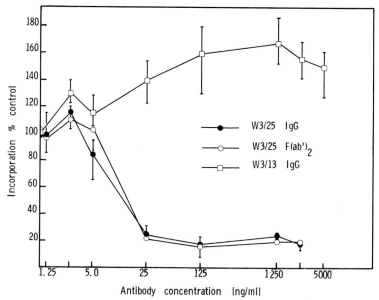

FIGURE 10. Effect of W3/25 and W3/13 antibody on the MLR. Lymph node cells (2×10^5) from PVG (RT1^c) were cultured with 5×10^5 irradiated spleen cells from HO.B2 (RT1^y) as described by Antczak et al. (1979). The monoclonal antibodies were added at the start of the culture period and [^{3}H]-Tdr at 72 hr. Incorporated counts were determined 18 hr later. All results have been normalized by putting the control MLR incorporation at 100%. The control values were 22×10^3 cpm for the experiments using W3/25 antibody or its F(ab')$_2$ fragment and 40×10^3 cpm for the W3/13 experiment.

FIGURE 11. (A) The ability of rat thymocytes but not rabbit thymocytes to absorb out the inhibitory action of W3/25 antibody on the rat MLR. W3/25 antibody was used unabsorbed or absorbed with rat or rabbit thymocytes. One absorption was done using enough cells to represent, for rat thymocytes, an approximate equivalence of antigen and antibody. The absorbed and unabsorbed preparations were examined for their ability to inhibit the rat MLR using the system described in the caption to Fig. 10. Results are expressed as a percentage of cpm from control cultures (54×10^3 cpm).

(B) Failure to inhibit the PHA-induced proliferation of rat lymph node cells by W3/25 antibody. PHA at $20 \mu g/ml$ was used to stimulate cultures of lymph node cells in the presence or absence of W3/25 antibody. Thymidine incorporation was determined 48 hr after initiation of culture. Control cultures, set at 100% in the figure, incorporated 35×10^3 cpm. Similar experiments (data not shown) were carried out using Con A; again no effect of W3/25 antibody was observed.

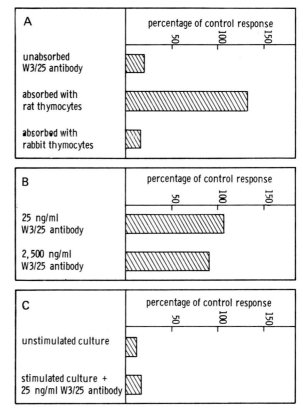

(C) The suppressive effect of W3/25 monoclonal antibody on the rat MLR using stimulator cells depleted of W3/25-positive cells. PVG rat TDL, depleted of W3/25-positive cells on the FACS, were irradiated and used as stimulators in the MLR with HO.B2 lymph node cells as responders. In the absence of W3/25 antibody the control cultures incorporated 18×10^3 cpm of [^{3}H]-Tdr and this has been taken as 100%. The figure shows the thymidine incorporation of unstimulated cultures and also of stimulated cultures in the presence of W3/25 antibody, expressed as percentages of the control response.

respond in a subsequent MLR. After 48 hr of preincubation a marked decrease in responsiveness was observed, which, however, was matched by a similar decrease in responsiveness by cells preincubated in the absence of W3/25 antibody. These observations make it unlikely that W3/25 antibody mediates its suppression by being cytotoxic. When the effect of W3/25 antibody on the response of rat lymph node cells to the T-cell mitogens Con A and phytohemagglutinin (PHA) was examined, no suppression was observed. Thus the suppression obtained in the MLR does not extend to mitogen-induced proliferation (Fig. 11).

Because W3/25-positive cells, in the above experiments, were present in both the responder and stimulator populations, the suppression of the MLR by W3/25 antibody could, in principle, be mediated by an interaction with either responder or stimulator cells. However, when unfractionated responders were cocultured with irradiated stimulators depleted of W3/25-positive cells, the subsequent MLR was strongly (90%) inhibited by W3/25 antibody (Fig. 11). This experiment unambiguously identified the W3/25-positive responder cell as the target for the inhibitory action of W3/25 antibody.

VII. Discussion

These studies establish the monoclonal antibodies W3/25 and MRC OX 8 as markers for thymocytes and peripheral T cells in the rat. In the thymus small but definite populations expressed one antigen to the exclusion of the other, but the great majority of thymocytes were labeled by both antibodies. Because peripheral T cells express one or other but not both markers, it seems probable that the small populations of singly marked cells in the thymus represent the mature elements that the thymus is known to contain (Cantor and Weissman, 1976). There can be no doubt that, since such a high proportion of thymocytes express both markers, the great majority of cortical thymocytes must be included in the population of W3/25-positive, MRC OX 8-positive cells. Whether these cells are precursors of the singly marked, presumably mature cells is not known. Nor is it known whether the subpopulation of W3/25-positive, MRC OX 8-positive cells that are also Ia-positive represents a different lineage from those that lack Ia or whether these subpopulations are different stages of the same differentiation sequence.

The spleens of congenitally athymic rats contained both W3/25-positive and MRC OX 8-positive cells, although the numbers present were much below those found in normal animals. No doubly marked cells were present so these cells resembled peripheral T cells rather than cortical thymocytes in their expression of antigens. The functional capacity of these cells remains to be established.

The functional studies of the W3/25-positive and MRC OX 8-positive peripheral T cells demonstrate that rat T cells are functionally heterogeneous. Cells that provided help for B cells and those mediating GVH and MLR were all W3/25-positive, MRC OX 8-negative. On the other hand, the suppression of antibody formation in the presence of an allogeneic interaction required the presence of W3/25-negative, MRC OX 8-positive cells. The phenotype of lymphocytes involved in cell-mediated immunity is not yet known. In view of the several functions ascribed to W3/25-positive cells, it may be reasonably anticipated that further cell-surface marker heterogeneity remains to be uncovered.

The MLR was remarkably sensitive to the inhibitory effect of W3/25 monoclonal antibody as it occurred at an initial antibody concentration such that there were only about 3 times as many molecules of antibody as antigen present in the assay. The mechanism of this inhibition, like the role of the W3/25 antigen itself, is not known. Cells that react in GVH assays do not demonstrably bind to monolayers of allogeneic cells (Chisholm and Ford, 1978) so it may not be possible to establish readily whether or not W3/25 antibody interferes with the recognition of alloantigens by responder cells. However, it is encouraging to find that a monoclonal antibody directed toward a T-cell-specific antigen has such a profound effect on a uniquely T-cell function.

VIII. Summary

Two mouse monoclonal antibodies called MRC OX 8 and W3/25 mark subsets of rat T lymphocytes. The antigens recognized were clearly identified on thymocytes and T lymphocytes but not on other tissues or hemopoietic cells. Most but not all thymocytes display both W3/25 and MRC OX 8 antigens, while in peripheral lymphoid tissues cells were either W3/25-positive, MRC OX 8-negative or W3/25-negative, MRC OX 8-positive. In normal rats the ratio of W3/25-positive to MRC OX 8-positive T cells was 80:20 in thoracic duct lymph, 70:30 in lymph node and 50:50 in spleen. In congenitally athymic rats neither cell type was significantly detected in TDL or bone marrow but spleen contained about 8% W3/25-positive, MRC OX 8-negative cells and a similar number of W3/25-negative, MRC OX 8-positive cells.

Activity for the helper, GVH, and MLR T cell functions was found in the W3/25-positive population but was absent in MRC OX 8-positive cells. The latter cell type, however, mediated an allogeneic suppressor function, which was not seen with w3/25-positive cells.

The MLR was inhibited by W3/25 antibody but this inhibition was not mediated via cytotoxic action of the antibody on the responding cells. This suggests that the W3/25 antigen may play a specific role in the MLR.

ACKNOWLEDGMENTS

R. Brideau was supported by the National Institute of Arthritis, Metabolism and Digestive Diseases, Grant No. AM 18530-05. W. R. McMaster was supported by an Exhibition of 1851 Scholarship.

References

Antczak, D. F., Brown, D., and Howard, J. C., 1979, Analysis of lymphocytes reactive to histocompatibility antigens. I. A quantitative titration assay for mixed lymphocyte interactions in the rat, *Cell. Immunol.* **43**:304.

Brideau, R. J., Carter, P. B., Mason, D. W., McMaster, W. R., and Williams, A. F., 1980, Two subsets of rat T lymphocytes defined with monoclonal antibodies, *Eur. J. Immunol.* (in press).

Cantor, H., and Boyse, E. A., 1976, Regulation of cellular and humoral immune responses by T-cell subclasses, *Cold Spring Harbor Symp. Quant. Biol.* **41**:23.

Cantor, H., and Weissman, I., 1976, Development and function of subpopulations of thymocytes and T lymphocytes, *Prog. Allergy* **20**:1.

Chisholm, P. M., and Ford, W. L., 1978, Selection of antigen-specific cells by adherence to allogeneic cell monolayers: Cytolytic activity, graft-vs.-host activity and numbers of adherent and nonadherent cells, *Eur. J. Immunol.* **8**:438.

Ford, W. L., Burr, W., and Simonsen, M., 1970, A lymph node weight assay for the graft-versus-host activity of rat lymphoid cells, *Transplantation* **10**:258.

Hunt, S. V., Mason, D. W., and Williams, A. F., 1977, In rat bone marrow Thy-1 antigen is present on cells with membrane immunoglobulin, and on precursors of peripheral B lymphocytes, *Eur. J. Immunol.* **7**:817.

Jensenius, J. C., and Williams, A. F., 1974, The binding of antiimmunoglobulin antibodies to rat thymocytes and thoracic duct lymphocytes, *Eur. J. Immunol.* **4**:91.

Köhler, G., and Milstein, C., 1976, Derivation of specific antibody-producing tissue culture and tumor lines by cell fusion, *Eur. J. Immunol.* **6**:511.

Letarte-Muirhead, M., Barclay, A. N., and Williams, A. F., 1975, Purification of the Thy-1 molecule, a major cell-surface glycoprotein of rat thymocytes, *Biochem. J.* **151**:685.

Loken, M. R., and Herzenberg, L. A., 1975, Analysis of cell populations with a fluorescence activated cell sorter, *Ann. NY Acad. Sci.* **254**:163.

McMaster, W. R., and Williams, A. F., 1979, Identification of Ia glycoproteins in rat thymus and purification from rat spleen, *Eur. J. Immunol.* **9**:426.

Mason, D. W., 1976, An improved autoradiographic technique for the detection of antibody-forming cells, *J. Immunol. Methods* **10**:301.

Mason, D. W., and Gallico, G. G., 1978, Tissue distribution and quantitation of Ia-like antigens in the rat, *Eur. J. Immunol.* **8**:741.

Mason, D. W., and Williams, A. F., 1980, The kinetics of antibody binding to membrane antigens in solution and at the cell surface, *Biochem. J.* **187**:1.

Möller, G., ed., 1969, Antigen sensitive cells, *Transplant. Rev.* **1**.

Nakayama, E., Shiku, H., Stockert, E., Oettgen, H. F., and Old, L. J., 1979, Cytotoxic T cells: Lyt phenotype and blocking of killing activity by Lyt antisera, *Proc. Natl. Acad. Sci. USA* **76**:1977.

Parish, C. R., and Hayward, J. A., 1974a, The lymphocyte surface. II. Separation of Fc receptor, C'_3 receptor and surface immunoglobulin-bearing lymphocytes, *Proc. R. Soc. Lond. [Biol.]* **187**:65.

Parish, C. R., and Hayward, J. A., 1974b, The lymphocyte surface. III Function of Fc receptor, C'_3 receptor and surface Ig bearing lymphocytes: Identification of a radio resistant B cell, *Proc. R. Soc. Lond. [Biol.]* **187**:379.

Piguet, P.-F., Dewey, H. K., and Vassalli, P., 1975, Study of the cells proliferating in parent versus F_1 hybrid mixed lymphocyte culture, *J. Exp. Med.* **141**:775.

Raff, M. C., 1971, Surface antigenic markers for distinguishing T and B lymphocytes in mice, *Transplant. Rev.* **6**:52.

Ritter, M. A., Gordon, L. K., and Goldschneider, I., 1978, Distribution and identity of Thy-1 bearing cells during ontogeny in rat hemopoietic and lymphoid tissues, *J. Immunol.* **121**:2463.

Scollay, R., Kochen, M., Butcher, E., and Weissman, I., 1978, Lyt markers on thymus cell migrants, *Nature* **276**:79.

Standring, R., McMaster, W. R., Sunderland, C. A., and Williams, A. F., 1978, The predominant heavily glycosylated glycoproteins at the surface of rat lymphoid cells are differentiation antigens, *Eur. J. Immunol.* **8**:832.

Sunderland, C. A., McMaster, W. R., and Williams, A. F., 1979, Purification with monoclonal antibody of a predominant leukocyte-common antigen and glycoprotein from rat thymocytes, *Eur. J. Immunol.* **9**:155.

Webb, M., Mason, D. W., and Williams, A. F., 1979, Inhibition of the mixed lymphocyte response with a monoclonal antibody specific for a rat T lymphocyte subset, *Nature* **282**:841.

White, R. A. H., Mason, D. W., Williams, A. F., Galfrè, G., and Milstein, C., 1978, T-lymphocyte heterogeneity in the rat: Separation of functional subpopulations using a monoclonal antibody, *J. Exp. Med.* **148:**664.

Williams, A. F., 1977, Differentiation antigens of the lymphocyte cell surface, in: *Contemporary Topics in Molecular Immunology,* Vol. 6 (G. L. Ada and R. R. Porter, eds.), Plenum, New York, pp. 83–116.

Williams, A. F., Barclay, A. N., Letarte-Muirhead, M., and Morris, R. J., 1976, Rat Thy-1 antigens from thymus and brain: Their tissue distribution, purification and chemical composition, *Cold Spring Harbor Symp. Quant. Biol.* **41:**51.

Williams, A. F., Galfre, G., and Milstein, C., 1977, Analysis of cell surfaces by xenogeneic myeloma-hybrid antibodies: Differentiation antigens of rat lymphocytes, *Cell* **12:**663.

16
Monoclonal Antibody Therapy of Mouse Leukemia

Irwin D. Bernstein, Robert C. Nowinski,
Milton R. Tam, Brian McMaster, L. L. Houston, and
Edward A. Clark

I. Introduction

Antibody treatment of neoplastic disease has long been of interest. Under certain limited conditions, significant inhibition of tumor growth has been achieved (reviewed in Wright and Bernstein, 1980). The therapeutic effects obtained with antisera have suggested a potential role for antibody therapy, but the success of this approach has so far not been impressive. Limitations in the effectiveness of serum treatment may have resulted from insufficient quantities of high-titered antibody of appropriate class, avidity, and specificity.

Conclusions about the ultimate utility of the antibody treatment of neoplasia may need to be reassessed as a result of the development of monoclonal antibody techniques (Köhler and Milstein, 1975, 1976). The availability of monoclonal antibody against tumor cell-surface antigens affords an opportunity heretofore unavailable to treat tumors with antibody in virtually unlimited amounts (Koprowski et al., 1978; Herlyn et al., 1979; Kennett and Gilbert, 1979; Yeh et al., 1979; Levy et al., 1979). The use of these antibodies of defined class, specificity,

Irwin D. Bernstein • Pediatric Oncology Program of the Fred Hutchinson Cancer Research Center, Seattle, Washington 98104, and Department of Pediatrics, University of Washington, Seattle, Washington 98195. Robert C. Nowinski • Tumor Virology Program of the Fred Hutchinson Cancer Research Center, Seattle, Washington 98104, and Department of Microbiology, University of Washington, Seattle, Washington 98195. Milton R. Tam and L. L. Houston • Tumor Virology Program of the Fred Hutchinson Cancer Research Center, Seattle, Washington 98104. Brian McMaster • Pediatric Oncology Program of the Fred Hutchinson Cancer Research Center, Seattle, Washington 98104. Edward A. Clark • Department of Genetics, University of Washington, Seattle, Washington 98195.

and avidity will also allow a precise characterization of antitumor effects *in vivo*. Although monoclonal antibodies against unique tumor cell-surface antigens have yet to be convincingly demonstrated, antibodies against differentiation antigens expressed by tumor cell surfaces are available (Kennett and Gilbert, 1979; Levy *et al.*, 1979). This latter type of antibody has provided the basis for the approach to serum therapy taken in our laboratories.

We have recently begun to evaluate the use of monoclonal antibodies against a normal differentiation antigen (Thy-1) for the treatment of murine leukemia. We have isolated hybrid cells producing monoclonal antibody of different immunoglobulin (Ig) classes against Thy-1.1. This chapter will summarize initial studies in which we have characterized the anti-Thy-1.1 monoclonal antibodies and studied their influence on transplantable AKR/J leukemia of spontaneous origin (Nowinski *et al.*, 1977) and normal T cells both *in vivo* and *in vitro*.

II. Characterization of Anti-Thy-1 Antibodies Used for Serum Therapy

The methods used to produce hybrid cells secreting IgG monoclonal anti-Thy-1.1 antibody are described elsewhere and in an accompanying chapter (Nowinski *et al.*, 1979, and this volume). For these purposes spleen cells used for hybridization were from strain 129 mice immunized with the transplantable AKR/J SL3 (Nowinski *et al.*, 1977) leukemia. Culture supernatants were screened in an antibody binding assay with Thy-1.1 antigen obtained as membrane fragments exfoliated by AKR/J SL3 cells into the tissue culture medium. Hybridomas secreting anti-Thy-1.1 antibody were cloned and established as tumors *in vivo* for the production of ascites fluids containing high-titered antibodies. The monoclonal antibodies used in these studies include: IgG2a antibodies designated 19-A10, 19-E12, and 19-F12(M); IgG3 antibodies designated 19-IXE8 and 19-XE5; and IgM antibodies designated T11D7 and T11A9. The development and characterization of the Thy-1.1-specific IgM antibodies have been described in a separate publication (Lake *et al.*, 1979).

Specificity of Anti-Thy-1.1 Monoclonal Antibodies. Specificity of the anti-Thy-1.1 monoclonal antibodies was examined by immunofluorescence and complement-dependent cytotoxicity assays. In each case the activities of the antibodies were examined on matched sets of thymus cells from congenic partners (AKR/J vs. AKR/Cum; A.Thy-1.1 vs. A). Results of immunofluorescence tests analyzed with the fluorescence-activated cell sorter (FACS II, Becton-Dickinson) are shown in Fig. 1. In these studies, thymocytes from AKR/J (Thy-1.1) and AKR/Cum (Thy-1.2) mice were incubated with each monoclonal antibody and then reacted with a fluorescein-conjugated goat anti-mouse immunoglobulin. As can be seen, intense fluorescence was associated with thymocytes from the AKR/J mice, but not with thymocytes of the AKR/Cum mice. Interestingly, thymocytes

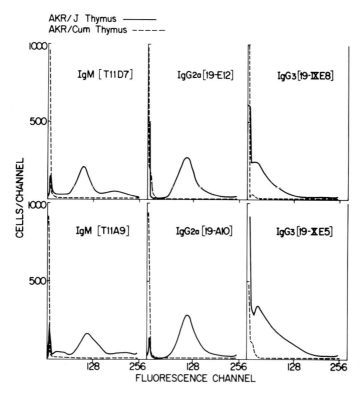

FIGURE 1. Specificity of monoclonal anti-Thy-1.1 antibodies. Thymocytes from AKR/J (Thy-1.1) and AKR/Cum (Thy-1.2) mice were treated with each of 6 ascites fluids containing monoclonal anti-Thy-1.1 antibodies. Following incubation with fluorescein-conjugated rabbit anti-mouse Ig serum, fluorescence activity per cell was determined with the FACS. Fluorescence was associated with Thy-1.1+ and not Thy-1.2+ cells (see text for additional details). Each histogram represents the analysis of 40,000 cells on the FACS II.

coated with the IgG3 antibodies appeared to show less fluorescence on a per cell basis. Moreover, analysis of the light-scatter properties of these cells showed the IgG3-coated thymocytes to be of smaller size. This was surprising since conventional fluorescence microscopic techniques showed that the IgG3 control thymocytes were equally fluorescent and of normal size as compared to cells that were coated with the IgG2a and IgM monoclonal antibodies. However, it was also noted by conventional microscopy that the IgG3 antibodies strongly agglutinated the thymocyte preparations. In fact, subsequent studies revealed that the apparent decrease in cell size that was observed with the FACS was an artifact that was due to the shearing of the aggregated AKR/J thymocytes on passage through the nozzle, and that much of the fluorescence detected was associated with cell fragments.

Complement-dependent cytotoxic tests demonstrated that each of the monoclonal antibodies (independent of isotype) mediated lysis of thymocytes from AKR/J and A. Thy-1.1 mice, but not from AKR/Cum and strain A mice. The titers of these ascites fluids ranged from 10^{-5} to 10^{-7} on the positive cells; these same ascites fluids showed virtually no activity at dilutions of 10^{-2} on the negative cells. Results of complement-dependent cytotoxicity against AKR/J SL2 leukemia cells are described in a later section.

In immune precipitation tests with NP40 lysates of ^{125}I-surface-labeled AKR/J SL2 cells, 19-E12, an IgG2a antibody, was shown to precipitate a 27,000-dalton protein (Fig. 2). A protein of identical molecular weight was also precipitated by conventionally prepared anti-Thy-1.1 antiserum. A similar protein has been precipitated by the antibodies TllD7, 19-IXE8, 19-XE5, and 19-A10.

III. Influence of Monoclonal Anti-Thy-1.1 Antibody on Murine Leukemia Cells

The effects of monoclonal antibodies on AKR/J SL2 cells were analyzed both *in vitro* and *in vivo*. Assays performed *in vitro* included antibody-induced cytolysis that was mediated by either complement (CDC) or by normal spleen cells (ADCC). In addition, we compared each of the monoclonal antibodies for antitumor activity against a transplant of the syngeneic AKR/J leukemia. These

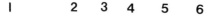

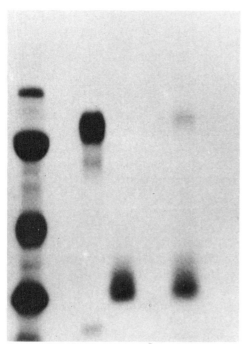

FIGURE 2. Immune precipitation assays with antisera against Thy-1.1 and gp70 antigens. Immune precipitation assays were performed with an NP40 lysate of ^{125}I-surface-labeled AKR/J SL2 leukemia cells and (2) goat anti-gp70 serum; (3) ascites fluid from hybrid cell 19-E12; (4) AKR/J anti-AKR/Cum thymus serum (detecting Thy-1.2); (5) AKR/Cum anti-AKR/J thymus serum (detecting Thy-1.1); and (6) normal mouse serum. Lane (1) contained ^{125}I-labeled molecular weight markers: phosphorylase b (97,000 daltons), bovine serum albumin (67,000 daltons), ovalbumin (45,000 daltons), and trypsin soybean inhibitor (25,000 daltons).

studies are described below, followed by a description of studies aimed at defining the mechanisms by which antibody inhibits tumor growth.

A. Antitumor Effects in Vitro

Ascites fluids containing monoclonal antibody were tested for CDC and ADCC activity against ^{51}Cr-labeled AKR/J SL2 leukemic cells. Results showed that antibody of each of the three isotypes tested, IgM, IgG2a, and IgG3, were lytic in CDC assays for the target cells at extremely high dilutions. The 50% titer endpoints ranged from approximately 2.6×10^5 to 3.2×10^7 (see Fig. 3). In contrast, in ADCC tests, only the IgG2a and IgG3 antibodies were effective. The titration curves of these antibodies were complex, the maximum ^{51}Cr release occurring approximately four double dilutions before a 20% lysis endpoint.

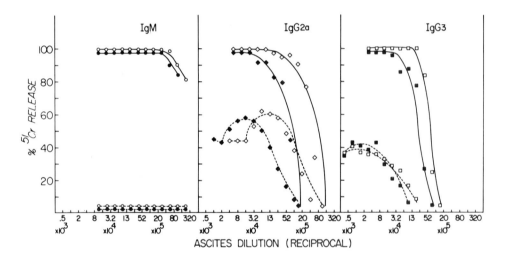

FIGURE 3. Complement- and cell-dependent lysis of AKR/J SL2 leukemia cells by monoclonal antibodies. Ascites fluids were tested in complement-dependent (CDC) (—) and antibody-dependent cell-mediated cytotoxicity assays (ADCC) (– – –). The ascites fluids contained either the IgM antibodies T11D7A (O—O) or T11A9 (●—●); the IgG2a antibodies 19-A10 (◆—◆) or 19-E12 (◇—◇); and the IgG3 antibodies 19-IXE8 (■—■) or 19-XE5 (□—□). For purposes of CDC, 50 μl of a target cell suspension (containing 10^4 ^{51}Cr-labeled AKR/J SL2 cells) was incubated for 45 min with 50 μl diluted antibody and 50 μl rabbit serum diluted 1/12 (as a source of complement). Intact cells were removed by centrifugation and an aliquot of the supernatant removed for counting. ^{51}Cr release was calculated relative to maximum release (determined by three cycles of freezing and thawing). ^{51}Cr release due to antibody or complement alone was generally less than 5% of the maximum release value. For purposes of ADCC assays, 50 μl of target cell suspensions (containing 10^4 ^{51}Cr-labeled AKR/J SL2 cells) were incubated for 4 hr with 50 μl effector cell suspensions (containing 10^6 spleen cells from normal nonimmunized 2-month-old C57BL/6 mice) and 50 μl diluted antibody. Intact cells were removed by centrifugation and the ^{51}Cr release relative to maximum release was determined. ^{51}Cr release seen with antibody or effector cells alone was generally below 10% of the maximum release values.

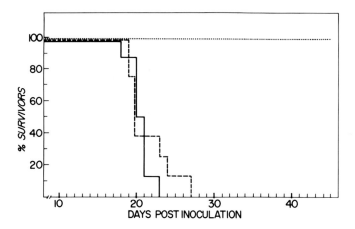

FIGURE 4. Treatment of AKR/J SL2 leukemia with IgG2a monoclonal anti-Thy-1.1 antibody. Three groups of AKR/J mice were inoculated s.c. with 10^5 AKR/J SL2 cells on day 0. Group 1(——), 8 untreated control mice; Group 2 (– – –), 8 control mice treated with rabbit serum alone; Group 3 (· · · · · ·), 6 test mice treated with 19-A10 ascites fluid and rabbit serum. Treatments were performed as follows: day 0, 100 μl 19-A10 ascites fluid and/or 100 μl rabbit serum i.v.; days 3, 7, 10, and 14, 50 μl 19-A10 ascites fluid and/or 100 μl rabbit serum i.p. [Reprinted from Bernstein *et al.*, 1980, by permission and copyright by American Association for the Advancement of Science, 1980.]

B. Antitumor Effects in Vivo

Initial experiments showed that passive immunization with IgG2a monoclonal antibody resulted in prolonged survival and, in a significant proportion of treated mice, cure of leukemia (Bernstein *et al.*, 1980). For example, in the treatment of AKR/J mice carrying a transplant of 10^5 AKR/J SL2 cells, a combination of 19-A10 ascites fluid and rabbit serum (used as source of complement) prevented tumor growth at the inoculum site and systemic leukemia in all mice. In contrast, control mice, either nontreated or treated with rabbit serum alone, all expired (Fig. 4).

C. Influence of Antibody Class

The following experiments were designed to compare the antitumor activity of monoclonal IgM, IgG2a, and IgG3 antibody *in vivo*. For this purpose, AKR/J mice were inoculated subcutaneously (s.c.) with 3 × 10^5 AKR/J SL2 cells, and antibody therapy initiated 1–2 hr later. Ascites fluids from the different hybridomas were adjusted in concentration* so that each mouse received approximately 1.5 mg of monoclonal antibody per dose. Since mice of the AKR/J strain were

---

*The quantity of antibody in ascites fluid was determined by electrophoresis on cellulose acetate membranes, followed by densitometric scanning of the stained membranes.

known to contain low levels of the complement component C′5, the mice in each treatment regimen were divided into two groups, one which received antibody alone and one which received antibody and 100 μl rabbit serum. In each case the complement was administered on the same day and, unless specified, by the same route as the antibody. The results of three such experiments are shown in Fig. 5.

Experiment I. In the first experiment (panel A), mice were treated with ascites fluid 19-E12 (IgG2a) or 19-XE5 (IgG3) alone or in combination with rabbit serum. Infusions were administered intravenously (i.v.) 1–2 hr after tumor inoculation, and then intraperitoneally (i.p.) on days 2, 4, and 7. In this particular experiment, significant prolongation of survival, but not cure, was observed due to the treatment with the IgG2a antibody. An intermediate effect due to the IgG3 antibody was observed, whereas no effect could be attributed to treatment with the rabbit serum alone.

Experiment II. In this experiment (panel B), the same 19-E12, and 19-XE5 ascites fluids were tested in comparison to the IgM-containing ascites fluid T11A9. Details of this study were the same as for the preceding one, except that the antibody/complement treatments were administered on days 0, 2, and 4 only. Prolonged survival and also a significant proportion of cures were attributed to the IgG2a antibody treatment. Again, a smaller effect was observed due to the IgG3 antibody. However, no effect whatsoever could be attributed to the IgM antibody.

Assessment of serum antibody in treated mice 1–2 hr after the final treatment showed that high cytotoxic titers (50% endpoint) were uniformly achieved in mice that received IgG2a antibody ($6.4–51.2 \times 10^{-3}$); mice treated with IgG3 antibody showed lower titers ($0.4–6.4 \times 10^{-3}$), whereas variable results were observed in IgM-treated mice ($1.6–102 \times 10^{-3}$). Importantly, however, 3 days after the final treatment only mice that had received the IgG2a antibody showed high cytotoxic titers ($0.8–12.8 \times 10^{-3}$); no activity was seen with the sera from mice that were treated with other antibodies.

Experiment III. On the chance that our failure to achieve an effect using the IgM antibody was a result of our choice of the i.p. route for most of the doses, or perhaps the use of a short treatment course, we administered the T11D7 ascites fluid i.v. every other day for 12 days. We infused approximately 3 mg of antibody on day 0, and 1.5 mg on subsequent days. Again, the results (panel C) failed to reveal an effect of the IgM antibody. This failure was somewhat surprising, especially since this monoclonal antibody was known to mediate complement-dependent lysis of AKR/J SL2 cells *in vitro* at extremely high dilutions. This failure could be explained in one of two ways: First complement-dependent cytotoxicity may not be an efficient antitumor mechanism *in vivo*. Rather, a cell-dependent cytotoxic mechanism, which was observed *in vitro* only with the IgG antibodies, may have been responsible for the antitumor effects *in vivo*. Second, it may be that IgM molecules are eliminated from the serum too rapidly to be effective under the conditions utilized here. We have begun to investigate this latter possibility and preliminary results are described below.

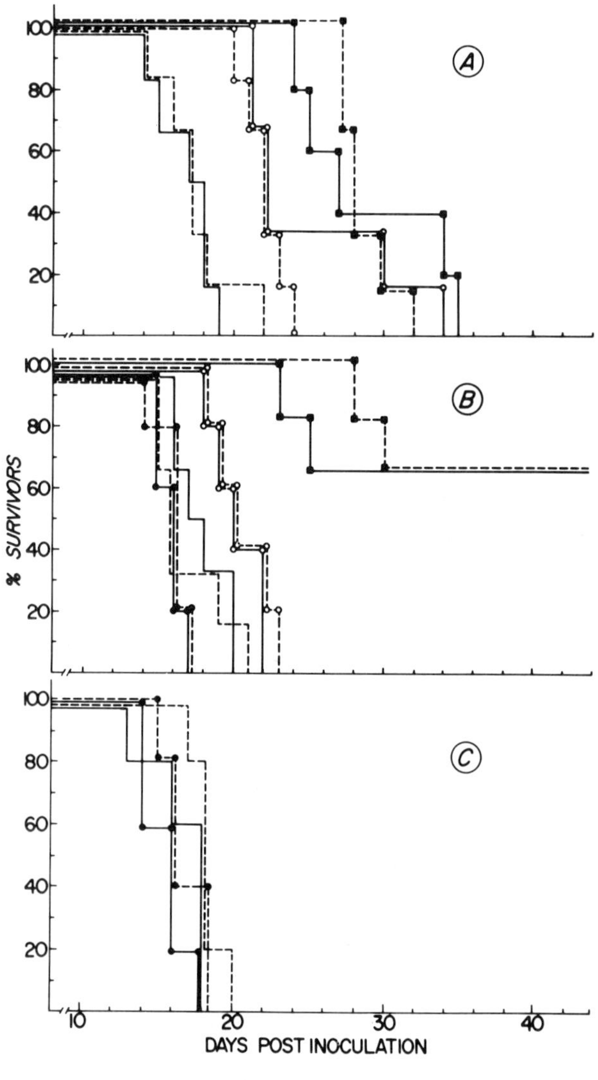

FIGURE 5. Treatment of leukemia transplants with monoclonal anti-Thy-1.1 antibody: effect of antibody subclass. Antibodies of the IgM, IgG2a, and IgG3 subclasses were compared for their ability to inhibit a subcutaneous transplant of 3×10^5 syngeneic AKR/J SL2 leukemia cells. In these experiments, approximately 1.5 mg of antibody and/or $100 \mu l$ rabbit serum was infused on each treatment day. Each of these experiments are described separately below:

Experiment I (panel A): Six groups of 6 AKR/J mice each were treated as follows: Group 1 (———), untreated controls; Group 2 (– – –), control mice treated with rabbit serum alone; Group 3 (O—O), mice treated with 19-XE5 (IgG3) ascites fluid alone; Group 4 (O- - -O), mice treated with 19-XE5 ascites fluid and rabbit serum; Group 5 (■—■), mice treated with 19-E12 (IgG2a) ascites fluid alone; and Group 6 (■- - -■), mice treated with 19-E12 ascites fluid and rabbit serum. Treatments were performed i.v. on day 0 and s.c. on days 2, 4, and 7.

Experiment II (panel B): Eight groups of AKR/J mice were treated as follows: Group 1 (———), 6 untreated mice; Group 2 (– – –), 6 control mice treated with rabbit serum alone; Group 3 (O—O), 5 mice treated with 19-XE5 (IgG3) ascites fluid;

Group 4 (O- - -O), 5 mice treated with 19-XE5 ascites fluid and rabbit serum; Group 5 (■—■), 6 mice treated with ascites fluid 19-E12 (IgG2a); Group 6 (■- - -■), 6 mice treated with ascites fluid 19-E12 and rabbit serum; Group 7 (●—●), 5 mice treated with T11A9 (IgM) ascites fluid; and Group 8 (●- - -●), 5 mice treated with T11A9 ascites fluid and rabbit serum. Treatments were performed i.v. on day 0 and i.p. on days 2 and 4.

Experiment III (panel C): Four groups of 5 AKR/J mice each were treated as follows: Group 1 (———), untreated controls; Group 2 (– – –), control mice treated with rabbit serum; Group 3 (●—●), mice treated with T11D7 (IgM) ascites fluid; and Group 4 (●- - -●), mice treated with T11D7 ascites fluid and rabbit serum. Treatments were performed on days 0, 2, 4, 6, 8, 10, and 12. The initial dose (day 0) was increased to approximately 3 mg of antibody. Ascites fluid was always administered i.v., while complement was infused i.v. on day 0 and i.p. thereafter.

IV. Pharmacokinetics of Monoclonal Antibodies

We have studied the half-life of ^{125}I-labeled monoclonal anti-Thy-1.1 IgM, IgG2a, and IgG3 antibodies in AKR/Cum mice. Each mouse was injected intravenously with 10×10^6 cpm of radiolabeled antibody, and the remaining cpm of antibody per mg of blood assessed following varying intervals. Calculations from the results shown in Fig. 6 indicated that the half-life of the monoclonal IgM antibody was significantly shorter than that of the IgG2a antibody. The IgM clearance curve was also more complex, with an initial rapid phase. Interestingly, the half-life of IgG3 was intermediate, correlating with its intermediate activity in the *in vivo* therapy studies. Although these studies suggest a potential correlation between antibody clearance and effects *in vivo*, it is still difficult to reconcile the complete susceptibility of mice that were treated for a full 12-day course.

Studies on the pharmacology of the monoclonal antibodies in AKR/J mice are presently in progress. Based on these results, experiments will be designed to achieve similar serum titers *in vivo* for each of the immunoglobulin classes. In this manner it should be possible to compare more precisely their antitumor activities *in vivo*. Nonetheless, our experiments to date have already demonstrated that, on a weight basis, IgG2a antibody is more effective than IgG3, and that IgM is relatively, or completely, ineffective in the treatment of leukemia.

V. Combined Surgical and Antibody/Complement Treatment

The studies presented in Fig. 5 demonstrated that IgG monoclonal anti-Thy-1.1 antibody can prolong the survival of leukemic mice. In instances where mice survived longer but were not cured as a result of antibody treatment, there

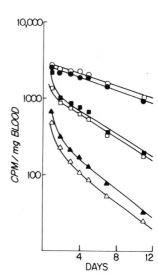

FIGURE 6. Clearance of ^{125}I-labeled monoclonal IgM, IgG2a, and IgG3 antibodies. ^{125}I-labeled monoclonal anti-Thy-1.1 antibodies (10^7 cpm per mouse) were infused i.v. into AKR/Cum mice and the amount of radioactivity in blood determined at intervals. Two mice were used for each antibody in the clearance assay; these are designated by the appropriate open or closed symbol on the graph. IgM (T11D7), ▲—▲ ; IgG2a (19-F12(M)), ●—● ; IgG3 (19-IXE8), ■—□ . The results were corrected for the rate of decay of ^{125}I.

was little or no effect of the treatment on local growth of tumor at the inoculum site. However, in all instances, when mice were cured of their leukemias by antibody treatments, complete inhibition of both systemic and local disease occurred. Thus, the monoclonal antibodies were effective primarily by retarding the development of systemic leukemia, and in most instances, they had a lesser effect on local tumor growth. In fact at the time the mice developed overt systemic leukemia, the size of tumors at the inoculum site was significantly larger in the treated as compared to the untreated mice. Presumably, the local tumor mass served as a reservoir for cells which subsequently metastasized and killed the host when effective antibody titers were no longer present. Based on this observation we have now used a combination of surgery to treat local disease and antibody/complement therapy to treat systemic disease in an attempt to achieve an increased cure rate (Bernstein et al., 1980). Accordingly, three groups of six (C57BL/6 × AKR/J)F_1 mice were challenged s.c. with 3×10^6 AKR/J SL2 leukemia cells. Two groups of mice were then treated with 50 μl 19-A10 antibody and 100 μl rabbit serum i.v. on day 0 and i.p. on days 3, 5, and 7. Tumors at the inoculum site were then excised from the mice in one of the treated and one of the control groups on day 10. The results showed 4 of 6 mice treated with a combination of surgery and antibody/complement were cured, whereas none of the mice treated with antibody/complement therapy or with surgery alone survived (data not shown).

VI. Mechanism of Antitumor Effects in Vivo

Collectively, the above-cited experiments demonstrated that monoclonal antibody treatment could dramatically influence the growth of syngeneic leukemia cells. However, the actual mechanism of this effect has still to be elucidated.

A. Does Antibody Affect Tumor in Vivo by Direct and/or Indirect Mechanisms?

The most likely explanation for the therapeutic effects of monoclonal anti-Thy-1.1 antibody is that the antibodies act directly by lysis of the leukemia cells. However, it is also possible that the anti-T cell antibodies act indirectly by modifying the host antileukemia immune response (e.g., by secondary effects on suppressor T cells).

In order to assess whether the antibodies act by direct mechanisms, we have asked whether the anti-Thy-1.1 antibody would inhibit tumor growth in mice where the antibody would not be expected to affect normal T cells. For this purpose the AKR/J SL2 leukemia was transplanted into AKR/Cum mice (Thy-1.2) and the tumor treated with 19-F12(M) antibody against Thy-1.1 antigen. As a control for the efficacy of the antibody treatment, a parallel group of AKR/J mice was also inoculated with the leukemia and treated with 19-F12(M) antibody in an identical manner. As shown in Fig. 7, inhibition of tumor growth was seen in both groups (AKR/J and AKR/Cum) of antibody treated mice. Since the anti-Thy-1.1 antibody was not reactive with the normal T cells of AKR/Cum mice, these results were considered evidence that a direct effect of antibody on the leukemia cells could affect tumor growth.

In order to determine whether there also was an indirect antitumor effect of antibody which was mediated by interaction of antibody with host T cells, we treated a transplant of 10^5 AKR/Cum leukemia cells (SL1) that was growing in AKR/J mice. In this instance the monoclonal antibodies would be expected to react with the normal T cells of the AKR/J mouse, but not with the transplant of AKR/Cum leukemia cells. For this purpose, the 19-A10 ascites fluid was administered in amounts equivalent in weight and cytotoxic activity to that used in the experiment in Fig. 4; it was infused along with rabbit serum on days 0, 2, 4, 6, 9, and 13. No inhibition of tumor growth was observed (data not shown), strongly

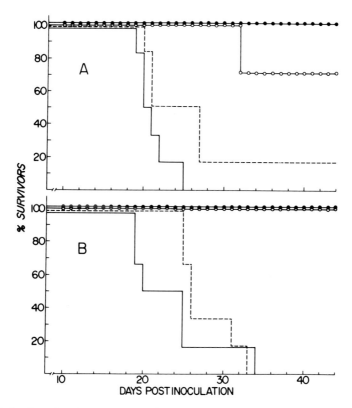

FIGURE 7. Mechanism of antitumor activity of anti-Thy-1.1 antibody. AKR/J (top panel) and AKR/Cum mice (bottom panel) were challenged s.c. with 10^5 AKR/J SL2 cells. Groups of 6 mice were treated as follows: Group 1 (———) untreated control mice; Group 2 (– – –) control mice treated with rabbit serum only; Group 3 (O—O) mice treated with 19-F12(M) ascites fluid only; and Group 4 (●—●) test mice treated with 19-F12(M) ascites fluid and rabbit serum. They were infused i.v. on day 0 and i.p. on days 3, 7, 10, and 14.

suggesting that indirect effects of the antibody on host T cells do not play a major role in the antitumor effect of serotherapy.

B. The Role of Complement

The above experiments suggested that antibody acts by the direct lysis of tumor cells. The two most obvious mechanisms by which this could occur were by a complement-dependent or a cell-dependent mechanism. Our experiments to date have suggested that infusion of antibody with complement resulted, overall, in an increased cure rate. The experiment in Fig. 8 represents one such example. In this experiment, $(129 \times AKR/J)F_1$ hybrid mice inoculated with 10^6 AKR/J SL2 cells were treated with 19-A10 ascites fluid on days 0, 2, 4, and 7. One half of the mice treated with antibody also received 100μl of rabbit serum at each treatment. Results showed that the antibody treatment with or without complement, led to a prolonged median survival of 33 days (as compared to 23 days for the controls). Three of eight mice were cured in the antibody-complement-treated group; no cures were achieved in the group treated with antibody alone. Cure was always associated with complete inhibition of tumor growth at the inoculum site, whereas local tumor invariably grew in all of the other mice, even when prolonged survival was observed. Thus, the major role of complement appeared to be amplification of the effect of antibody on local tumor growth.

There was also evidence to suggest that complement influences the effect of

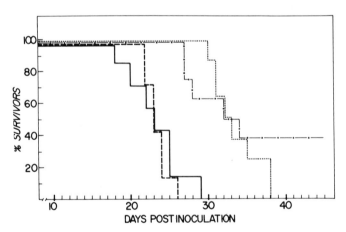

FIGURE 8. Serum therapy of AKR/J SL2 leukemia with monoclonal anti-Thy-1.1 antibodies: effect of complement. Four groups of $(129 \times AKR/J)F_1$ hybrid mice were inoculated s.c. with 10^6 AKR SL2 cells on day 0. Group 1 (———), 7 untreated control mice; Group 2 (– – –), 7 control mice treated with rabbit serum (as a source of complement) alone; Group 3 (· · · · · · ·), 8 test mice treated with 19-A10 ascites fluid alone; Group 4 (· – · – ·), 8 mice treated with 19-A10 ascites fluid and rabbit serum. Treatments were performed as follows: day 0, 100 μl 19-A10 ascites fluid and/or 100 μl rabbit serum i.v.; days 2, 4, and 7, 50 μl 19-A10 ascites fluid and/or 100 μl rabbit serum i.p. [Reprinted from Bernstein et al., 1980, by permission and copyright by American Association for the Advancement of Science, 1980.]

antibody on local tumor growth, but may not significantly affect treatment of the metastatic disease. This was suggested by the failure of IgM antibody (which mediated complement-dependent, but not cell-dependent lysis *in vitro*) to affect tumor growth. It is conceivable therefore that the complement-dependent mechanism plays a significant role in the inhibition of local tumor, while other mechanisms, presumably involving ADCC, may be of importance in preventing systemic disease.

VII. Influence of Monoclonal Antibody on Normal T Cells in Vivo

Since the anti-Thy-1.1 antibody used to treat leukemia was also reactive with normal AKR/J cells, we were also concerned about the effects of antibody on host T lymphocytes. Effects on host immunity were not grossly apparent, since treated mice generally remained healthy if they were rendered tumor free or until they suffered from overt systemic leukemia.

A. Enumeration of T Cells

The extent of T-cell elimination or alteration in AKR/J mice given monoclonal anti-Thy-1.1 antibody and exogenous complement was determined. We estimated the proportion of thymus, spleen, or lymph node cells bearing T- or B-cell markers, and in addition any cells coated with IgG2a antibody. In order to do so, we used the FACS for analysis of cells stained with the following reagents: First, T-cell Thy-1.1 antigen was investigated using the fluorescein-conjugated anti-Thy-1.1 antibody 19-E12. Second, the proportion of T cells bearing adsorbed IgG2a antibody 19-E12 (which presumably was blocking the Thy-1.1 sites in most cases) was identified using a fluorescein-conjugated rabbit anti-mouse IgG2a antibody. In addition, a very small number of B cells was expected to stain with the anti-IgG2a reagent. Third, the proportion of B cells was examined using a biotin-conjugated monoclonal anti-IgD antibody in combination with an avidin–fluorescein label. The fluorescein- and biotin-conjugated antibodies used in this study were a gift of Dr. J. Ledbetter, Stanford University.

In these experiments, groups of mice were treated with 50 μl of 19-E12 ascites fluid i.v., and 50 μl complement i.v. on days 0, 2, 4, 7, and 10; 24 hr later and then 7, 14, and 21 days later, thymus and lymph node were examined (Fig. 9). The results showed a significant diminution of the number of cells brightly stained with the fluorescent anti-Thy-1.1 antibody in both lymph node and thymus 24 hr after the last treatment; analysis with the anti-IgG2a antibody showed a small increase of stained cells in lymph node, and a larger increase in the thymus. These anti-IgG2a-stained cells may therefore include cells with Thy-1.1 antigenic sites partially or completely blocked by the infused antibody. Studies with the anti-IgD antibody showed that the proportion of B cells in the lymph

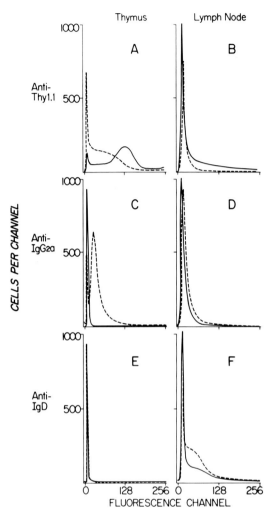

FIGURE 9. Enumeration of T cells in the thymus and lymph nodes of AKR/J mice treated with anti-Thy-1.1 monoclonal antibody and rabbit complement. Lymphoid cells from the thymuses and lymph nodes of AKR/J mice (———), or AKR/J mice treated (- - - - -) with 19-E12 (IgG2a) anti-Thy-1.1 monoclonal antibody (on days 0, 2, 4, 7, and 10), were examined on day 11 for potential changes in the populations of T or B cells. Immunofluorescence reactions were performed with (i) fluorescein-conjugated 19-E12 antibody (to measure Thy-1.1 positive cells), (ii) fluorescein-conjugated rabbit anti-mouse IgG2a immunoglobulin (to measure cells coated with 19-E12 antibody used in the treatment), and (iii) a biotin-conjugated monoclonal anti-IgD antibody in combination with an avidin–fluorescein label (to measure IgD-bearing B cells). Each histogram represents the analysis of 40,000 cells on the FACS II.

node was increased in the treated mice. This suggests that antibody treatment greatly reduced the number of T cells from lymph node, but thymocytes were, to a great extent, coated with the anti-Thy-1.1 antibody. The extent to which thymocytes may have been eliminated was not defined.

Results of similar analyses at subsequent time points showed that significant recovery in the number and proportion of T cells in lymph node was not evidenced 21 days following cessation of treatment. The level of available thymus Thy-1.1 surface antigen was still depressed on day 7, but returned to normal by 14 days after cessation of treatment. Increased detection of Thy-1.1 presumably resulted from loss of IgG2a antibody that previously blocked the Thy-1.1 cell surface sites, since a decreased number of thymocytes bearing surface IgG2a was detected at days 7 and 14.

Since a large proportion of thymocytes was coated with the anti-Thy-1.1

antibody, we assessed whether the coated lymph node or thymus cells were primed for lysis upon interaction with complement. We infused AKR/J mice with 50 μl 19-A10 antibody and 100 μl complement on days 0, 2, 4, and 7. On day 9 thymocytes and lymph node cells were obtained, incubated *in vitro* with or without complement, and assayed for viability using a trypan blue cytotoxicity test. The results showed that addition of complement alone to thymocytes of treated mice caused essentially complete lysis; no lysis was seen when thymocytes from normal mice were incubated with complement. This suggested that although the IgG2a antibody could enter the thymus and coat thymocytes, it failed to lyse the cells. In contrast, lymph node cells from treated mice did not show significant lysis upon incubation *in vitro* with either complement alone or in combination with anti-Thy-1.1 antibody. Thus, treatment may have eliminated the lymph node T cells *in vivo* because sufficient complement or effector cells were present. Presumably, sufficient amounts of effector cells or complement were not available within the thymus.

B. T-Cell Function

In one experiment, spleen cells were obtained from AKR/J mice treated with 50 μl 19-A10 ascites fluid and 100 μl rabbit serum on days 0, 2, 4, and 7. Two days after the last treatment spleen cells were obtained from these and control mice. The results (Table I) showed that the proliferative response of spleen cells from treated mice to the T cell mitogen Con A was impaired, whereas the response to the B cell mitogen LPS was similar to that seen with control cells. Cells from treated mice were also cultured with stimulating allogeneic cells. The proliferative response was significantly less than that seen in the control mice; when these cells were also tested for cytotoxic activity against ^{51}Cr-labeled allogeneic cells, an impaired cytotoxic cell response was also seen. Thus, treatment with monoclonal anti-Thy-1.1 antibody and complement appears to significantly depress T-cell function. These results also demonstrate another potential use for monoclonal antibody, i.e., as a highly effective anti-T-cell reagent.

VIII. Concluding Remarks

The results of studies presented here strongly suggest a clinical usefulness of monoclonal antibodies for treatment of leukemia. These experiments are of particular importance since the therapy was directed at a normal differentiation antigen, analogous to those expressed by certain human leukemias and lymphomas (Borella and Sen, 1973; Kersey *et al.*, 1973; Brovet *et al.*, 1976; Roberts *et al.*, 1978). In some instances antibody could directly cure mice, while in others, antibody was capable of curing established disease in combination with surgery. Although the mechanism of action of anti-Thy-1 antibody has not as yet been

TABLE I

Cellular Responses by AKR/J Spleen Cells following in Vivo Infusions of Monoclonal Anti-Thy-1.1 Antibody and Complement

Responding spleen cells from mice treated with[a]	Proliferative response to mitogen[b]			Response to B10.Sn allogeneic stimulating cells[c]		
				Proliferative response[b]		Cytotoxic response: % specific cytotoxicity
	Con A	LPS	Control	Stimulated	Unstimulated	
Antibody + complement	7.0	19.0	2.8	9.5	1.1	29.5
Untreated controls	27.8	21.6	2.4	63.3	2.2	55.2

[a]Mice were treated with $50\,\mu$l 19-A10 ascites fluid and $100\,\mu$l rabbit serum i.v. on day 0 and i.p. on days 2, 4, and 7. Spleens were removed and cells tested on day 9.

[b]Responding cells (2×10^5) were cultured with concanavalin A (Con A; Pharmacia, Uppsala) at a concentration of $0.3\,\mu$g/ml, with lipopolysaccharide W (LPS; *E. coli* 055-BS, Difco Laboratories, Detroit) at a concentration of $50\,\mu$g/ml, or alone in a volume of 0.1 ml serum-free EHAA medium in wells of a microtiter plate (Cooke No. 1-221-24). Following 72 hr of incubation, $0.25\,\mu$ Ci [^{3}H]thymidine was added to each culture. After an additional 16-hr incubation, counts per minute (cpm) [^{3}H]thymidine incorporated per culture was determined. Results are shown as cpm $\times 10^3$.

[c]Responding cells (5×10^5) were cultured with 7.5×10^5 X-irradiated stimulating spleen cells in 0.1 ml medium supplemented with 0.5% syngeneic mouse serum. Following a 5-day culture period, proliferative activity was determined as above and cytotoxicity determined by adding 5×10^3 ^{51}Cr-labeled, LPS-stimulated B10.Sn spleen cells to each well. Following an additional 4-hr incubation period, the amount of ^{51}Cr release into the supernatant fluid was determined. Percent cytotoxicity was determined using the formula $(S_e - S_0/S_m - S_0) \times 100$, where S_e is ^{51}Cr release in experimental cultures, S_m is the maximal release due to multiple freeze–thaw cycles, and S_0 is the spontaneous release by labeled cells in medium or excess unlabeled target cells. Percent specific cytotoxicity was calculated as the difference between the cytotoxicity observed with antigen-stimulated and unstimulated AKR/J spleen cells.

defined, it appears to do so by a direct, presumably lytic mechanism and does not involve a host T-cell response. Whether lysis is mediated by a complement-dependent and/or cell-dependent mechanism remains to be defined. Data thus far suggest that although complement appears to play a role in amplifying antibody effects on tumor cells at a local site, it may not play a role in antibody effects against metastasizing cells. Alternative mechanisms such as ADCC may be operating to prevent metastases.

Our future studies will be directed toward a careful analysis of antibody treatment of transplanted as well as spontaneous leukemias. Information regarding the influence of antibody class, the requirement for exogenous complement, the pharmacology of monoclonal antibody, and the possible emergence of Thy-1.1-negative transplanted or spontaneous leukemias in antibody-treated mice will provide guidelines for future clinical studies. Additionally, studies on the ability of monoclonal antibody to specifically deliver cytotoxic compounds or radioactive labels to tumor deserves special attention in the near future. Hopefully, information accrued from studies such as these will allow us to avoid pitfalls inherent in past empirical approaches in clinical trials using other forms of immunotherapy. Finally, it should be noted that these exciting possibilities will only be fully realized when cell lines are developed that allow production of monoclonal human antibodies against similar types of antigens on human tumor cells.

ACKNOWLEDGMENT

This investigation was supported by Grant CA 26386 awarded by the National Cancer Institute, Department of Health, Education, and Welfare.

References

Bernstein, I. D., Tam, M. R., and Nowinski, R. C., 1980, Mouse leukemia: Therapy with monoclonal antibodies against a thymus differentiation antigen, *Science* **207**:68.

Borella, L., and Sen, L., 1973, T cell surface markers on lymphoblasts from acute lymphocytic leukemia, *J. Immunol.* **111**:1257.

Brovet, J. C., Valensi, F., Daniel, M. T., Flandrin, O., Preudhomme, J. L., and Seligmann, M., 1976, Immunological classification of acute lymphoblastic leukemias: Evaluation of its clinical significance in a hundred patients, *Br. J. Haematol.* **33**:319.

Herlyn, M., Steplewski, Z., Herlyn, D., and Koprowski, H., 1979, Colorectal carcinoma-specific antigen: Detection by means of monoclonal antibodies, *Proc. Natl. Acad. Sci. USA* **76**:1438.

Kennett, R. H., and Gilbert, F., 1979, Hybrid myelomas producing antibodies against a human neuroblastoma antigen present on fetal brain, *Science* **203**:1120.

Kersey, J. C., Sabad, A., Gajl-Peczalska, K., Hallgren, H. M., Yunis, E. J., and Nesbit, M. E., 1973, Acute lymphoblastic leukemic cells with T (thymus-derived) lymphocytic markers, *Science* **182**:1355.

Köhler, G., and Milstein, C., 1975, Continuous cultures of fused cells secreting antibody of predefined specificity, *Nature* **256**:495.

Köhler, G., and Milstein, C., 1976, Derivation of specific antibody-producing tissue culture and tumor lines by cell fusion, *Eur. J. Immunol.* **6**:511.

Koprowski, H., Steplewski, Z., Herlyn, D., and Herlyn, M., 1978, Study of antibodies against human melanoma cells produced by somatic hybrid cells, *Proc. Natl. Acad. Sci. USA* **75**:3405.

Lake, P., Clark, E. A., Khorshidi, M., and Sunshine, D. H., 1979, Production and characterization of cytotoxic Thy-1.1 antibody-secreting hybrid cell lines, *Eur. J. Immunol.* **9**:875.

Levy, R., Dilley, J., Fox, R. I., and Warnke, R., 1979, A human thymus leukemia antigen defined by hybridoma monoclonal antibodies, *Proc. Natl. Acad. Sci. USA* **76**:6552.

Nowinski, R. C., Hays, E. F., Doyle, T., Linkhart, S., Medieros, E., and Pickering, R., 1977, Oncornaviruses produced by murine leukemic cells in culture, *Virology* **81**:363.

Nowinski, R. C., Lostrom, M. E., Tam, M. R., Stone, M. R., and Burnette, W. N., 1979, The isolation of hybrid cell lines producing monoclonal antibodies against the p15(E) protein of ecotropic murine leukemia viruses, *Virology* **93**:111.

Roberts, M. Greaves, M., Janossy, G., Sutherland, R., and Pain, C., 1978, Acute lymphoblastic leukemia (ALL) associated antigen. Expression in different haematopoietic malignancies, *Leuk. Res.* **2**:105.

Wright, P. W., and Bernstein, I. D., 1980, Serotherapy of malignant disease, *Prog. Exp. Tumor Res.* **25**:140.

Yeh, M. Y., Hellström, I., Brown, J. P., Warner, G. A., Hansen, J. A., and Hellstrom, K. E., 1979, Cell surface antigens of human melanoma identified by monoclonal antibody, *Proc. Natl. Acad. Sci. USA* **79**:2927.

PART V
MONOCLONAL ANTIBODIES TO MICROORGANISMS

17
Mapping of Viral Proteins with Monoclonal Antibodies

Analysis of the Envelope Proteins of Murine Leukemia Viruses

ROBERT C. NOWINSKI, MARY R. STONE, MILTON R. TAM,
MARK E. LOSTROM, W. NEAL BURNETTE, AND
PAUL V. O'DONNELL

I. Introduction

The mouse leukemia viruses (MuLV) are a highly polymorphic group of agents that occur as endogenous infections in inbred and feral mice. All mice contain some genetic equivalents of MuLV, although considerable variation occurs in the particular viruses that are inherited by one mouse strain or another. On the basis of host range characteristics the endogenous MuLV have been classified into three major groups: (1) ecotropic MuLV efficiently infect murine cells, but not cells of other species (Hartley *et al.*, 1970), (2) xenotropic MuLV efficiently infect the cells of other species, but not murine cells (Levy, 1973), and (3) amphotropic MuLV efficiently infect cells of both murine and heterologous origin (Rasheed *et al.*, 1976; Hartley and Rowe, 1976). Viruses of each of these groups can be further subclassified by more defined biological characteristics [e.g., N-ecotropism vs. B-ecotropism (Hartley *et al.*, 1970) and inducible vs. noninducible xenotropic properties (Barbacid *et al.*, 1978)] and recombinant viruses with the prop-

ROBERT C. NOWINSKI • Tumor Virology Program of the Fred Hutchinson Cancer Research Center, Seattle, Washington 98104, and Department of Microbiology, University of Washington, Seattle, Washington 98195. MARY R. STONE, MILTON R. TAM, MARK E. LOSTROM, AND W. NEAL BURNETTE • Tumor Virology Program of the Fred Hutchinson Cancer Research Center, Seattle, Washington 98104. PAUL V. O'DONNELL • Memorial Sloan-Kettering Cancer Center, New York, New York 10021.

erties of two different parental viruses have also been found to occur at high frequency *in vivo* (Hartley *et al.*, 1977; Elder *et al.*, 1977).

The actual induction of leukemia in mice is a complex process that probably involves multiple viruses (Hartley *et al.*, 1977; Elder *et al.*, 1977; Nowinski *et al.*, 1977; Nowinski and Hays, 1978). In fact the *de novo* generation of unique recombinant viruses with expanded host range (polytropic) in individual mice is probably a direct event that precedes the transformation of thymocytes to leukemia cells (Elder *et al.*, 1977). Since these recombinant viruses are known to contain intragenic rearrangements in the *env* gene, there is speculation that the envelope proteins of these agents serve as transforming gene products.

This complexity associated with the numerous endogenous and recombinant viruses of the mouse makes it particularly difficult to study these events *in vivo*. It would therefore be desirable to develop specific probes that are capable of efficiently identifying and quantitating the expression of individual viruses within this multicomponent system. For this purpose we have isolated a series of hybrid cell lines that produce monoclonal antibodies that react with the viral envelope proteins of MuLV (Nowinski *et al.*, 1979). These hybrid cells were prepared by the method of Köhler and Milstein (1975, 1976), utilizing lymphocytes from mice that were immunized against MuLV-producing leukemia cells. Since our previous studies (Nowinski *et al.*, 1974) had shown that mice develop a vigorous immune response to the envelope proteins [gp70 and p15(E)] of MuLV, it was assumed that the majority of hybrid cells would produce monoclonal antibodies primarily against these antigens. This expectation has been realized, and we describe here studies performed with a panel of antibodies against the gp70 and p15(E) proteins. Exploiting the known reactivity of these monoclonal antibodies to only limited segments (epitopes) of the protein antigens, we have mapped the sites of five different epitopes on the viral envelope polypeptides.

II. Isolation of Hybrid Cell Lines Producing Monoclonal Antiviral Antibodies

Hybridizations were performed between BALB/c MOPC 21 NS1 myeloma cells and the lymphocytes of C57BL/6 (B6) or 129 strain mice that were immunized with viable cells of the MuLV-producing AKR SL3 leukemia. The NS1 myeloma cell line was kindly provided by C. Milstein (Molecular Research Council, Cambridge). In certain fusions (No. 9, 16, 19) the spleen and lymph node cells were obtained from B6 or 129 mice 3 days after their third weekly intraperitoneal challenge with 10^7 AKR SL3 cells. In fusion 26, 129 mice were immunized with mink cells (CCL64) that had been purposefully infected with either xenotropic (e.g., BALBv.2, NZB, or AT124), amphotropic (e.g., feral mouse), or recombinant polytropic (e.g., AKR MCF 13) MuLV. The procedures for hybridization of the spleen and myeloma cells have been described in detail (Nowinski *et al.*, 1979); briefly, the NS1 cells and lymphocytes were fused at a 1:4 ratio with 50% polyethylene glycol (PEG) and the cell mixtures plated in RPMI 1640 medium supplemented with 15% fetal calf serum (FCS) into the 96 wells of a Microtest II plate (Falcon Plastics, Inc.) at a concentration of 10^6 cells/well. Following selection in hypoxanthine–aminopterin–thymidine (HAT) medium the hybrid cells were isolated and their antibody products assayed by an antibody binding (AB) test utilizing ^{125}I-labeled protein A (IPA) from *Staphylococcus aureus* (Greenwood *et al.*, 1963; Kessler, 1975).

For the AB assay, $2\,\mu$g of MuLV (density-gradient purified) in $50\,\mu$l of phosphate-buffered saline (PBS, pH 7.2) was adsorbed to the individual wells of a microtest plate by incubation overnight at 37°C. The following morning the wells of the plate were blocked from further nonspecific protein adsorption by a 2-hr incubation with $150\,\mu$l of 5% bovine serum albumin (BSA) in PBS. The AB assay was performed in three steps:

1. $50\,\mu$l of culture fluid was incubated in each of the virus-adsorbed wells for 45 min at 37°C. Nonbound immunoglobulins were then removed from the original plate of wells by washing $3 \times$ with PBS containing 1% BSA.
2. 10^5 cpm of IPA in $50\,\mu$l PBS containing 1% BSA was added to each of the virus-adsorbed wells for 45 min at 37°C. The residual nonbound IPA was then removed from the wells by washing $4\times$ with PBS.
3. The immune reactions were detected by autoradiography for 24 hr at -70°C on Kodak NS-2T film with enhancement by X-ray intensifying screens (Swanstrom and Shank, 1978).

Culture fluids from fusions 9 and 16 were tested in AB assays with AKR ecotropic MuLV as antigen. This procedure was then modified, and in fusions 19 and 26, the culture fluids were tested in the AB assay on a panel of six different viruses. This latter procedure was accomplished by replicate-plating of the culture fluids onto virus-adsorbed Microtest plates that contained either ecotropic (AKR), recombinant polytropic (AKR MCF 13 or AKR MCF 247), or xenotropic (AKR, BALBv.2, or NZB) MuLV. Culture fluids from approximately 15% of the wells contained antibodies that reacted with at least one, or possibly several, of the viruses. Of particular interest was the observation that culture fluids from certain hybrids contained antibodies that reacted with only a limited number of viruses. In fact we observed some culture fluids that reacted with only a single virus of the panel (e.g., antibodies that were AKR ecotropic MuLV-specific).

Since our initial studies (Nowinski *et al.*, 1979) indicated that immunoglobulin synthesis was unstable in the majority of hybrid cells, we attempted to prevent the overgrowth of immunoglobulin-producing cells through the combined use of low-density passage and cell cloning. For this purpose the hybrid cells were initially passaged at low density and then twice cloned. Culture fluids from individual hybrids were retested at each step to assure the continued production of antibody. Cloning was accomplished by endpoint dilution in Microtest plates (one cell seeded per three wells) with a "feeder cell" suspension of thymocytes (3 $\times 10^6$/ml) in order to increase the plating efficiency of the hybrid cells. After 10 weeks of cell growth, and continued selection for antibody-producing cells, 30 stable antibody-producing cell lines were obtained. Each of the hybrid cell lines was then inoculated (2–5×10^6 cells intraperitoneally) into syngeneic ($129 \times$ BALB)F_1 or (B6 $\times$ BALB)F_1mice for the production of ascites fluids containing high-titered antibodies. Cellulose acetate electrophoresis (Microzonal System, Beckman Instruments) of ascites fluids from individual mice demonstrated that a single monoclonal immunoglobulin (at a concentration of 5–20 mg/ml) was associated with each hybridoma.

In addition, immunoglobulins in the culture fluid from each of the hybrid cell lines were concentrated by ammonium sulfate precipitation (40% saturation) and tested in immunodiffusion assays with heterologous antisera prepared against purified mouse immunoglobulins; this enabled the determination of isotype for each monoclonal antibody. To assess further the homogeneity of the monoclonal antibodies each of the immunoglobulins were examined by two-dimensional gel electrophoresis. For this purpose the hybrid cell lines were grown overnight in [^{35}S]methionine and their antibody products isolated from the culture fluid by adsorption to formalin-fixed *S. aureus*. Following elution into sample buffer the antibodies were separated into their constituent chains by sequential isotachophoresis and sodium dodecyl sulfate (SDS)–polyacrylamide gel electrophoresis (PAGE) (O'Farrell, 1975; Nowinski *et al.*, 1979). Each of the antibodies contained one heavy chain, composed of multiple charge variants, and one or two light chains. Since the NS1 cell did not produce heavy chains, it was concluded that the single heavy chain in each of the monoclonal antibodies was encoded by the lymphocyte parent of the hybrid; this was also considered to be formal evidence for the monoclonal origins of these antibodies.

III. Serological Characteristics of Antiviral Monoclonal Antibodies

A. Reactions of Anti-MuLV Antibodies with a Panel of Murine and Nonmurine Retraviruses

A total of 30 independent cloned hybrid cell lines that produced antibody against MuLV were isolated from four fusions. Ascites fluids from hybridomas of each of these cell lines were tested in AB assays against a panel of different retraviruses of murine and nonmurine origin. The results of these tests with 19 representative ascites fluids are summarized in Table I. Nine patterns of reactivity were observed, with the antibody products from several different hybrids yielding similar reactions.

These results can be summarized as:

1. Antibody from hybrid 16-E4 reacted with the endogenous N-ecotropic MuLV of AKR mice, but not with other representatives of the panel of murine and nonmurine retraviruses.
2. Antibodies from hybrids 16-B7, 16-G10, and 16-D7 had a common pat-

TABLE I

Reactions of Monoclonal Antibodies in AB Assays with Retroviruses of Murine and Nonmurine Origin

Viral antigen	Pattern of reaction								
Hybrids:	I 16-E4	II 16-B7; 16-G10; 16-D7	III 16-C1; 19C4	IV 19A2	V 9-E8; 9-E9; 16-G2	VI 19VIIIE8; 19-H6; 19-C11	VII 19-F8	VIII 26-A10; 26-F6	IX 26-G10; 26-H3; 26-D1
Endogenous N-ecotropic MuLV									
AKR	+	+	+	+	+	+	+	–	–
BALB/c	–	+	–	+	+	+	+	–	–
Endogenous B-ecotropic MuLV									
AKR	–	+	+	+	+	+	+	–	–
BALB/c	–	–	–	+	+	+	+	–	–
Endogenous xenotropic MuLV									
AKR	–	–	–	–	–	+	+	+/–	–
BALB	–	–	–	–	–	+	+	+/–	+
NIH	–	–	–	–	–	+	+	+/–	–
Endogenous amphotropic MuLV									
Feral mouse	–	–	–	–	+	+	+	–	–
Exogenous NB-ecotropic MuLV									
Friend	–	–	–	+	+	+	+	–	–
Rauscher	–	–	–	+	+	+	+	–	–
Exogenous polytropic MuLV									
AKR MCF 247	–	–	+	+	+	+	+	–	–
AKR MCF 13	–	–	–	–	+	+	+	–	–
Heterologous retroviruses									
Rat (NRK) endogenous virus	–	–	–	–	–	–	–	–	–
Feline FeLV	–	–	–	–	–	–	+	–	–
Feline endogenous RD114 virus	–	–	–	–	–	–	–	–	–
Mink endogenous virus	–	–	–	–	–	–	+	+/–	–
Wooley monkey (SSV/SSAV) virus	–	–	–	–	–	–	+	–	–
Baboon endogenous virus	–	–	–	–	–	–	–	–	–
Gibbon endogenous virus	–	–	–	–	–	–	–	–	–
Rhesus M-PMV virus	–	–	–	–	–	–	–	–	–

tern of reaction. These antibodies reacted with the endogenous N-ecotropic MuLV of AKR and BALB/c mice. Although the antibodies also reacted with the endogenous B-ecotropic MuLV of AKR mice, they did not react with the endogenous B-ecotropic MuLV of the BALB/c strain. Furthermore, these antibodies did not react with endogenous amphotropic or xenotropic MuLV, or with a variety of exogenous ecotropic and polytropic MuLV, and with a panel of nonmurine retraviruses.

3. Antibodies from hybrids 16-C1 and 19-C4 had a common pattern of reaction. These antibodies reacted with the endogenous N- and B-ecotropic MuLV of AKR mice, and with the recombinant AKR MCF 247 polytropic virus. They did not react, however, with the endogenous N- or B-ecotropic viruses of BALB/c mice, the recombinant AKR MCF 13 polytropic virus, or with an additional panel of endogenous amphotropic and xenotropic MuLV. Similarly, these antibodies did not react with a variety of exogenous MuLV, or with a panel of nonmurine retraviruses.

4. Antibody from hybrid 19-A2 reacted with the endogenous N- and B-ecotropic MuLV of AKR and BALB/c mice, with AKR MCF 247 polytropic virus, and with the exogenous Friend and Rauscher viruses. This antibody was not reactive with other endogenous or exogenous ecotropic, amphotropic, or xenotropic MuLV, or with the panel of nonmurine retraviruses.

5. Antibodies from hybrids 9-E8, 9-E9, and 16-G2 had a common pattern of reaction. These antibodies reacted with all ecotropic and amphotropic MuLV tested, but not with xenotropic MuLV or with retraviruses of nonmurine origin. The broad pattern of reaction of these antibodies indicates that they identified a "class-specific" antigen of the ecotropic and amphotropic murine retraviruses.

6. Antibodies from hybrids 19-VIIIE8, 19-H6, and 19-C11 had a common pattern of reaction. These antibodies showed yet a broader pattern of reaction and identified all MuLV isolates tested, regardless of host range. They did not, however, react with retraviruses of nonmurine origin. As a result, they were considered to identify a "group-specific" antigen of the murine retraviruses.

7. Antibody from hybrid 19-F8 reacted in a group-specific fashion with all MuLV tested. In addition, this antibody also reacted with feline leukemia virus (FeLV). Although showing "interspecies-specific" reactivity with FeLV, this antibody did not show cross-reaction with six other retraviruses of nonmurine origin, including the feline endogenous RD114 virus.

8. Antibodies from hybrids 26-A10 and 26-F6 had a common pattern of reaction. These antibodies reacted strongly with viruses of the sarcoma/leukosis (SSV/SSAV) complex of the woolley monkey, weakly with the endogenous xenotropic MuLV of BALB/c and NIH mice and the endogenous feline RD114 virus, and not at all with other retraviruses of murine or nonmurine origin.

9. Antibody from hybrids 26-G10, 26-H3, and 26-D1 reacted exclusively with the endogenous xenotropic MuLV of BALB/c mice; they did not

react with other representatives of the diverse panel of retraviruses of either murine or nonmurine viruses.

Although the 19 antibodies listed in Table I have been broadly separated into nine distinct groups according to their reactions in AB assays, it has become apparent that with continued analysis subtle differences can be demonstrated in the specificity of different antibodies within a single serological group. In fact early in these experiments we were occasionally misled in our efforts to define the relatedness of one monoclonal antibody to another. For example, it was originally thought that the 19-F8 and 19-VIIIE8 antibodies detected the same antigenic specificity, as they reacted comparably on a panel of eight different MuLV. However, upon the inclusion of FeLV into the panel of viruses used for screening (see Table I and Fig. 1) a difference in specificity between these two antibodies was found. As a result of these difficulties in classification (i.e., one could imagine the continued splitting of serological groups upon additional testing with new viruses), the decision was made to designate the antibody product of a *single* hybrid cell line as the marker for a *single* antigen epitope.

Accordingly, nine hybrid cell lines were selected as prototypes for further characterization. The criteria used for the selection of these prototype cell lines were (1) the pattern of reactivity of their antibody products with different viruses, (2) the phenotypic stability of the hybrid cell line, (3) the isotype of immunoglobulin produced by the hybrid cell, and (4) the quantitative yield of monoclonal antibody in the ascites fluids of hybridoma-bearing mice. The nine prototype hybrids selected were 16-E4, 16-B7, 16-C1, 19-A2, 9-E8, 19-VIIIE8, 19-F8, 26-F6, and 26-G10.

In Fig. 1 are shown the patterns of reactions of ascites fluids from six of these prototype hybrid cell lines in AB assays with a panel of eight different viruses. Each of these antibodies demonstrated a characteristically different pattern of reaction. These patterns of reactivity reproduced those described in Table I. As shown here, the ability of these antibodies to discriminate antigenic differences between individual viruses was most striking. In some cases the ascites fluids demonstrated 100,000-fold differences in their titers of reaction with different viral isolates.

B. Identification of Viral Proteins Detected by the Monoclonal Antibodies

Monoclonal antibodies produced by the prototype cell lines were examined in radioimmune precipitation (RIP) assays with the proteins of AKR MuLV that were radiolabeled with either ^{125}I, $[^3H]$leucine, or $[^{35}S]$methionine. In parallel, RIP reactions were performed with goat or rabbit antisera that were prepared against purified proteins [gp70, p15(E), p30] of MuLV. Immune complexes were collected on formalin-fixed *S. aureus,* washed extensively to remove nonspecifically bound radioactivity, and then eluted into SDS-containing sample buffer for analysis by SDS-PAGE.

Immune precipitation of the viral proteins was readily accomplished with the goat and rabbit polyvalent antisera. The monoclonal antibodies, however,

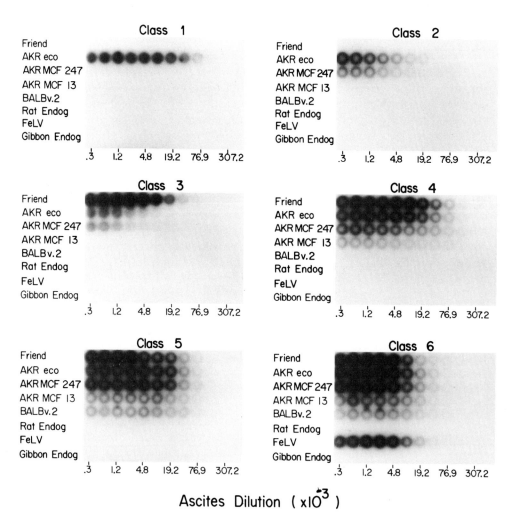

FIGURE 1. Antibody-binding assays with ascites fluids from mice bearing hybridomas. Serial twofold dilutions of ascites fluids (starting at 1/300 dilution) were incubated in the wells of virus-absorbed microtest plates. Immune reactions were detected by the addition of ^{125}I-labeled protein A and subsequent autoradiography. Prototype antibodies for each of the classes of reaction were Class 1, 16-B7; Class 2, 16-C1; Class 3, 19-A2; Class 4, 9-E8; Class 5, 19-VIIIE8; and Class 6, 19-F8.

showed some variation in their ability to precipitate viral proteins in the standard RIP assay.* As a result of this variation, the RIP assays were performed under a variety of conditions (e.g., in the presence or absence of disulfied-reducing agents) and with viruses that were radiolabeled with different isotopes. By the combined use of these different procedures a coherent pattern of reaction of

*The reason for the low precipitating activity of certain of the monoclonal antibodies was not determined, although it was hypothesized that either some of the antigenic determinants on the viral proteins were labile to the solubilization procedure, or that the physical location of these determinants in the viral proteins conferred steric constraints on the formation of precipitates.

seven of the nine prototype monoclonal antibodies emerged. Representative gels from two of these experiments are shown in Fig. 2.

The RIP assays shown in Fig. 2A were performed with [35S]methionine-labeled AKR MuLV. In this instance the virus was dissociated in 0.5% NP40 under reducing conditions (0.1% dithiothreitol) and the immune precipitates from these reactions solubilized in sample buffer containing mercaptoethanol just prior to analysis by SDS-PAGE. The inclusion of dithiothreitol in the lysis buffer resulted in the dissociation of the disulfide-linked gp70:p15(E)/p12(F) complex (gp90env) that occurs in detergent-lysed virus (Pinter and Fleissner, 1975) and prevented the coprecipitation that commonly occurred with these proteins. As shown in this gel, the goat anti-gp70 serum precipitated a single protein of 70,000 daltons, while the monoclonal antibody 9-E8 precipitated two antigenically related proteins, p15(E) and p12(E), which migrated as bands of 15,000 and 12,000 daltons. In contrast, control reactions performed with normal mouse serum or with the ascites of hybrid 19-E12 (containing antibody against Thy-1.1 antigen) did not result in the precipitation of either gp70 or the p15(E)/p12(E) proteins.

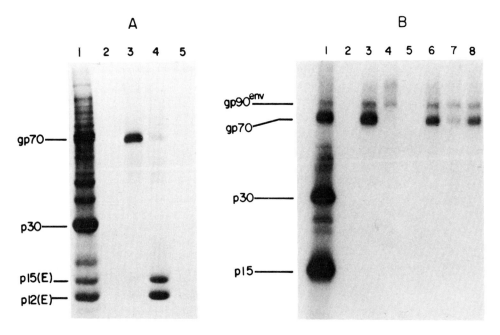

FIGURE 2. Radioimmune precipitation of viral proteins. (A) [35S]methionine-labeled AKR MuLV dissociated with PBS containing 0.5% NP40 and 0.1% dithiothreitol. (B) 125I-labeled AKR MuLV dissociated with PBS containing 0.5% NP40. Immune precipitation reactions were performed with 1/500 dilutions of: (2) normal mouse serum; (3) goat anti-gp70 serum; (4) ascites fluid 9-E8; (5) ascites fluid 19-E12; (6) ascites fluid 16-B7; (7) ascites fluid 16-C1; and (8) ascites fluid 19-A2. Lane (1) contained a nontreated virus preparation. Immune precipitates were collected on formalin-fixed *S. aureus* and eluted into SDS-containing buffer for PAGE. Autoradiography of gel A was enhanced by fluorography; autoradiography of gel B was enhanced by an X-ray-intensifying screen.

An alternative precipitation system is shown in Fig. 2B. In this case the RIP assays were performed with ^{125}I-labeled AKR MuLV. It should be noted that with this labeling procedure the gp70 protein of the virus was heavily labeled by ^{125}I, while the p15(E)/p12(E) proteins, which each contained only a single tyrosine residue, were poorly labeled. Since it was not possible to directly visualize the p15(E)/p12(E) proteins in these gels, a strategy was developed to indirectly monitor their presence in immune precipitates. For this purpose we utilized ^{125}I-labeled virus that was solubilized without reducing agents. Under these conditions the p15(E)/p12(E) proteins remained complexed to radiolabeled gp70 and could be detected as a single band migrating with an apparent mass of 90,000 daltons. Accordingly, the RIP assays presented in Fig. 2B were performed with ^{125}I-labeled virus that was dissociated with 0.5% NP40 in the absence of dithiothreitol. The immune precipitates from these reactions were then solubilized in sample buffer without mercaptoethanol and analyzed by SDS-PAGE. As shown in Fig. 2B the goat anti-gp70 serum precipitated both the 70,000-dalton monomer of gp70, and the 90,000-dalton gp90^{env} complex. In contrast, the monoclonal antibody 9-E8 precipitated only the gp90^{env} complex, demonstrating the selective reactivity of this antibody for the p15(E)/p12(E) proteins. On this same gel are shown the reactions of ^{125}I-labeled AKR MuLV with the monoclonal antibodies from hybrids 16-B7, 16-C1, and 19-A2, all of which yielded results similar to that observed with the goat anti-gp70 serum. Controls run in these gels included RIP reactions performed with normal mouse serum and the ascites fluid from hybrid 19-E12, neither of which precipitated gp70, p15(E), or their disulfide-linked gp90^{env} complex.

On the basis of these and other gels (data not shown) it was concluded that antibodies from the prototype cell lines 16-E4, 16-B7, 16-C1, and 19-A2 reacted with antigenic determinants on gp70, while antibodies from the prototype cell lines 9-E8, 19-VIIIE8, and 19-F8 reacted with antigenic determinants on p15(E). To date we have not had success in precipitation assays with antibodies from the 26-F6 and 26-G10 cell lines; therefore, the detailed specificity of these antibodies remains unknown.

C. Nomenclature for Monoclonal Antiviral Antibodies

Considering the complexity of serological reactions detected by this initial catalogue of nine reagents, it would be advantageous to have a standardized system for the analysis and nomenclature of monoclonal antibodies and their corresponding antigenic determinants. Since it is unlikely that it will be possible to define chemically the actual antigenic determinants on the viral proteins (owing to the fact that some of these determinants will reflect spatial as well as primary structural properties), it is suggested that the antibody product of a single hybrid clone be used to identify a single antigenic determinant. Implicit in this proposal is the premise that each monoclonal antibody reacts with only a single antigenic determinant. Although it is recognized that the affinity and avidity of each antibody will vary for a variety of different antigenic conformations, the selected use of antibodies and antigens with strong binding characteristics should generally satisfy this premise.

In the construction of a nomenclature we have considered two biologically significant factors: (1) the antigenic determinant that is detected by the antibody, and (2) the nature of the monoclonal antibody itself. For this purpose the first portion of the nomenclature states the viral protein on which the antigenic determinant resides. This is performed according to existing nomenclature [e.g., gp70 or p15(E)]. The specific epitope detected by the antibody is designated by an appended superscript letter above the designation of the viral protein (e.g., gp70^a, gp70^b, gp70^c). The appended superscript letter for each epitope is decided according to the pattern of reaction of the antibody with a panel of antigenically distinct viruses or by competition antibody-binding assays. The second portion of the nomenclature concerns the origin and properties of the monoclonal antibodies. This information contains both a description of the host in which the antibody was produced (e.g., strain of mouse) and the immunoglobulin isotype of the antibody. In Table II are listed the nomenclature and characteristics of the nine prototype monoclonal antibodies described in this report.

IV. Mapping of Viral Proteins with Monoclonal Antibodies

As has been described by other investigators (Galfrè et al., 1977; Oi et al., 1978; Lemke et al., 1978) and ourselves (Stone and Nowinski, 1980) the availability of monoclonal antibodies provides a new level of precision in the serological analysis of complex polymorphic protein antigens. The antibodies produced by cloned hybrid cells in culture are chemically homogeneous and react with constant avidity to single epitopes. As such these antibodies are remarkably specific probes for small regions of complex proteins. We have recently exploited these unique properties of monoclonal antibodies to investigate the arrangement of seven epitopes on the envelope proteins of MuLV. For this purpose we have used two techniques—one involving topological mapping by competition antibody-binding assays, and the other involving genetic mapping through the use of viral recombinants. In the following sections we describe results from both analyses; furthermore, since the results of these studies suggest a simple arrangement for the seven epitopes, we also present a hypothetical map for the order of these epitopes on the gp70 and p15(E) proteins of AKR MuLV.

A. Topological Mapping of Epitopes by Competition Antibody-Binding Assays with Monoclonal Antibodies

Although different isolates of MuLV varied in their antigenic profiles (see Table I), the AKR N-ecotropic MuLV was found to contain seven of the known antigen epitopes on its envelope proteins. In RIP assays, four of these epitopes were identified on gp70, while three other epitopes were identified on p15(E).

TABLE II

Summary of Nine Prototype Monoclonal Antibodies That React with the Envelope Proteins of MuLV and Nonmurine Retroviruses

Prototype hybrid cell	Antibody characteristics				Distribution of the epitope on murine and nonmurine retroviruses
	Epitope	Strain of origin	Isotype of immunoglobulin	Formal designation of monoclonal antibody	
16-B7	gp70[a]	129	γ2a	gp70[a]/129(γ2a)	Type-specific: N-endogenous ecotropic MuLV, also some endogenous B-ecotropic MuLV
16-C1	gp70[b]	129	γ2a	gp70[b]/129(γ2a)	Type-specific: Certain N- and B-endogenous ecotropic MuLV, AKR MCF 247 polytropic MuLV
19-A2	gp70[c]	129	γ3	gp70[c]/129(γ3)	Type-specific: Certain N- and B-endogenous ecotropic MuLV, AKR MCF 247, Friend and Rauscher MuLV
16-E4	gp70[d]	129	γ2a	gp70[d]/129(γ2a)	Type-specific: AKR endogenous N-ecotropic MuLV
9-E8	p15(E)[a]	C57BL/6	γ2a	p15(E)[a]/B6(γ2a)	Class-specific: Ecotropic and amphotropic MuLV
19-VIIIE8	p15(E)[b]	129	γ2b	p15(E)[b]/129(γ2b)	Group-specific: Ecotropic, amphotropic, and xenotropic MuLV
19-F8	p15(E)[c]	129	γ2b	p15(E)[c]/129(γ2b)	Interspecies-specific: Ecotropic, amphotropic, and xenotropic MuLV, exogenous feline FeLV
26-F6	Unknown	129	γ2a	Information not available for complete designation	Type-specific: Endogenous BALB/c and NIH xenotropic MuLV, endogenous feline RD114, SSV/SSAV wooley monkey viruses
26-G10	Unknown	129	γ2a	Information not available for complete designation	Type-specific: endogenous BALB/c xenotropic MuLV

This occurrence of multiple epitopes on the individual proteins of the AKR virus presented the unique opportunity to investigate the actual spatial arrangement of epitopes within a single molecule.

It was reasoned that if two epitopes were closely located on a viral protein, their corresponding monoclonal antibodies would demonstrate (as a result of steric hindrance) competitive binding properties. On the other hand, if the two epitopes were at sufficiently distant sites on the protein, their corresponding antibodies would not bind competitively. To examine these possibilities further we have developed a competition antibody-binding (CAB) assay.

This CAB assay was a modified form of the AB assay described in Section II. In this case, however, two antibodies, one nonlabeled and one radiolabeled, were tested in sequential fashion for binding to viral antigens adsorbed in the wells of Microtest II plates. For this purpose, monoclonal antibodies from six of the prototype cell lines were purified by affinity chromatography with protein A of *S. aureus* (Stone and Nowinski, 1980). The purified antibodies were then radiolabeled with ^{125}I by the chloramine-T method and tested in competitive AB assays with nonlabeled antibodies from ascites fluids or antisera.

In preliminary studies on the conditions required for CAB assays, it was found that the monoclonal antibodies from different hybridomas varied in their avidity of binding to the proteins of the AKR virus. This variation in antibody avidity was examined in detail by the methods of Frankel and Gerhard (1979), and by this means it was possible to classify individual monoclonal antibodies as having "low" or "high" avidity for a particular antigen. In subsequent analyses, these differences in antibody avidity were found to be of primary importance. For example, when two antibodies of similar specificity and avidity were compared in CAB assays, mutual competition was observed. However, if the CAB assay was performed with two antibodies of similar specificity, but of different avidities, the competition reactions invariably favored the binding of the antibody with higher avidity. Therefore, without careful consideration of these factors it was possible to misinterpret the results of CAB assays. With these potential artifacts in mind, CAB assays were performed between ^{125}I-labeled monoclonal antibodies and the antibodies that were contained in the ascites fluids of hybridoma-bearing mice.

CAB assays were performed between each of six ^{125}I-labeled prototype monoclonal antibodies and the nonlabeled ascites fluids from a panel of 14 hybridomas. In addition, each of the ^{125}I-labeled monoclonal antibodies was also tested in CAB assays with three polyvalent antisera that were prepared in goats or rabbits against purified viral proteins. The results of these tests are shown in Table III and Fig. 3, and are described below in two parts:

1. The initial set of experiments examined the specificity of the CAB assay. For this purpose we utilized the antibodies in polyvalent antisera as competitors for the binding of ^{125}I-labeled monoclonal antibodies.
2. The second set of experiments was designed to investigate the spatial arrangements of the different epitopes on individual viral proteins. These particular assays were performed with pairs of monoclonal anti-

TABLE III

Results of CAB Assays of ^{125}I-Labeled Monoclonal Antibodies with Polyvalent Antisera and Ascites Fluids from Hybridomas

Source of competitor [specificity]	Competition reaction with ^{125}I-labeled monoclonal antibody[a]					
	16-B7	16-C1	19-A2	9-E8	19-VIIIE8	19-F8
Polyvalent antiserum						
Goat anti-gp 70	−	+	+	−	−	−
Goat anti-p15(E)	−	−	−	+	+	+
Goat anti-p30	−	−	−	−	−	−
Ascites fluid [anti-gp70[a]]						
16-B7	+	−	−	−	−	−
16-D7	+	−	−	−	−	−
16-G10	+/−	−	−	−	−	
Ascites fluid [anti-gp70[b]]						
16-C1	−	+	+/−	−	−	−
19-C4	−	+	+/−	−	−	−
Ascites fluid [anti-gp70[c]]						
19-A2	−	+/−	+	−	−	−
Ascites fluid [anti-p15(E)[a]]						
9-E8	−	−	−	+	−	−
9-E9	−	−	−	+	−	−
Ascites fluid [anti-p15(E)[b]]						
19-VIIIE8	−	−	−	−	+	+
19-H6	−	−	−	−	+/−	+/−
19-C11	−	−	−	−	+	+/−
Ascites fluid [anti-p15(E)[c]]						
19-F8	−	−	−	−	+	+

[a]+, >90% competition of antibody binding at 1/40 dilution of the competitor; +/−, 50–90% competition of antibody binding at 1/20-1/40 dilution of the competitor; −, <10% competition of antibody binding at 1/20 dilution of the competitor.

bodies that had been grouped into different serological classes according to their reactions with a panel of viruses. Since these antibodies were known to react with serologically distinct epitopes, it was assumed that competitive reactions would be indicative of steric hindrence that resulted from closely spaced epitopes.

1. CAB Assays with Polyvalent Antisera

CAB assays were performed with six different ^{125}I-labeled monoclonal antibodies and three polyvalent antisera that were prepared in goats or rabbits against purified gp70, p15(E), or p30 viral proteins. The results of these CAB assays (Table III) confirmed the previously described specificities of the monoclonal antibodies in RIP assays (see Section III.B).

Three representative CAB assays with polyvalent antisera are shown in Fig. 3. Note that the binding of ^{125}I-labeled 19-A2 antibody (which detected the

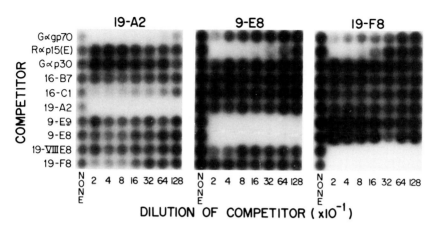

FIGURE 3. CAB assays with polyvalent antisera, hybridoma ascites fluids, and ^{125}I-labeled mono-clonal antibodies. Polyvalent antisera prepared in goats (G) and rabbits (R) against the purified proteins of Rauscher MuLV were tested as competitors for the binding of ^{125}I-labeled antibodies 19-A2, 9-E8, and 19-F8. In parallel, the ascites fluids from hybridomas 16-B7, 16-C1, 19-A2, 9-E9, 9-E8, 19-VIIIE8, and 19-F8 were tested as competitors for the same panel of radiolabeled antibodies. Fifty μl of serial twofold dilutions of antisera or ascites fluids (starting at 1/20 dilution) were incubated in the wells of virus-absorbed microtest plates (0.5 μg AKR MuLV per well). ^{125}I-labeled monoclonal antibody (2 × 10^5 cpm) was then added to each well, and the extent of binding determined (16 hr) by autoradiography of the test plate.

gp70^c epitope) was competed by the antiserum against gp70, but not by the antisera against p15(E) or p30. In contrast, the binding properties of ^{125}I-labeled 9-E8 antibody [which detected the p15(E)^a epitope] and 19-F8 antibody [which detected the p15(E)^c epitope] were competed by the antiserum against p15(E), but not by the antisera against gp70 or p30.

2. CAB Assays with Monoclonal Antibodies from Different Serological Classes

The results of CAB assays performed between the prototype monoclonal antibodies are summarized in Table III. In general, noncompetition was observed between all antibodies that reacted with epitopes on *different* viral proteins. Thus antibodies directed against epitopes of p15(E) did not compete with the binding of antibodies directed against epitopes of gp70, and reciprocally. In contrast, both noncompetitive and competitive interactions were observed between antibodies that reacted with epitopes on a *single* viral protein. Representative autoradiograms of these assays are shown in Fig. 3.

In the left panel of Fig. 3 is shown a CAB assay with ^{125}I-labeled 19-A2 antibody and the ascites fluids from seven different hybridomas. The 19-A2 antibody was competed completely by its homologous (19-A2) ascites fluid, partially by 16-C1 ascites fluid, and not at all by ascites fluids containing antibodies that identified other epitopes of gp70 or p15(E). As shown in Table III, the binding of the 19-A2 antibody was also competed by ascites fluids 19-C4, which showed the same serological reactivity with the panel of retraviruses as did 16-C1. Furthermore, the partial competition that occurred between the binding of 19-A2 and 16-C1 antibodies was also found in CAB assays where the reactants were tested in the reciprocal direction (i.e., ^{125}I-labeled 16-C1 antibody vs. 19-A2 ascites fluid).

In the middle panel of Fig. 3, the binding of ^{125}I-labeled 9-E8 antibody was competed completely by both its homologous (9-E8) ascites fluid and by another ascites fluid (9-E9) that showed the same pattern of reaction with the panel of retraviruses. However, the binding of 9-E8 antibody was not competed by either the 19-VIIIE8 or 19-F8 ascites fluids (which identified other epitopes on p15(E)), or by ascites fluids that contained antibodies reactive with three different epitopes of gp70. As shown in Table III, the binding of 9-E8 antibody was also competed by the ascites fluids from two other antibodies with the same serological specificity, but not by the ascites fluids from two antibodies that showed similar reactivity to 19-VIIIE8. Also shown in Table III, the noncompetition between 9-E8 antibody and either 19-VIIIE8 or 19-F8 antibodies was confirmed in CAB assays where the reactants were tested in the reciprocal direction.

In the right panel of Fig. 3, the binding of ^{125}I-labeled 19-F8 antibody was inhibited completely by its homologous (19-F8) ascites fluid and by the ascites fluid of the 19-VIIIE8 hybridoma. The binding of 19-F8 antibody, however, was not competed by the 9-E8 or 9-E9 ascites fluids, or by other ascites fluids that contained monoclonal antibodies directed against three epitopes of gp70. In other CAB assays (Table III) the binding of 19-F8 antibody was also competed by the ascites fluids of two other antibodies that had similar reactivity to 19-VIIIE8. Furthermore, the competitive interactions between the binding of 19-F8 and 19-VIIIE8 antibodies was confirmed where the reactants were tested in the reciprocal direction (Table III).

The collective data presented in Table III and Fig. 3 led to the conclusion that the gp70 and p15(E) proteins each contained at least two distinct antigen sites. With the gp70 protein, the gp70[b] and gp70[c] epitopes were clustered together into one of these sites, while the gp70[a] epitope was located at a distant second site. The structure of p15(E) showed analogous features. In this case the p15(E)[b] and p15(E)[c] epitopes were clustered together in one site, while the p15(E)[a] epitope was located at a distant second site.

It was further noted in the CAB assays that the extent of the competition reaction varied considerably with different pairs of monoclonal antibodies. For example, the competition reactions observed between the anti-p15(E)[b] and anti-p15(E)[c] antibodies were stronger than the competition reactions that were observed between the anti-gp70[b] and anti-gp70[c] antibodies. Since the extent of these competition reactions appeared to be independent of the bindings avidities of the reactants for the viral proteins, it was thought that they were reflections of the distances that existed between a particular pair of epitopes. On this basis, it was speculated that the p15(E)[b]/p15(E)[c] epitopes were physically closer to each other on the p15(E) protein than were the gp70[b]/gp70[c] epitopes on the gp70 protein.

B. Genetic Mapping of Epitopes on Recombinant Viruses with Monoclonal Antibodies

The precise serological typing of viruses with monoclonal antibodies (e.g., see Fig. 1) also points to their utility in the genetic analysis of viral recombinants. For this purpose, the naturally occurring recombinant MuLV of AKR mice (referred to as MCF viruses, Hartley et al., 1977) are of particular interest. These viruses, which arise by genetic recombination between N ecotropic and xenotropic MuLV, appear to contain genetic substitutions within the *env* gene (Hartley et al., 1977; Elder et al., 1977). Since the extent of this genetic substitution within the *env* gene varies from one recombinant MCF virus to another, it should be possible to use these viruses to perform a linkage analysis of epitopes that are present selectively in either the ecotropic or xenotropic parent virus.

As shown in Table I, our early data indicated that the monoclonal antibodies were, in fact, capable of distinguishing antigenic subtleties among different viruses of AKR mice. Thus, the phenotype of the AKR N-ecotropic MuLV was found to be $gp70^{a+}:gp70^{b+}:gp70^{c+}:gp70^{d+}:p15(E)^{a+}:p15(E)^{b+}:p15(E)^{c+}$, while the phenotype of the AKR xenotropic MuLV was $gp70^{a-}:gp70^{b-}:gp70^{c-}:gp70^{d-}:p15(E)^{a-}:p15(E)^{b+}:p15(E)^{c+}$. The AKR recombinant MCF 247 virus, on the other hand, had the phenotype $gp70^{a-}:gp70^{b+}:gp70^{c+}:gp70^{d-}:p15(E)^{a+}:p15(E)^{b+}:p15(E)^{c+}$. On the assumption that the recombination events which occurred in the AKR MCF viruses were essentially a single genetic substitution in the *env* gene, these findings suggested that in MCF 247 the $gp70^a$ and $gp70^d$ epitopes were coded within the region of recombination; furthermore, it appeared from this finding that either the $gp70^b$ or the $gp70^c$ epitope served as a marker for the border of the recombination site.

As a result of these initial findings it was reasoned that a continued analysis of a series of recombinant viruses (each containing different genetic substitutions in the *env* gene) would yield both a "serological" map of the viral envelope protein, as well as information concerning the genetic structure of the *env* gene. For this purpose, one of us (PVO) has established a panel of mink fibroblast cell cultures that are each infected with a cloned isolate of recombinant polytropic MuLV. These cell lines, as well as control cells infected with cloned AKR ecotropic or xenotropic MuLV, have now been tested in fixed-cell immunofluorescence IF tests with seven of our prototype monoclonal antibodies.

The results of IF tests with 12 recombinant polytropic MuLV and two control parent-type (ecotropic and xenotropic) MuLV are shown in Table IV. In initial tests on the control viruses, five of the seven monoclonal antibodies were found to react specifically with cells infected with the AKR ecotropic MuLV; two of the antibodies, however, had group specificity and reacted with both the ecotropic and xenotropic isolates. As a result of their reactions with both parental viruses, the two group-specific antibodies were excluded from the panel, and the analysis was continued with the five ecotropic-specific antibodies.

In IF tests with cell lines infected with recombinant viruses, several of the ecotropic-specific monoclonal antibodies showed negative results (Table IV). In fact, the "nonreactions" of these monoclonal antibodies with recombinant vi-

Table IV
Reactions of Monoclonal Antibodies in Fixed-Cell Immunofluorescence Tests with Mink Cells Infected with Polytropic MuLV Isolated from AKR Mice[a]

Virus		Monoclonal antibodies						
		Anti-gp70				Anti-p15(E)		
Host range	Isolate no.	19-A2 [gp70^c]	16-C1 [gp70^b]	16-E4 [gp70^d]	16-B7 [gp70^a]	9-E8 [p15(E)^a]	19-VIIIE8 [p15(E)^b]	19-F8 [p15(E)^c]
Polytropic	247, SC37	+	+	−	−	+	+	+
Polytropic	134-2	+	−	−	−	+	+	+
Polytropic	13, Akv-1-C36	−	−	−	−	+	+	+
Polytropic	69L1, SC30, 2169-12	+	+	−	−	−	+	+
Polytropic	28-7, 30-2, 26-4, 47-1	−	−	−	−	−	+	+
Ecotropic	Akv-1	+	+	+	+	+	+	+
Xenotropic	AKR X6	−	−	−	−	−	+	+

[a]Control reactions included NIH cells infected with ecotropic MuLV and mink cells infected with xenotropic MuLV.

ruses occurred with distinct patterns, suggesting that this was a consequence of the "deletion" of a cluster of ecotropic epitopes from the viral envelope protein. Presumably the site of this "deletion" was the region of the viral protein in which new epitopes coded by the xenotropic parent were substituted. This clustered "deletion" or substitution of ecotropic epitopes in the envelope proteins of these viruses led us to speculate on linkage relationships that existed between the nucleic acid sequences that coded for certain epitopes. For example, in 17 of 18 recombinant viruses the gp70^c and gp70^b epitopes segregated in a coordinate manner. Thus, these epitopes appeared closely linked. This could be contrasted to the relationship between the gp70^c and gp70^a epitopes, where only 12 of 18 recombinants demonstrated a coordinate segregation of these markers. Similar linkage relationships between other epitopes on the gp70 and p15(E) proteins could also be deduced. On the basis of these findings, and as shown in Table IV, sequences coding for these epitopes have been tentatively ordered on the viral genome as: 5′ end:gp70^c:gp70^b:[gp70^a:gp70^d]:p15(E)^a:[p15(E)^b:p15(E)^c]: 3′ end.*

C. A Proposed Serological Map for Epitopes on the Viral Envelope Proteins

With the collective data obtained from topological and genetic studies we have proposed a map for seven of the epitopes on the AKR MuLV *env* gene products. This map, shown in Fig. 4, contains four major regions. Two regions

*The order of epitopes within the brackets is presently unknown.

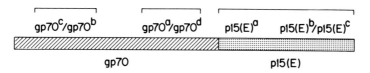

FIGURE 4. A proposed map for the orientation of seven epitopes on the envelope proteins of ecotropic AKR MuLV. The precise orientation of epitopes within the brackets are presently unknown, as are the actual physical distances between individual epitopes.

on the gp70 protein contain the gp70^c/gp70^b and gp70^a/gp70^d epitope clusters, while two regions on the p15(E) protein contain the p15(E)^a and p15(E)^b/p15(E)^c epitopes.*

Several features of the proposed map are of interest:

1. The region of gp70 containing the gp70^a/gp70^d epitopes was deleted or genetically substituted by xenotropic information in 18 recombinants tested (including 4 isolates not shown in Table IV). This view of a "hot spot" in the gp70 region of the recombinant polytropic viruses conforms with the oligonucleotide mapping studies of Rommelaere et al. (1978) that were performed with another panel of MCF viruses of AKR and C58 origin.

2. In contrast to this finding of a gp70 hot spot, regions of the *env* gene coding for the gp70^c/gp70^b and p15(E)^a epitopes were variably deleted or genetically substituted in different recombinant viruses. This suggested that the left-hand and right-hand termini of the recombination site varied from one viral isolate to another. These particular findings differed from those of the previously quoted studies of Rommelaere et al. (1978), where in addition to their conclusion of a recombination hot spot in gp70, these authors also proposed a common left-hand terminus to the recombination site.

3. The region of genetic substitution in certain recombinant MuLV included portions of the p15(E) protein. This demonstrated that the recombination events influenced viral proteins other than gp70, a fact which was hitherto unknown.

4. Due to the group specificity of the monoclonal antibodies that were reactive with the p15(E)^b/p15(E)^c epitopes, it was not possible to demonstrate

*Recently, we have performed a test of this hypothesis with another monoclonal antibody (35/56) against the gp70 protein of ecotropic MuLV. This antibody was kindly provided by Dr. U. Hammerling (Sloan-Kettering Institute). In CAB assays the 35/56 antibody competed with the binding of ^{125}I-labeled 19-A2, but not with the binding of ^{125}I-labeled 16-B7. This suggested that the location of the 35/56 epitope was closer to the gp70^c/gp70^b region of gp70 than to the gp70^a/gp70^d region. This conjecture was further supported by genetic mapping. In this case, the 35/56 epitope showed noncoordinate segregation with gp70^c in 7/18 recombinants; in the same analysis, the 35/56 epitope segregated noncoordinately with gp70^a in 11/18 recombinants. Since the 35/56 epitope cosegregated with gp70^c in the recombinant viruses 26-4 and 47-1, but not in the recombinant viruses 28-7, 30-2, 13, or Akv-1-C36, it was concluded that the sequences encoding the 35/56 epitope mapped to the 5' side of gp70^c.

genetic recombination in this area of the genome—in addition, the precise orientation of the three epitopes in the p15(E) region remained an open question. In fact, it should be emphasized that the map presented in Fig. 4 does not indicate the actual physical distances between epitopes on the viral proteins. It is conceivable, for instance, that all four of these newly described epitope clusters are representative of only a small portion of the total *env* gene.

5. The observation that the topological and genetic maps were in close agreement suggested that major segments of the envelope proteins were in an extended conformation, and that the structure of individual epitopes was determined by genomic sequences that were either contiguous, or in close proximity, to each other. Otherwise, if the epitopes were formed by complex tertiary structures (which were coded by noncontiguous regions of the genome), one would expect that the topological and genetic maps would not be concordant.

Finally, it should be possible in the near future to extend our methods to include an actual physical mapping of epitopes on the viral proteins. Assuming that the majority of epitopes are generated as contiguous regions of the protein it should be possible to perform a serological analysis with fragments of the virion polypeptides. For example, utilizing a set of fragments of various lengths (generated by cyanogen bromide or limited enzymatic cleavage) the minimal distances between two epitopes could be measured. Furthermore, the order of these epitopes on the polypeptide could be established following the alignment of protein fragments with conventional sequencing methods. This should then enable a direct test of the map that has been generated by topological and genetic methods.

D. Speculations on the Utility of a Serological Map for Biological and Biochemical Analysis of Murine Leukemia Viruses

As shown in Sections III and IV the monoclonal antibodies provide a unique opportunity to investigate discrete segments of protein structure with unusually high precision. By a combined approach one can envisage the construction of a serological map that can be used to relate protein primary structure, protein topology, and protein function. The practical aspects of such a map can be illustrated by two examples:

1. The classification and typing of recombinant MuLV. Although the polytropic recombinant MuLV have been demonstrated to be a heterogeneous population, there has not been, to date, a simple method for determining subtle differences between individual members of this broad family of viruses. As shown in Table IV, monoclonal antibodies against epitopes of the viral envelope proteins now provide a solution to this problem. With a panel of five monoclonal antibodies we have already subclassified 18 isolates of recombinant polytropic MuLV into five distinct serological groups. It is apparent that an extension of our present

collection of monoclonal antibodies (with specificity for epitopes of either ecotropic or xenotropic MuLV) will permit further subdivision of these agents. In this manner it should be possible to monitor, both *in vivo* and *in vitro,* the expression of individual viruses. In addition, this approach also enables a rapid determination of the extent of genetic recombination that has occurred within an individual viral isolate. This will prove to be of particular interest when we begin to compare the biological properties (e.g., oncogenicity, host range) of these viruses to their serological (and genetic) profiles.

2. As probes for the tertiary structure of viral proteins. Present methods for the analysis of protein tertiary structure require large amounts of highly purified proteins. Serological methods with monoclonal antibodies (e.g., CAB assays) provide an additional approach that requires relatively small amounts of protein that can be performed within the natural biological setting. In fact once a defined physical and topological map for a series of epitopes on a single protein become available, it should be possible to relate specific conformational changes within proteins to serological changes that occur in their antigenic profiles. More specifically, Ihle *et al.* (1976) have shown with ferritin-labeled antisera that the gp70 protein of MuLV has at least two serologically distinct forms—one present on the cell surface and the other within the envelope of assembled virions. With an appropriate panel of monoclonal antibodies it should be possible to investigate this phenomenon in detail. Similarly, monoclonal antibodies could be used to examine other viral and cellular proteins that are associated with cellular transformation. In this regard, the temperature sensitive *src* product of Rous sarcoma virus would be a most attractive candidate for study. With a panel of monoclonal antibodies against the *src* product it should be possible to investigate conformational changes associated with the loss of transforming function.

References

Barbacid, M., Robbins, K. C., Hino, S., and Aaronson, S. A., 1978, Genetic recombination between mouse type C RNA viruses: A mechanism for endogenous viral gene amplification in mammalian cells, *Proc. Natl. Acad. Sci. USA* **75:**923.

Elder, J. H., Gautsch, J. W., Jensen, F. C., Lerner, R. A., Hartley, J. W., and Rowe, W. P., 1977, Biochemical evidence that MCF murine leukemia viruses are envelope (env) gene recombinants, *Proc. Natl. Acad. Sci. USA* **74:**4676.

Frankel, M., and Gerhard, W., 1979, The rapid determinations of binding constants for antiviral antibodies by a radioimmunoassay. An analysis of the interaction between hybridoma proteins and influenza virus, *Mol. Immunol.* **16:**101.

Galfrè, G., Howe, S. C., Milstein, C., Butcher, G. W., and Howard, J. C., 1977, Antibodies to major histocompatibility antigens produced by hybrid cell lines, *Nature* **266:**550.

Greenwood, F. C., Hunter, W. M., and Glover, J. S., 1963, The preparation of I-131-labelled human growth hormone of high specific radioactivity, *Biochem. J.* **89:**114.

Hartley, J. W., and Rowe, W. P., 1976, Naturally occurring murine leukemia viruses in wild mice: Characterization of a new "amphotropic" class, *J. Virol.* **19:**19.

Hartley, J. W., Rowe, W. P., and Huebner, R. P., 1970, Host-range restrictions of murine leukemia viruses in mouse embryo cell cultures, *J. Virol.* **5**:221.

Hartley, J. W., Wolford, N. K., Old, L. J., and Rowe, W. P., 1977, A new class of murine leukemia viruses associated with the development of spontaneous lymphomas, *Proc. Natl. Acad. Sci. USA* **74**:789.

Ihle, J. W., Lee, J. C., Longstreth, J., and Hanna, M. G., 1976, Characterization of virion and cell surface reactivities of natural immune sera to murine leukemia viruses, in: *Tumor Virus Infections and Immunity* (R. L. Crowell, ed.), University Park Press, Baltimore, p. 197.

Kessler, S. W., 1975, Rapid isolation of antigens from cells with staphylococcal protein A–antibody adsorbent: Parameters of the interaction of antibody–antigen complexes with protein A, *J. Immunol.* **115**:1617.

Köhler, G., and Milstein, C., 1975, Continuous cultures of fused cells secreting antibody of predefined specificity, *Nature* **256**:495.

Köhler, G., and Milstein, C., 1976, Derivation of specific antibody-producing tissue culture and tumor lines by cell fusion, *Eur. J. Immunol.* **6**:511.

Lemke, H., Hammerling, G. J., Hohman, C., and Rajewsky, K., 1978, Hybrid cell lines secreting monoclonal antibody specific for major histocompatibility antigens of the mouse, *Nature* **271**:249.

Levy, J. A., 1973, Xenotropic viruses: Murine leukemia viruses associated with NIH Swiss, NZB, and other mouse strains, *Science* **182**:1151.

Nowinski, R. C., and Hays, E. F., 1978, Oncogenicity of AKR endogenous leukemia viruses, *J. Virol.* **27**:13.

Nowinski, R. C., Kaehler, S. L., and Burgess, R. R., 1974, Immune response in the mouse to endogenous leukemia viruses, *Cold Spring Harbor Symp. Quant. Biol.* **39**:1123.

Nowinski, R. C., Hays, E. F., Doyle, T., Linkhart, S., Medieros, E., and Pickering, R., 1977, Oncornaviruses produced by murine leukemia cells in culture, *Virology* **81**:363.

Nowinski, R. C., Lostrom, M. E., Tam, M. R., Stone, M. R., and Burnette, W. N., 1979, The isolation of hybrid cell lines producing monoclonal antibodies against the p15(E) protein of murine leukemia viruses, *Virology* **93**:111.

O'Farrell, P. H., 1975, High resolution two-dimensional electrophoresis of proteins, *J. Biol. Chem.* **250**:4007.

Oi, V. T., Jones, P. P., Goding, J. W., Herzenberg, L. A., and Herzenberg, L. A., 1978, Properties of monoclonal antibodies to mouse Ig allotypes, H-2, and Ia antigens, *Curr. Top. Microbiol. Immunol.* **81**:115.

Pinter, A., and Fleissner, E., 1975, The presence of disulfide-linked gp70-p15(E) complexes in AKR murine leukemia virus, *Virology* **83**:917.

Rasheed, S., Gardner, M. B., and Chan, E., 1976, Amphotropic host range of naturally occurring wild mouse leukemia viruses, *J. Virol.* **19**:13.

Rommelaere, J., Faller, D. V., and Hopkins, N., 1978, Characterization and mapping of RNase T1-resistant oligonucleotides derived from the genomes of AKv and MCF murine leukemia viruses, *Proc. Soc. Natl. Acad. Sci. USA* **75**:495.

Stone, M. R., and Nowinski, R. C., 1980, Topological mapping of murine leukemia virus proteins by competition-binding assays with monoclonal antibodies, *Virology* **100**:370.

Swanstrom, R., and Shank, P. R., 1978, X-ray intensifying screens greatly enhance the detection by autoradiography of the radioactive isotopes ^{32}P and ^{125}I, *Anal. Biochem.* **86**:184.

18

Monoclonal Antibodies against Influenza Virus

WALTER GERHARD, JONATHAN YEWDELL,
MARK E. FRANKEL, A. DWIGHT LOPES, AND LOUIS STAUDT

I. Introduction

Influenza virus (Kilbourne, 1975) is an enveloped, segmented single-stranded RNA virus. The virus derives its lipid envelope during the process of maturation (budding) from the plasma membrane of the host cell. Two types of viral glycoproteins, the hemagglutinin (HA) and the neuraminidase (NA), form a dense array of surface projections (spikes) on the outside of the lipid envelope. Inside the envelope are five virus-coded proteins: the matrix (M) protein, which is thought to form an internal protein sheet beneath the lipid envelope; the nucleoprotein (NP), which is associated with the viral RNA; and three proteins of large molecular weight with proven or suspected polymerase activity (P1, P2, P3). The viral proteins constitute 70–75% of the dry weight of the virion and are present in the following approximate proportions: M (40%), HA (32%), NP (21%), NA (5%), P1, -2, -3 (2%). In addition to these seven structural proteins, two nonstructural viral proteins are produced in the infected cell. Furthermore, the initial virus inoculum contains components (glycolipids, carbohydrates) that are not coded for by the viral genome but are intimately associated with the virion. Although present in small quantity, the immunogenicity of these components is often potentiated as a result of their association with the virus (Lindenmann, 1977). Consequently, infection or immunization with influenza virus elicits highly heterogeneous and polyspecific immune sera that are not suitable, in general, for studies concerned with the delineation of the antigenic structure of individual viral components.

WALTER GERHARD, JONATHAN YEWDELL, MARK E. FRANKEL, A. DWIGHT LOPES, AND LOUIS STAUDT • Wistar Institute of Anatomy and Biology, Philadelphia, Pennsylvania 19104.

The polyspecificity of antiinfluenza antisera has been reduced in the past (1) by using appropriate pairs of recombinant viruses as immunogen and test virus, (2) by absorption of undesired antibody specificity, or (3) by using a purified viral protein as immunogen. However, apart from the fact that the production of "monospecific" antisera by any of the above methods is a time-consuming task, it is often difficult to ascertain completely the monospecificity of these antisera. Moreover, any "monospecific" antiserum remains polyspecific with respect to the individual antigenic sites of the given protein and is not suitable, therefore, for the delineation of the fine antigenic composition of individual viral proteins. Also, if such antisera are used in functional antiviral assays (e.g., neutralization, antibody-dependent cell-mediated or complement-dependent lysis of virus-infected cells) it cannot be determined to what extent individual virus–antibody interactions contribute to the observed activity. For these reasons, monoclonal antibodies, generated by somatic cell hybridization, have become valuable tools in the analysis of influenza and may provide new basic immunological as well as virological information.

II. The Generation of a Diverse Panel of Antiinfluenza Hybridomas

A previous analysis of the humoral antiinfluenza immune response of BALB/c mice performed under clonal conditions in the splenic fragment culture system (Gerhard, 1977), showed that 183 monoclonal anti-HA (PR8) antibodies were able to differentiate 44 antigenic determinants ("epitopes," Jerne, 1960) present on the HA molecule of PR8 and of one or several virus strains of the serologically related HON1 and H1N1 subtypes (see the Appendix to this chapter). Those findings implied that any randomly selected monoclonal antibody provides only a very restricted view of the overall antigenic structure of the HA molecule and, consequently, that a relevant assessment of its antigenic structure would require a large and diverse panel of monoclonal antibodies.

The present section analyzes the effect of some experimental procedures on the diversity of the hybridoma antibodies generated. The factors considered include the number of cells seeded per initial hybrid culture, variations of the immunization protocol, variations of the time interval between last immunization and sacrifice of the mice used as lymphocyte donors, and the organ source of the donated lymphocytes.

A. Frequency of Antiviral Hybrids

We have found that individual hybrid cultures, when cloned, yield one and rarely two clearly distinguishable antiviral clones. This finding was attributed to rapid overgrowth of the initial hybrid cultures by a few hybrid cell lines (Gerhard et al., 1978). Thus, in order to make the selection of hybridomas independent of their growth rate, and to decrease the chance of overgrowth of an antiviral hybridoma by an undesired hybrid, the initial hybrid cultures were routinely seeded, immediately following fusion with polyethylene glycol (PEG)-1000 (see volume Appendix), with approximately 100,000 donor lymphocytes per culture. Under these conditions, 500–1000 hybrid cultures could be set up per donor spleen.

The number of antiviral hybrid cultures obtained with the procedure depended on the ratio of splenocytes to myeloma cells during fusion. For instance, roughly 4 times more antiviral antibody-secreting hybrid cultures (approximately $1/10^5$ splenocytes) were obtained when immune spleen cells were fused with P3/X63-Ag8 (Köhler and Milstein, 1976) at a ratio of 2:1 instead of 10:1. Yet, the number of non-antiviral hybrids increased at the same time by more than 12-fold. Thus, the chance of an undesired hybrid overgrowing the antiviral hybrid increased considerably at the fusion ratio of two splenocytes per one myeloma cell. Although the latter could be overcome by further decreasing the seeding cell density (e.g., 10,000–20,000 splenocytes/well) this would make the size of individual experiments prohibitively large. For these reasons we have chosen a ratio of approximately 7:1 and a seeding density of approximately 10^5 in our standard fusion protocol with P3/X63-Ag8. However, individual myeloma cells seem to exhibit quite different fusion efficiencies. Thus, with the nonsecretor myeloma Sp2/0-Ag14 (Shulman et al., 1978), we have found the ratio of two splenocytes per one myeloma cell to be optimal.

TABLE I

The Specificity of Antiviral Hybridomas in Relation to Various Fusion Protocols[a]

Fusion protocol			Number of antiviral hybridomas specific for				
Route of immunization (priming/ boost)	Origin of lymphocytes	Days after boost	HA	NA	NP	M	Not determined
i.p./i.v.	Spleen	3	39	1			3
i.n./i.v.	Spleen	3	14		1		2
i.n./i.n.	Spleen	3	2				3
	LN	3			2		
	Spleen	5	1		2		1
	LN	5	8	1	5		2
	Spleen	7	14			2	5
	LN	7	1	1			6
	Spleen	9			5		7
	LN	9			3	1	1

[a]All fusions were performed according to the standard procedure using P3/X63-Ag8 myeloma cells. LN, mediastinal lymph nodes; i.p., intraperitoneal; i.v., intravenous; i.n., intranasal. The specificity of hybridomas was determined as described in the appendix to this chapter. Not included in Table I are many hybridomas that cross-reacted in the radioimmunoassay (RIA) with various egg-grown viruses believed to express serologically unrelated viral proteins. At present, these hybridomas are assumed to be directed against an immunogenic and antigenic carbohydrate moiety derived from the chicken host during virus replication in the allantoic cavity of embryonated hen's eggs.

B. The Specificity of Antiviral Hybridoma Antibodies

Influenza infection induces, in general, a strong immune response to the viral proteins HA, NA, and NP and, less frequently, to the M protein (Cretescu *et al.*, 1978). In contrast to this polyspecific immune response *in vivo*, hybridomas derived from 5 different mice that were primed by an intraperitoneal (i.p.) injection and boosted, 3 days prior to fusion, by an intravenous (i.v.) injection of influenza virus seemed to be directed almost exclusively against the HA molecule (Table I, first line).

This apparent overrepresentation of HA-specific hybridomas may have been due to the particular immunization or fusion protocol used. Therefore, a series of experiments were performed according to various protocols. BALB/c mice infected intranasally (i.n.) were boosted either i.v. or i.n. with virus. The fusions of the lymphocytes from the spleen and draining lymph nodes were performed at various times after challenge (Table I). Fusion of splenic lymphocytes of i.n.-infected mice 3 days after antigenic challenge by the i.v. route yielded predominantly HA-specific hybrids. However, fusion of lymphocytes from tracheobronchial lymph nodes or spleen from i.n.-primed and i.n.-challenged mice resulted in many hybridomas against the internal viral proteins. These experiments indicate that both the time interval after challenge and the source of the lymphocytes affect the relative frequency of hybrids against internal vs.external virus proteins.

A variety of different factors may explain the relationship between fusion protocol and hybrid specificity. First, i.v. immunization may selectively recruit precursor B cells committed for the viral surface glycoproteins into the spleen. Second, the route of primary infection (i.p. vs. i.n.) may influence antigen processing and/or antigen presentation. Third, the immune response to the different viral antigens may proceed asynchronously. For instance, the early immune response may involve predominantly B cells committed to the viral surface antigens, whereas the late immune response may be directed more against internal viral proteins, possibly as a result of their release from lysed, virus-infected host cells or presentation on accessory cell surfaces.

Although these preliminary experiments do not provide conclusive evidence concerning the relative importance of the various factors, they clearly indicate that it is advisable to vary the fusion protocol if one aims at generating a diverse repertoire of hybridomas comparable to the polyspecific immune response occurring *in vivo*.

C. The Heavy Chain of Antiviral Hybridoma Antibodies

It is well established that different biological properties of immunoglobulin (Ig) molecules are associated with the constant region of the various Ig heavy-chain isotypes. It was of interest, therefore, to examine whether each Ig isotype could be generated by somatic cell hybridization and whether certain Ig isotypes could be generated selectively. Since the isotype composition of the antiviral

Table II

The Distribution of Heavy-Chain Isotypes of Antiviral Hybridomas[a]

	Antiviral heavy-chain isotype											
	μ		a		$\gamma 1$		$\gamma 2a$		$\gamma 2b$		$\gamma 3$	
Days after boost	SP	LN	SP	LN	SP	LN	SP	LN	SP	LN	SP	LN
3	22	0	0	0	17	0	28	2	6	0	9	0
5	1	0	0	1	1	3	2	8	0	1	0	0
7	5	0	0	1	6	2	6	3	3	0	0	0
9	4	1	0	0	2	2	3	2	2	1	1	0
Total	32	1	0	2	26	7	39	15	11	2	10	0

Comparison of Splenic Hybridomas and Splenic Fragment Clones

	μ	a	$\gamma 1$	$\gamma 2 + \gamma 3$
Splenic hybridomas, no.	32	0	26	60
Splenic hybridomas, %	27	0	22	51
Splenic fragment, no.	60	73	58	133
Splenic fragment clones, %	19	23	10	41

[a]The isotypes were determined in a double-sandwich RIA and/or a competition RIA (see Section V, Appendix). The isotype composition of 177 antiinfluenza antibody clones obtained in the splenic fragment culture system was analyzed. Splenic fragment clones show very frequently a switch in isotype. The total number of isotypes is therefore larger than the total number of clones analyzed. SP, spleen; LN, mediastinal lymph nodes.

immune response in the respiratory tract (IgM low or not detectable, IgA > IgG) differs from the immune response observed in the serum (IgM variable depending on the interval after primary or secondary immunization, IgA < IgG) the number of hybridomas of a given isotype is presented in Table II in relation to the time interval after challenge and to the origin of the lymphocytes used for fusion. In addition, the isotype distribution of splenic hybridomas is compared in Table II to the isotypes of antiinfluenza antibody clones observed in the splenic fragment culture system after adoptive transfer of virus-primed spleen cells (Cancro *et al.*, 1978, and unpublished observations).

The following major points are evident. First, the time interval after challenge does not influence significantly, as might have been expected, the isotype of the resulting hybridomas. However, the origin of the lymphocytes used for fusion has a clear-cut effect on the resulting hybrids. Thus, 32 of 118 splenic and only 1 of 27 lymph node hybridomas were of the IgM isotype, and no splenic but 2 lymph node hybridomas were of the IgA isotype. Second, comparison of the splenic hybridomas to splenic fragment antibody clones shows a good correlation between the expression of IgM and IgG isotypes, but a discrepancy with regard to the expression of the IgA isotype. It is reasonable to assume that the splenic fragment antibody clones represent an unbiased cross section of the humoral

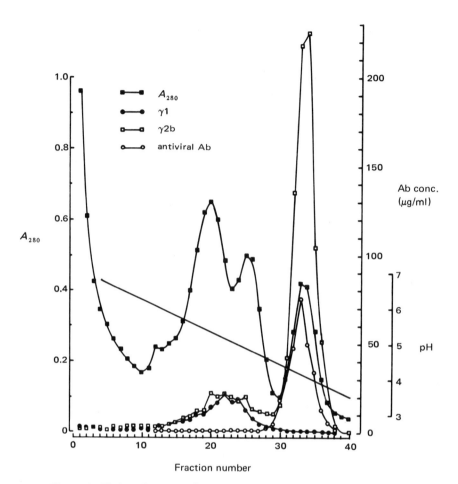

FIGURE 1. Elution of H16-S53 from Sepharose–protein A by pH gradient.

antiviral immune repertoire. The underrepresentation of the IgA isotype in hybridomas, however, is not understood. It may be related to the particular myeloma parent (P3/X63-Ag8) used in these experiments and might change with a different myeloma parent. Furthermore, the screening radioimmunoassay (RIA) used for selection of antiviral hybrid cultures may be biased against IgA-producing hybrids.

All antiviral hybrids tested so far (that were derived from (P3/X63-Ag8) secrete antiviral as well as the parental (γ1) Ig heavy chain. In the case of hybridomas of γ2a, γ2b, and γ3 isotype, the dimeric parental IgG1 molecule can be separated readily from dimeric antiviral Ig's by fractionation of the hybridoma culture fluid in a pH gradient on a Sepharose–protein A column (Ey et al., 1978). Also this procedure often provides a good separation of parental/antiviral heavy-chain hybrid molecules from dimeric antiviral Ig molecules (Fig. 1). We are currently investigating (1) the extent of "scrambling" between the parental and antiviral Ig molecules based on their light chains, and (2) methods to further separate the various Ig molecules based on their light chains. It is clear, however, that the use of nonsecreting parental myeloma cells (Shulman *et al.*, 1978) ultimately represents the best solution for obtaining homogeneous Ig molecules.

III. Study of Viral Antigens

A. Fine Antigenic Analysis of the Hemagglutinin Molecule

The HA molecule (HA spike) of influenza virus is a glycoprotein of approximate molecular weight 220,000. The molecules of infectious egg-grown virions are trimers of disulfide-linked HA1 (MW 50,000)–HA2 (MW 25,000) polypeptides. From an epidemiological point of view, the molecule is of paramount importance, since anti-HA antibodies (in contrast to antibodies against other viral proteins) neutralize viral infectivity *in vitro* and consequently protect against infection *in vivo*. However, as demonstrated by the recurrence of influenza epidemics and pandemics, influenza virus has been able to bypass the immunological defense mechanisms established against the influenza virus strains that circulated previously in the host population.

For the purpose of anticipation of major influenza epidemics and for effective vaccine production, human influenza isolates are continuously surveyed for the extent of antigenic change occurring in the HA molecule. Antiviral antisera used for this analysis disclosed the existence of two groups of antigenic determinants, one strain-specific, and one shared among several virus strains (Schild, 1970; Laver *et al.*, 1974; Virelizier *et al.*, 1974). However, the heterogeneity of these antisera prevented further dissection of the antigenic structure of the HA molecule. In the splenic focus system, one third of all monoclonal anti-PR8 antibodies tested were directed against strain-specific HA determinants, while two thirds were directed against determinants shared by PR8 and several heterologous viruses. The latter antibodies allowed the description of over 50 epitopes on the HA molecule of A/PR8/34 (HON1) (Cancro *et al.*, 1978). However, it was not possible to further dissect the strain-specific group of determinants. In addition, although separate epitopes on the HA could be identified, it was not possible to relate one to another in either a structural or functional sense, i.e., it remained unknown whether they represented overlapping antigenic structures of the same site or belonged to several antigenic sites with distinct nonoverlapping boundaries.

Mutant viruses with single amino acid changes localized in individual HA epitopes would allow a concerted analysis of the HA molecule. We have attempted to obtain such strains via selection of variant viruses by titrating cloned parental PR8 virus in the presence of an overneutralizing amount of an anti-HA hybridoma antibody. Under these experimental conditions only mutant viruses with antigenic changes in the epitope complementary to the combining site of the selecting antibody were able to grow. Although these changes are sufficient

TABLE III

Antigenic Analysis of PR8 Mutant Viruses Selected with Antibody PEG-1[a]

Hybridoma antibody	Parental PR8	Binding of antibody in RIA to			
		PR8 mutants			
		PV1	PV3	PV9	PV12
PEG-1	+	−	−	−	−
Y8-2C6	+	−	−	−	−
Y8-3B3	+	−	−	−	+
Y8-4C5	+	−	−	+	+
H9-B20	+	+	−	+	+
H17-L19	+	+	+	+	+
H18-S48	+	+	+	+	+

[a] The hybridoma antibodies tested in the indirect RIA for their binding capacity to 20 hemagglutinating units of the indicated purified viruses in the form of solid phase immunoadsorbents (Frankel and Gerhard, 1979). The binding capacity of the antibody to the HA molecule of the mutant(s) is significantly decreased (usually below limit of detectability) (−) or indistinguishable (+) from its binding to the parental HA molecule.

to prevent neutralization by the selecting antibody, these viruses exhibit a virtually unchanged overall antigenic structure (Gerhard and Webster, 1978). Peptide mapping experiments have indicated that these viruses are identical to the parental virus except for one or at most two amino acid substitutions (Laver *et al.*, 1979a,b).

An example of a selection experiment is shown in Table III. All mutants are characterized by decreased (usually not detectable) binding to the antibody used for their selection (in the present example PEG-1). Antigenic analysis of the mutants with other hybridoma antibodies allows identification of three types of patterns: (1) some heterologous antibodies (e.g., Y8-2C6) "recognize" the antigenic change of all mutants, i.e., these antibodies are similar to the selecting antibody in that they no longer bind to any of the mutants; (2) other antibodies (e.g., Y8-3B3, Y8-4C5, H9-B20) recognize the antigenic change exhibited by some but not all of the mutants, and (3) some antibodies (H17-L19, H18-S48) recognize none of the antigenic changes. The first two groups of antibodies thus appear to identify epitopes which coincide or partially overlap with the epitope of PEG-1. On the other hand, the third group of antibodies seem to delineate epitopes that do not share the modified antigenic areas with PEG-1.

Additional groups of mutant viruses have been selected with seven different antibodies. Anti-HA antibodies could, thus, be arranged in specificity families based on their reaction with these mutant viruses. Several observations can be made at this time concerning these reactivities (Table IV). First, the seven mutant groups comprise four independently mutating sets of antigenic determinants. The P, D, and L mutant groups can be paired with the C, N, and A groups, respectively. For example, the P and C group are paired because antibodies that delineate antigenic changes in the P mutant group also distinguish variations in the C group. These four groups of determinants, therefore, repre-

Table IV
Epitope Map[a]

Hybridoma antibody		Parent PR8	Mutant group			
			B	P-C	D-N	L-A
H2-6C4	(B)	+	−	+	+	+
H-6A5		+	+/−	+/−	+	+
H2-4B3	(C)	+	+	−	+	+
H2-4B1	(D)	+	+	+	−	+
H9-D3	(L)	+	+	+	+	−
H18-S28		+	+	+	+	+

[a]The construction of the HA-epitope map is exemplified with 6 hybridoma antibodies, four of which have been used for the selection of the various HA-mutant groups. The B,P-C, D-N, and L-A mutant groups comprise 6, 9, 3, and 3 antigenically distinct mutants, respectively. The symbols indicate that the given hybridoma antibody exhibits, compared to the parental virus, a significantly decreased binding (−) or unchanged binding (+) to all mutants of the given mutant group. The only exception is H2-4B1 (D) which does not differentiate one mutant (selected with antibody N) from the parental virus. (+/−) indicates that the antibody differentiates some but not all mutants from the parental virus.

sent four clusters of antigenic epitope markers. Second, one family of antibodies cannot distinguish variations in any of the four determinant groups thus indicating the presence of at least one additional independent epitope group (X). Subsequent selection of mutants with the latter antibodies should allow further characterization of this antigenic area. Third, when the antibodies are tested against heterologous viruses and grouped as to strain-specific or cross-reactive, it is seen that determinant groups B and P-C are predominantly strain-specific while L-A, D-N, and the as yet undefined X groups are shared among several other virus strains. Finally, at least two antibodies have been tested that distinguish variations in both the B and P-C determinant groups, suggesting a "closer" relationship between these two groups than between any of the other groups. However, further analysis of new hybridoma antibodies may allow the establishment of linkages between these other groups.

B. Analysis of the Mechanism of Antigenic Drift

As mentioned above, the prevention of influenza infection has been shown to be mediated, *in vitro* and *in vivo*, by anti-HA antibodies. Thus, the recurrence of influenza in nature can be attributed primarily to changes in the antigenicity of the HA. Two types of antigenic alterations have been identified in influenza: the major change, or antigenic shift, results from the sporadic introduction (presumably by the mechanism of gene reassortment) of a serologically novel HA molecule (subtype) into the human influenza virus pool and, as a consequence, leads in general to worldwide influenza pandemics. On the other hand, antigenic drift leads to minor changes of the HA molecule which are, in part, responsible for the recurrent epidemics within an interpandemic period. In

TABLE V

The Frequency of Antigenic Variation in Different HA Epitopes of A/PR/8/34[a]

Epitope	Number of parental virus preparations analyzed	Number of variants per infectious unit of parental virus		
		Mean ($\log_{10}$)		SD ($\log_{10}$)
B	4	−5.57	±	0.65
C	4	−5.57	±	0.37
D	5	−5.27	±	1.09
N	5	−5.56	±	0.56
L	4	−6.26	±	0.25

[a]Individual plaque-cloned preparations of PR8 were titrated in the presence and absence of hybridoma antibody in the allantois on shell culture system. Variant frequency (*VF*) was determined by the formula:

$$VF = \frac{\text{Titer of virus in presence of anti-PR8 hybridoma Ab}}{\text{Titer of virus in absence of Ab}}$$

nature antigenic drift is thought to result from the selection of spontaneously arising mutant viruses that exhibit (due to an antigenic change in the HA molecule) an increased growth potential in the partially immune host population. Both mechanisms make an effective vaccination of the human population difficult or impossible.

Using monoclonal hybridoma antibodies, we have attempted to model antigenic drift with three goals in mind: (1) to search for antigenic HA determinants which are "resistent" to drift, thus making the production of a "drift-proof" vaccine possible, (2) to examine, in detail, the molecular basis for drift, and (3) to evaluate the feasibility of anticipating antigenic drift.

Using the allantois on shell culture system (Yewdell *et al.*, 1979) we have determined the frequency of antigenic variation in each of the independent epitope groups described in the previous section. Several conclusions can be drawn from these data (Table V). First, the frequency of antigenic variation at individual epitopes is in line with point mutation rates reported for other systems and is perfectly compatible with the idea that the variants selected *in vitro* represent genomic point mutations resulting in single amino acid changes in the HA molecule (Laver *et al.*, 1979). Second, the variant frequency seems to be independent of the fine specificity of the selecting hybridoma antibody, i.e., variants arise as frequently in PR8-specific as in cross-reactive epitope groups. Thus, the latter epitopes do not constitute "drift-proof" antigenic HA determinants as could have been expected from the observation that they underwent considerably less drift in nature than the PR8-specific epitope groups. The reason for the relative conservation of cross-reactive epitope groups in nature remains unknown. Possible explanations are that (1) the cross-reactive epitope groups are of low immunogenicity for the human immune system, or (2) antibodies directed against these epitope groups are less effective in protecting against virus infection. Both cases would result in a decreased selection pressure for mutations in the cross-reactive epitope groups. Third, since there are at least five independently mutating HA epitope groups (each capable of mediating virus neutralization), and since the frequency of antigenic variation in each of these epitopes is of the order of $10^{-5.5}$, the frequency of a quintuple variant capable of escaping neutralization by antisera possessing all 5 antibody specificities would be of the order of 10^{-27}. This frequency is far too low to account for naturally occurring antigenic drift. One must consider, therefore, that (1) rare single-point mutations occur, which alter many of the epitopes simultaneously by inducing an extensive conformational change, (2) the mutation rate of human virus (before adaptation to experimental host systems) or during replication in human respiratory tract is higher than that observed with egg-adapted virus during replication in eggs, or (3) some individuals of the human population exhibit a restricted anti-HA response, thus allowing drift to occur in a sequential manner.

In order to examine these possibilities, it must be determined first to what extent antigenic change constitutes epidemiologically significant antigenic drift. To this end we have isolated variant viruses by sequential selection with various antibodies. Analysis of these sequential variants with ferret sera (which are routinely used to survey antigenic drift in nature) should show how many sequential mutation steps are required until the ferret antisera detect "significant" drift in the variants compared to the original parental virus and whether the experimental selection system results in drift toward an epidemic virus strain originally isolated from human patients after (or before) the prevalence of PR8. Presently, however, several points can be made concerning these sequential variants. For instance, seven sequential selections have been made each resulting in a new variant that retained the antigenic character of its immediate predecessor except for the epitope in which mutants were selected. Furthermore, the sequential selections did not decrease the growth potential of the virus nor change the mutability of the HA molecule. For instance, the quintuple variant BCLDN and the original parental virus PR8 gave rise to variants at a similar frequency in the presence of an antibody that reacted with both variant and parental virus. Thus, these findings demonstrate the remarkable plasticity of the HA molecule.

C. Expression of Viral Proteins on Infected Cells

It is generally accepted that the NP and M proteins are located exclusively inside the viral envelope. However, based on the binding of "monospecific" antisera to virus-infected cells it has been claimed that NP (Virelizier et al., 1977) as well as M protein (Biddison et al., 1977; Braciale, 1977; Ada and Yap, 1977) are expressed on the virus-infected cell surface. The monoclonal nature of hybridoma antibodies makes them the ideal reagent for such studies because artifacts due to contamination of antisera with antibodies directed against proteins other than the one under consideration are eliminated unless, of course, some viral proteins are actually antigenically crossreactive.

Using hybridoma antibodies directed against four of the influenza virus

TABLE VI

Expression of Viral Proteins on Surface of Infected Cells[a]

| Antibody | Specificity | Binding (cpm) of antibody in RIA to P815 cells infected with | | | |
| | | A/PR8 | | B/Lee | |
		Intact	Disrupted	Intact	Disrupted
M2-2B3	M	27	1569	32	110
M2-1C6	M	22	2575	23	115
H17-L13	NP	97	2613	14	107
H2-4B1	HA	1921	3481	25	79
H18-L17	NA	603	2728	17	95
TC-2C6	HN (Sendai)	20	87	16	84

[a] 8 hours after infection, viable P815 cells were assayed via indirect RIA in which cells are first incubated with hybridoma antibody, washed, and incubated with [^{125}I]rabbit anti-mouse F(ab')$_2$, washed and counted in a gamma counter. Disrupted cells were assayed similarly but only after cells were freeze/thawed, sonicated, and dried onto polyvinyl wells. Entries represent quadruplicate samples. TC-2C6, an anti-Sendai hybridoma, was included as control for nonspecific binding by hybridoma culture fluid.

structural proteins (HA, NA, NP, M), we have looked at surface expression of viral antigens in P815 cells 8 hr after infection with influenza virus A/PR8 or B/Lee (B/Lee infected cells serving as control cells, since influenza type A and B viruses are not antigenically cross-reactive) (Yewdell and Gerhard, submitted for publication). As can be seen in Table VI, the sensitive RIA used clearly indicates that anti-NA and anti-HA antibodies bind well to viable infected cells. (The anti-NP antibody binds to a considerably lesser extent and the anti-M antibodies show no binding above control values.) That NP and M proteins are expressed in infected cells is clearly shown by the RIA performed on disrupted cells in which all four proteins are detected.

While this experiment provides strong evidence that M is not expressed on the surface of the infected P815 cells, it can only be conclusively stated that the epitopes to which the anti-M hybridoma antibodies bind are not accessible to antibody in the cellular RIA employed. Thus, absolute proof of the absence or presence of any protein at the cell surface can come only from the use of a large number of hybridoma antibodies combined with supportive evidence obtained using other techniques, such as lactoperoxidase iodination of infected cells followed by immunoprecipitation with hybridoma antibody.

IV. Study of the Antiviral Immune Response

The previous sections have dealt with applications of the antiviral hybridoma antibodies for the study of some virological aspects of influenza that require the use of monoclonal (and thus monospecific) antibodies. On the other

TABLE VII

Relationship between Fine Specificity and Biological Activity
of Anti-HA Hybridoma Antibodies

HA-epitope group	Antibody activity	
	Inhibition of hemagglutination	Effect on neuraminidase activity
B	High	Enhance
P-C	High	Enhance
N-D	High	No Effect
L-A	Low	Decrease
X	Low	Decrease
Y	Absent	(Not tested)

hand, using the virus as the tool, the same experimental system is being applied to study basic immunological questions.

A. The Biological Activity of Antiviral Antibodies

It is well established that antibodies can express various biological functions that allow the humoral immune system to influence the outcome of the virus–host relationship at many different stages (virus neutralization, virus–antibody complex formation, lysis of virus-infected cells in conjunction with complement or effector cells, interference with antiviral T-cell function, modulation of the immune response). If the biological activities of the humoral immune system are studied with heterogeneous antisera one is confronted again with the fact that the observed activity represents the sum of many individual activities, i.e., it remains unknown to what extent individual antibodies contribute, in a synergistic or antagonistic way, to the observed activity.

We have, therefore, initiated experiments aimed at delineating the relationship between the fine specificity and biological activity of anti-HA hybridoma antibodies in vitro. Preliminary experiments (Table VII) indicate that hybridoma antibodies directed against the B, P-C and N-D epitope groups exhibit, independent of their isotype, a 5- to 10-fold higher HI activity than antibodies directed against the L-A and X epitope groups. It is evident also that these functional experiments allow us to define an additional epitope group(s) (Y) on the HA molecule through which antibodies are unable to mediate HI activity. Furthermore, the anti-HA antibodies influence also, though to a small extent (2- to 3-fold enhancement or inhibition compared to control) the viral neuraminidase activity. Again, the effect is related to the fine specificity of the anti-HA antibodies.

Another example of a difference in biological activity of anti-HA antibodies, possibly related to their fine specificity, has been observed in antibody mediated blocking of antiviral cytotoxic T-cell activity. Thus, two anti-HA antibodies were shown to inhibit partially ^{51}Cr release by cytotoxic T cells restricted to killing WSN-infected P815 cells (K^dD^d) in the context of the D^d haplotype. In contrast, cytotoxic T cells restricted to the K^d haplotype were inhibited by one (H15C5) but not the other (H9-D3) hybridoma antibody (Frankel *et al.*, 1979).

Thus, these analyses may ultimately allow us to characterize individual portions of the HA molecule through which antibodies mediate different biological activities.

B. The Use of Hybridomas to Analyze the Anti-HA B-Cell Repertoire

The panel of anti-HA hybridomas is a sampling from the BALB/c anti-HA B-cell repertoire which can be used to analyze that repertoire, provided the sampling is representative. Previous studies of the anti-HA repertoire have used the splenic focus culture system (Cancro *et al.*, 1978, 1979) to generate small quantities of monoclonal anti-HA antibodies. The diversity of these antibodies was studied using the general method of fine specificity analysis. Briefly, the antibodies were tested for their reactivities with a panel of different influenza viruses isolated from nature. Two antibodies that differed in their reactivity with a virus were said to have different "reactivity patterns" (RP) and were thus distinct clonotypes. A similar fine specificity analysis of the anti-HA hybridomas has been greatly extended using the virus mutants. For example, eight hybridomas that had indistinguishable RPs on the panel of viruses isolated from nature were all clearly distinguishable by their reactivities with the mutant viruses. Nevertheless, it is not known whether hybridomas which possess identical RPs can be distinguished by a different method of clonotype analysis. To this end, antiidiotype antisera have been made against anti-HA hybridoma antibodies.

Antiidiotypic antisera were made in rabbits by immunization with hybridoma antibody purified from culture fluid. The rabbit antisera were absorbed extensively with myeloma antibodies of the same isotype as the immunizing antibody to remove all antiisotype reactivity. A competitive RIA for idiotype was set up by adsorbing an antiidiotypic antiserum to the wells of a polyvinyl microtiter plate. The purified hybridoma antibody used for immunization was iodinated with ^{125}I and the binding of this labeled antibody to the antiidiotype-coated microtiter well was measured in the presence of culture fluids from the other anti-HA hybridomas in the panel. Using the antiidiotype serum made against the hybridoma H2-4B3, 41 of 43 hybridoma culture fluids tested gave less than 20% inhibition of binding of labeled H2-4B3 to the antiidiotype serum. However, culture fluids from two hybridomas gave 100% inhibition in the idiotype assay. These hybridomas, HI6-S53 and HI6-S19, have the same RP as H2-4B3 and are thus, by two criteria, equivalent clonotypes. Furthermore, none of the hybridomas that were negative in the idiotype assay had the same RP as H2-4B3. These three cross-reactive hybridomas were derived from fusions involving two individual animals. Further, such observations of repeated clonotypes in different individuals will allow us to calculate the number of distinct anti-HA clonotypes in BALB/c mice.

V. Appendix

A. Classification of Influenza Type A Viruses

Influenza type A viruses are grouped into four subtypes (H0N1, H1N1, H2N2, H3N2), each characterized by the serotype of their HA (H0, H1, H2, H3) and NA (N1, N2) molecule. Except for H0 and H1, individual H serotypes exhibit no or only very slight cross-reaction in the hemagglutinin inhibition (HI) test. Within each serotype, antigenic drift has generated a considerable number of distinct yet antigenically more or less cross-reactive HA molecules which are characteristic for individual virus strains. The antiviral hybridomas described in the present study were produced against A/PR/8/34 (H0N1) and A/WSN/31 (H0N1).

B. Determination of the Specificity of Antiviral Hybridoma Antibodies

Due to its segmented genome, mixed infection of a host cell allows us to generate "recombinant" viruses that contain a mixed assortment of RNA genes derived from either one of the parental viruses. Thus, using recombinants of PR8 (H0N1) and HK (H3N2) of known genotype (which were kindly provided by Dr. P. Palese, Mt. Sinai Hospital, New York) the specificity of all antibodies that reacted with a viral protein of PR8 but not of HK could be determined on the basis of the antibody reactivity with the appropriate PR8-HK recombinants.

C. Isotype Assay

The isotypes of the monoclonal hybridoma antibodies are determined by either a double antibody or competitive binding radioimmunoassay. For both assays, isotype-specific antisera were made by immunizing rabbits with purified mouse myeloma proteins of known isotype. When possible, the rabbits were boosted with another myeloma of the same isotype in order to minimize antiidiotype responses. Each antiserum was extensively absorbed with myeloma proteins of the other isotypes to render it isotype-specific.

In the double antibody assay, 10 hemagglutinating units of purified influenza virus are dried in each well of a 96-well flexible polyvinyl microtiter plate (Cooke Engineering, Alexandria, VA). Dilutions of hybridoma culture fluid are then incubated in these wells for 90 min (all incubations are performed at room temperature). The wells are then washed three times with phosphate buffered saline containing 0.08% sodium azide and 1% gamma globulin free horse serum. Isotype-specific rabbit antisera are added, the plates are incubated and washed as before, and finally developed with an [125I]goat anti-rabbit gamma globulin antibody preparation. The amount of [125I]goat anti-rabbit antibody bound correlates to the amount of the given isotype bound to the viral immunoadsorbent. This assay will only detect hybridoma clones which produce antiviral antibody; however, hybrid antibody molecules comprised of heavy chains from both parent genomes will bind antiserum specific for both isotypes.

The competitive binding assay uses purified [^{125}I]mouse myeloma proteins of known isotype. Isotype-specific antisera at appropriate dilutions are incubated overnight in the flexible microtiter plates. The wells are then incubated with phosphate buffered saline containing 0.08% sodium azide and 1% bovine serum albumin for 1 hr. The assay consists of incubating labeled myeloma proteins in these isotype specific wells in the presence of varying amounts of cold competitors. Unlabeled myeloma proteins as cold competitors are used to standardize the assay. The amount of [^{125}I]myeloma protein bound to the wells is determined by gamma counting. This assay does not require the competing Ig to express any specific antibody activity. In fact, hybridoma clones resulting from fusion of spleen cells with the secretor cell line P3/X63-Ag8 always express the Y1 isotype in this assay as well as the isotype of the antibody from the spleen cell parent.

References

Ada, G. L., and Yap, K. L., 1977, Matrix protein expressed at the surface of cells infected with influenza viruses, *Immunochemistry* **14**:643.

Biddison, W. E., Doherty, P. C., and Webster, R. G., 1977, Antibody to influenza virus matrix protein detects a common antigen on the surface of cells infected with type A influenza viruses, *J. Exp. Med.* **146**:690.

Braciale, T. J., 1977, Immunologic recognition of influenza virus-infected cells. II. Expression of influenza A matrix protein on the infected cell surface and its role in recognition by crossreactive cytotoxic T cells, *J. Exp. Med.* **146**:643.

Cancro, M. P., Gerhard, W., and Klinman, N. R., 1978, The diversity of the influenza-specific primary B cell repertoire in BALB/c mice, *J. Exp. Med.* **147**:776.

Cancro, M. P., Wylie, E., Gerhard, W., and Klinman, N. R., 1979, Patterned acquisition of the antibody repertoire: The diversity of the hemagglutinin-specific-B cell repertoire in neonatal BALB/c mice, *Proc. Natl. Acad. Sci. USA* **76**:6577.

Cretescu, L., Beare, A. S., and Schild, G. C., 1978, Formation of antibody to matrix protein in experimental influenza A virus infections, *Infect. Immun.* **22**:322.

Ey, P. L., Prowse, S. J., and Jenkin, C. R., 1978, Isolation of pure IgG1, IgG2a and IgG2b immunoglobulins from mouse serum using protein A-Sepharose, *Immunochemistry* **15**:429.

Frankel, M. E., and Gerhard, W., 1979, The rapid determination of binding constants for antiviral antibodies by a radioimmunoassay, *Mol. Immunol.* **16**:101.

Frankel, M. E., Effros, R., Doherty, P. C., and Gerhard, W., 1979, A monoclonal antibody to viral glycoprotein blocks virus immune effector T cells operating at H-2D^d but not at H-2K^d, *J. Immunol.* **123**:2438.

Gerhard, W., 1977, The delineation of antigenic determinants of the hemagglutinin of influenza A viruses by means of monoclonal antibodies, *Top. Infect. Dis.* **3**:15.

Gerhard, W., and Webster, R. G., 1978, Selection and characterization of antigenic variants of A/PR/8/34(H0N1) influenza virus with monoclonal antibodies, *J. Exp. Med.* **148**:383.

Gerhard, W., Croce, C. M., Lopes, D., and Koprowski, H., 1978, Repertoire of antiviral antibodies expressed by somatic cell hybrids, *Proc. Natl. Acad. Sci. USA* **75**:1510.

Jerne, N. K., 1960, Immunological speculations, *Annu. Rev. Microbiol.* **14**:341.

Kilbourne, E. D., ed., 1975, *The Influenza Viruses and Influenza,* Academic Press, New York.

Köhler, G., and Milstein, C., 1976, Derivation of specific antibody-producing tissue culture and tumor lines by cell fusion, *Eur. J. Immunol.* **6**:511.

Laver, W. G., Downie, J. C., and Webster, R. G., 1974, Studies on antigenic variation in influenza virus. Evidence for multiple antigenic determinants on the hemagglutinin subunits of A/Hong Kong/68(H3N2) and the A/England/72 strains, *Virology* **59**:230.

Laver, W. G., Gerhard, W., Webster, R. G., Frankel, M. E., and Air, G. M., 1979a, Antigenic drift in type A influenza virus: Peptide mapping and antigenic analysis of A/PR/8/34(H0N1) variants selected with monoclonal antibodies, *Proc. Natl. Acad. Sci. USA* **76**:1425.

Laver, W. G., Air, G. M., Webster, R. G., Gerhard, W., Ward, C. W., and Dopheide, T. A. A., 1979b, Antigenic drift in type A influenza virus: Sequence differences in the hemagglutinin of Hong Kong(H3N2) variants selected with monoclonal hybridoma antibodies, *Virology* **98**:226.

Lindenmann, J., 1977, Host antigens in enveloped RNA viruses, in: *Virus Infection and the Cell Surface* (G. Poste and G. L. Nicolson, eds.), North-Holland, Amsterdam.

Schild, G. C., 1970, Studies with antibody to the purified hemagglutinin of an influenza AO virus, *J. Gen. Virol.* **9**:191.

Shulman, M., Wilde, C. D., and Kohler, G., 1978, A better cell line for making hybridomas secreting specific antibodies, *Nature* **276**:269.

Virelizier, J. L., Postlethwaite, R., Schild, G. C., and Allison, A. C., 1974, Antibody responses to antigenic determinants of influenza virus hemagglutinin, *J. Exp. Med.* **140**:1559.

Virelizier, J. L., Allison, A. C., Oxford, J. S., and Schild, G. C., 1977, Early presence of nucleoprotein antigen on surface of influenza virus infected cells, *Nature* **266**:53.

Yewdell, J. W., Webster, R. G., and Gerhard, W., 1979, Antigenic variation in three distinct determinants of an influenza type A hemagglutinin molecule, *Nature* **279**:246.

19
Monoclonal Antibodies against Rabies Virus

Hilary Koprowski and Tadeusz Wiktor

I. Introduction

The study of rabies virus and its components with hybridoma antibodies is of particular importance for several reasons. First, rabies, a rhabdovirus, is unique in its ability to infect all warm-blooded animals, including man. It is a strictly neurotropic virus, replicating in neurons and spreading through axons and nerve cells from the site of infection to the central nervous system; the virus is never detected in the blood of infected animals. Transmission occurs in most cases by bites or scratches and only on very rare occasions by inhalation.

Second, rabies is part of the Lyssavirus group, which comprises three other rhabdoviruses classified as rabies-related viruses. However, the antigenic relationship between rabies-related viruses and rabies virus has not been clearly determined; it is evident that the study of serologic reactions with antibodies in sera from immunized animals has been inadequate for the clarification of this relationship. Furthermore, over the course of decades of research, only minor antigenic differences have been detected within the rabies group itself, among strains of the virus isolated in many parts of the world and studied in many different laboratories. The immunization of humans with vaccine containing live fixed virus has led in the past to several cases of postvaccinal disease in the people exposed; however, because of the minimal ability of immune sera to detect strain variations, it was not possible to determine whether the disease had been caused by the vaccine virus or by the street virus (uncloned field virus obtained from cases of rabies in man and animals) they had also been exposed to.

Finally, it is tacitly assumed but has not been proven that the few strains of fixed virus (virus adapted to laboratory animals) used for the production of

Hilary Koprowski and Tadeusz Wiktor • Wistar Institute of Anatomy and Biology, Philadelphia, Pennsylvania 19104.

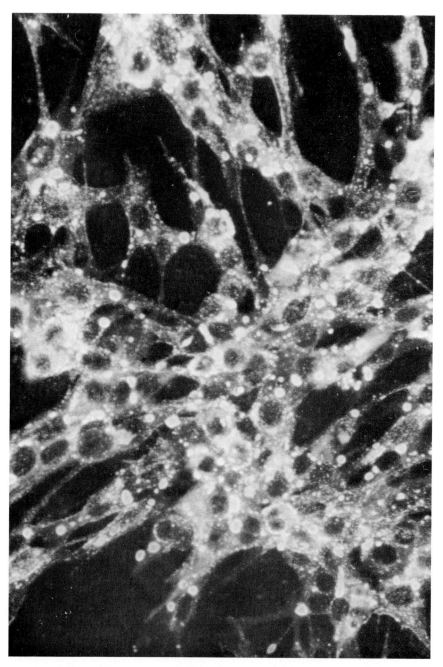

Figure 1. Indirect fluorescent antibody staining of rabies (ERA)-infected BHK-21 cells. Left: fixed

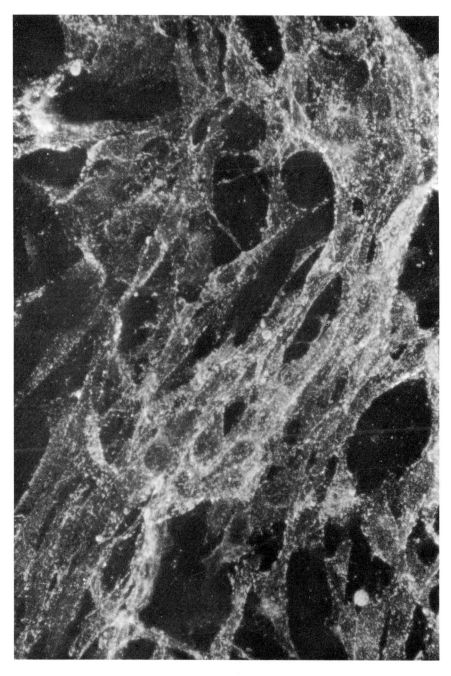

cells; membrane fluorescence (×250). Right: unfixed cells; nucleocapsid fluorescence (×250).

human vaccines show sufficient cross-reactivity with the street viruses present in a given area to convey protection to exposed individuals.

II. Monoclonal Antibodies against Rabies Virus

A. Production and Screening

Table I shows the number of hybridomas produced through the fusion of P3/X63-Ag8 cells with splenocytes obtained from BALB/c mice immunized against several strains of rabies and rabies-related viruses (see Wiktor *et al.*, 1980, for description of origin and history of virus strains). Mice were inoculated twice at 4- to 8-week intervals with betapropiolactone-inactivated virus suspension, with isolated nucleocapsids (in the case of the ERA strain) or with live virus (in the case of street virus). Three to four days after the second injection, mouse splenocytes were fused with mouse myeloma cells according to the technique described in the Appendix. Observation, selection, and cloning of hybridomas produced by the fusion of the two types of cells followed patterns described in the Appendix.

Specificity of the antibodies produced by the hybridomas was determined by (1) radioimmunoassay (RIA) for binding to rabies-infected cells, (2) indirect immunofluorescence (FA) test with live or acetone-fixed virus-infected cells (Fig. 1), (3) plaque reduction test, and (4) neutralization test in mice (Wiktor and Koprowski, 1978), as shown in Table II.

Rabies virus consists of a nucleocapsid surrounded by a lipidic envelope. Five major polypeptide components of different molecular sizes form the protein moiety of the virion (Sokol *et al.*, 1971): two nucleoproteins (N and L), a

TABLE I

Production of Hybridomas from P3/X63-Ag8 Mouse Myeloma Cells and Splenocytes from Mice Immunized against Rabies

Immunization of mice			
Lyssavirus group	Strain of virus[a]	Material[b]	Ratio of hybridomas secreting rabies antibodies
Rabies	ERA	V-BPL	56/95
	ERA	N	3/12
	CVS	V-BPL	26/52
	Kelev	V-BPL	45/74
	Street	Live virus	5/18
Rabies-related	Lagos bat	V-BPL	3/18
	Mokola	V-BPL	9/24

[a]ERA, infected target cells.
[b]V-BPL, virus inactivated by β-propiolactone. N, nucleocapsid.

Table II

Specificity Determination for Rabies Virus Hybridoma Antibodies

						Testing procedure				
		Infected cells								
			Immunofluorescence staining[a]			Virions				
Definition of antibody specificity		Immuno-		Acetone-	Formalin-	Neutral- ization		Viral components (RIA)		
	RIA	lysis	Live	fixed	fixed	(PFU $\log_{10}$)	RIA	N[b]	G[c]	NS[d] or M[e]
Anti-N	+	−	−	INC	INC	−	+	+	−	?
Anti-G	+	+	ME	ME	ME	+ (≥4.0)	+	−	+	?
Anti-NS	+	−	−	−	INC	−	+	−	−	?
Anti-M	+	+	ME	ME	ME	− (1.3 − 1.7)	+	−	−	?

[a]INC, cytoplasmic inclusions; ME, membrane of infected cells.
[b]N, nucleocapsid.
[c]G, glycoprotein.
[d]NS, nonstructural protein.
[e]M, matrix protein.

glycoprotein (G) and two membrane proteins (M1 and M2). However, it was recently reported that the M1 protein may be part of the nucleocapsid (Zaides *et al.*, 1979) and equivalent to the "nonstructural" (NS) protein of the vesicular stomatitis virus (VSV).

The number of hybridoma antibodies showing different specificities for rabies virus components is shown in Table III. Hybridomas produced from mice that had been immunized with the inactivated (V-BPL) ERA, CVS, Kelev, or Mokola strain viruses secreted antibodies that reacted with each of the components of the virus. In contrast, of the three hybridomas produced from mice immunized with street virus, antibodies secreted by one reacted with the glycoprotein of the virus, and those secreted by the other two reacted with either the NS or the M protein. The immunization of mice with Lagos bat virus resulted in the production of hybridomas which secreted antibodies binding only to the glycoprotein of the virus. Finally, as expected, hybridomas produced from mice that had been immunized with the purified nucleocapsid of the ERA virus secreted antibody directed only against the nucleocapsid components of the virus. Examples of the classification of hybridoma antibodies by specificity in RIA for glycoproteins, nucleocapsids or other components of the virus are shown in Table IV.

B. *Antinucleocapsid Antibodies*

Table V shows the results of RIA with antibodies produced by seven hybridoma clones that reacted with nucleocapsid preparations of four fixed rabies

TABLE III
Reactivity of Hybridomas with Various Viral Components

Immunizing material		Number of hybridomas reacting with viral components		
Strain of virus	Material	$G^{a,b}$	$N^{c,d}$	NS^e or $M^{b,f}$
ERA	V-BPL^g	8	6	2
	N	0	3	0
CVS	V-BPL	4	7	15
Kelev	V-BPL	8	7	14
Street	Live virus	1	0	2
Lagos bat	V-BPL	3	0	0
Mokola	V-BPL	1	2	7

^{a}G, glycoprotein. ^{e}NS, nonstructural protein.
^{b}RIA with ERA-infected cells as target. ^{f}M, matrix protein.
^{c}N, nucleocapsid. ^{g}V-BPL, virus inactivated by β-propiolactone.
^{d}Target is isolated nucleocapsid from ERA.

viruses and three rabies-related viruses, with the exception of the Kelev strain (Flamand *et al.*, 1980a,b). Hybridoma antibody 502-3 showed binding to the nucleocapsids of all rabies and rabies-related viruses; hybridoma antibody 377-7 and 103-7 reacted only with rabies viruses and, even then, only weakly with CVS; hybridoma antibody 422-5 reacted only with rabies-related viruses. Hybridoma antibodies 222-9, 237-3, and 389 did not bind the nucleocapsids of rabies virus HEP but did react with the nucleocapsids of all other rabies viruses. The nucleocapsids of the three rabies-related viruses can be distinguished from one another through binding with the appropriate antinucleocapsid hybridoma antibodies.

Table VI shows the number and the specificities of antinucleocapsid hybri-

TABLE IV
Reactivity of Hybridomas with Viral Antigens^a

Hybridoma	Antigen			
	Virus	N^b	G^c	Background
Anti-G	5932^d	2	810	20
	6107	10	800	40
Anti-N	4145	1357	22	22
	3920	1247	22	70
Other specificity	1737	72	7	25
	1682	75	57	25

^{a}From Flamand *et al.* (1980a). ^{c}G, glycoprotein.
^{b}N, nucleocapsid. ^{d}cpm Bound in RIA.

TABLE V

Immunoreactivity of Hybridoma Antibodies with Nucleocapsid Antigens[a]

Target virus strains	Results of RIA with hybridoma antibodies (cpm)						
	502-3[b]	103-7[c]	422-5[d]	377-7[b]	222-9[e]	237-3[e]	389[b]
ERA	3748	2457	177	4638	2265	2581	2037
Kelev	6607	5894	140	5517	5709	6375	4720
CVS-11	6364	3276	223	1486	2221	3947	3323
HEP	3752	3403	180	4688	32	14	245
Duvenhage	7287	431	1773	745	12	14	2361
Lagos bat	5212	0	3462	41	2498	8	2615
Mokola	4911	0	3030	52	1398	2465	220

[a]Except in the case of the Kelev strain, when purified virus was used. From Wiktor *et al.* (1980).
[b]Mice immunized with Kelev virus.
[c]Mice immunized with ERA virus.
[d]Mice immunized with Mokola virus.
[e]Mice immunized with CVS.

doma antibodies reacting with nucleocapsids of different members of the rabies-fixed and rabies-related groups of viruses. By far the largest number of hybridomas secreted antibodies that reacted with the four fixed and the HEP rabies viruses. One hybridoma antibody, 502-2, reacted with all rabies and rabies-related viruses; another hybridoma antibody, 422-5, reacted only with rabies-related viruses. Antibodies secreted by seven hybridomas did not bind to the nucleocapsids of HEP but did react with the nucleocapsids of all other fixed rabies viruses. Of these, three reacted with the three rabies-related viruses as well. The specificities displayed by 389, 237-3, and 222-9 hybridomas allowed us to distinguish among the three rabies-related viruses.

Since the production of street viruses in concentrations sufficient for the isolation and purification of nucleocapsid proteins presents considerable difficulties, assays of the specificities of antinucleocapsid hybridomas for street virus nucleocapsids were performed in an FA test on impression smears of cells of mouse brains infected with street virus (Wiktor *et al.*, 1980). The results, shown in Table VII, may be summarized as follows. Antibodies secreted by 17 of 21 hybridomas mediated FA of cells of brain tissue infected with all street viruses and with the standard laboratory strain CVS. The Sodja virus, isolated in Europe, the NH virus, isolated in Africa, and four viruses isolated in South America (all except 91) were identical to one another and to the laboratory CVS in their binding of hybridomas 364-11, 377-7, 102-27, and 193. The two viruses isolated in Western Europe (France and Germany) were identical to one another in reactivity and differed from all other viruses. The two viruses isolated in the USSR, the two viruses isolated in Burundi, and the NYC virus, isolated in the USA, showed the same binding pattern. Finally, hybridoma antibody 193 stained the antigens of only one of four North American viruses but, with only one exception (91), reacted with all other viruses. The results obtained with antinucleocapsid hybridoma antibodies enabled us to construct two panels of anti-

TABLE VI
Classification of Nucleocapsid Hybridomas[a]

| Hybridomas | | | Virus strain[b] | | | | | Hybrid-doma[c] group |
| | | | Rabies | | Rabies-related | | | |
Immunizing virus	Number in the group	Representative	CVS ERA Kelev Flury-LEP	Flury-HEP	Mokola	Lagos bat	Duvenhage	
ERA ⎫ CVS ⎬ Kelev ⎭	11	590.2	+	+	−	−	−	A
Kelev	1	510	+	+	−	−	+	B
Kelev	1	522.2	+	+	+	+	+	C
ERA	3	104-7	+	−	+	+	+	D
CVS	2	222-9	+	−	+	+	−	E
CVS	1	237-3	+	−	+	−	−	F
Kelev	1	389	+	−	−	+	+	G
Mokola	1	422-5	−	−	+	+	+	H

[a]From Flamand et al. (1980a).
[b]+, Positive in binding assay; −, no detectable binding.
[c]These groups were established on the basis of various cross-reactivities.

nucleocapsid antibody clones. Using these panels in FA staining of infected cells, we have been able to diagnose regularly the infection of animal tissue with rabies and rabies-related viruses and to distinguish among individual viruses within each group. As shown in Table VIII, antibodies of clone 502-3 mediate the staining of nucleocapsids of all rabies and rabies-related viruses; antibodies of clone 103-7 stained antigens of rabies viruses only; and antibodies of clone 422-5 stained antigens of rabies-related viruses only. Using the antibodies secreted by the remaining four hybridoma clones, we have been able to distinguish (1) the rabies viruses CVS and HEP both from one another and from other members of the rabies virus group, and (2) the three rabies-related viruses from one another.

C. Antiglycoprotein Antibodies

The presence of these antibodies was determined in RIA with purified virions (Flamand et al., 1980b) from fixed rabies and rabies-related viruses (Table IX). On the basis of their specificities, hybridoma antibodies were classified into 14 distinct groups. Group III, the largest group, consists of hybridomas which reacted with all viruses of the rabies group and cross-reacted with the Duvenhage virus of the rabies-related group. Antibodies of the two hybridomas in Group I cross-reacted with all rabies and rabies-related viruses, and antibodies of hybridomas from Groups II, III, and IV cross-reacted with all rabies viruses

TABLE VII

Immunofluorescence (FA) with Nucleocapsid Hybridoma Antibodies of Impression Smears from Mouse Brains Infected with Rabies Virus[a]

Virus strains				FA of cells exposed to hybridoma antibodies				
Continent	Country	Strain	Origin	17[b]	364-11	377-7	102-27	193
Europe	France	AF	Fox	+	−	+	+	−
	FRG	SF	Fox	+	−	+	+	+
	Czecho-slovakia	Sodja	Mouse	+	+	−	+	+
	USSR	SV	Man	+	+	+	+	+
	USSR	REZ	Man	+	+	+	+	+
Africa	Burundi	RD	Dog	+	+	+	+	+
	Burundi	UG	Goat	+	+	+	+	+
	Nigeria	NH	Horse	+	+	−	+	+
S. America	Chile	51	Dog	+	+	−	+	+
	Chile	91	Man	+	+	−	+	−
	Brazil	AG	Man	+	+	−	+	+
	Brazil	ARE	Vaccine	+	+	−	+	+
	Brazil	DR	Vampire bat	+	+	−	+	+
N. America	USA	NYC	Dog	+	+	+	+	+
	USA	GEO	Dog	+	+	+	+	−
	USA	ATF	Fox	+	+	+	+	−
	USA	UD	Bat	+	+	+	−	−
Standard control	CVS 11,24,26			+	+	−	+	+

[a]From Wiktor *et al.* (1980).
[b]Antibodies secreted by 17 hybridomas reacted with nucleocapsids of all strains listed in this table.

TABLE VIII

Differential Diagnosis of Members of the Lyssavirus Group by FA Staining with Nucleocapsid Hybridoma Antibodies[a]

Viruses		FA staining with hybridoma antibodies						
		Basic panel			Subdividing panel			
Group	Strains	502-3	103-7	422-5	337-7	222-9	237-3	389
Rabies	Street and fixed	+	+	−	+	+	+	+
	CVS-11	+	+	−	−	+	+	+
	HEP	+	+	−	+	−	−	−
Rabies-related	Duvenhage	+	−	+	−	−	−	+
	Lagos bat	+	−	+	−	+	−	+
	Mokola	+	−	+	−	+	+	−

[a]From Wiktor *et al.* (1980).

TABLE IX

Immunoreactivity of Antiglycoprotein Hybridoma Antibodies against Rabies and Rabies-Related Viruses[a]

Hybridoma Origin	No.	Rabies[b] CVS	PM	ERA	HEP	Kelev	Rabies-related[b,c] DUV	LAG	MOK	Hybridoma group
Kelev	523-1	+	+	+	+	+	0	0	0	I
	505-2	0	+	0	+	+	0	0	0	I
ERA	120-61	0	+	+	+	+	0	0	−	II
ERA	110-10	0	+	+	+	+	0	−	−	III
	176	0	+	+	+	+	0	−	−	III
Kelev	507-1	+	+	+	+	+	0	−	−	III
	509-6	+	+	+	+	+	0	−	−	III
	528-2	0	+	+	+	+	0	−	−	III
AF[d]	613-2	+	+	+	+	+	+	−	−	III
ERA	193-9	0	+	+	+	+	−	−	−	IV
Kelev	503	+	+	+	+	+	−	−	−	IV
	522-3	0	+	0	+	+	−	−	−	IV
CVS	231-22	+	+	+	+	−	−	−	−	V
ERA	194-2	+	+	+	−	−	0	−	−	VI
ERA	101-1	+	−	+	+	−	−	−	−	VII
	162	+	−	+	+	−	−	−	−	VII
CVS	248-9	+	+	+	−	−	−	−	−	VIII
Kelev	514-2	−	−	−	+	+	0	−	−	IX
Kelev	504-1	−	−	−	+	+	−	−	−	X
ERA	127-5	−	−	+	−	+	−	−	−	XI
CVS	220-8	+	−	−	−	−	−	−	−	XII
	240	+	−	−	−	−	−	−	−	XII
Kelev	359-2	−	−	−	−	+	−	−	−	XIII
	508-9	−	−	−	−	+	−	−	−	XIII
Mokola	419-1	−	−	−	−	−	−	−	+	XIV

[a]From Flamand *et al.* (1980b).
[b]+, Positive results in RIA and in neutralization test; 0, positive results in RIA and negative results in neutralization test; −, no binding in RIA.
[c]DUV, Duvenhage; LAG, Lagos bat; MOK, Mokola.
[d]AF, street virus; all other rabies strains are fixed viruses.

and, with the exception of antibodies from Group IV, with either one or two rabies-related viruses.

Antibodies produced by hybridomas from the remaining groups cross-reacted with a lesser number of viruses. Three hybridoma groups showed a single specificity each: Group XII for CVS, Group XIII for Kelev, and Group XIV for Mokola. As in the case of antinucleocapsid antibodies, none of the hybridomas produced from mice immunized with rabies-related viruses secreted antibodies that cross-reacted with rabies viruses. Hybridoma antibody obtained through the immunization of mice with the AF street virus cross-reacted with all rabies viruses and with the Duvenhage virus of the rabies-related group.

The 25 antiglycoprotein hybridomas listed in Table IX were evaluated for neutralizing activity against the eight virus strains listed in the same table. A complete correlation between binding activity in RIA and virus neutralization was obtained for HEP and Kelev viruses. However, the Duvenhage virus, which reacted positively in RIA with 11 hybridomas, was neutralized by one hybridoma only, 613–2. Mokola virus was also neutralized by only one hybridoma, 419-1, even though it had reacted positively with two additional hybridomas in the RIA test. Lagos bat virus was not neutralized by any of the three hybridomas with which it had shown binding in RIA. Of 19 hybridomas which showed binding in RIA to CVS virus, 12 neutralized the virus. Finally, the ERA virus was neutralized by all but two of 19 and PM viruses by all but one of 15 hybridomas positive in RIA. We are at present not able to offer any satisfactory explanation for this puzzling observation.

Nine rabies viruses originally isolated in the field from humans and from different species of animals on four continents were tested in a neutralization test with nine hybridoma antibodies. As shown in Table X, viruses AF and SF, isolated from foxes in France and Germany, respectively, showed identical patterns of cross-reactivity with neutralizing hybridoma antibodies. The two viruses isolated from humans in the USSR also showed identical patterns of cross-reactivity. Each of the remaining viruses had distinctive specificities, the UD virus isolated from a bat being the only one which was not neutralized by hybridoma antibody produced from mice immunized with the AF street virus. Since

TABLE X

Neutralization of Various Field Strains of Rabies Virus by Hybridoma Antibodies[a]

Hybridoma antibody		Neutralization of rabies virus isolated from humans and animals in various geographical regions[b]								
Origin	Code	UD USA (bat)	DR Brazil (vampire bat)	91 Chile (man)	DUV South Africa (man)	RD Central Africa (dog)	AF France (fox)	SF Germany (fox)	SV USSR (man)	REZ USSR (man)
CVS-11	220-8	0	0	0	0	0	0	0	0	0
	231-22	0	+	0	0	+	+	+	+	+
	248-2	0	+	+	0	0	+	+	+	+
ERA	101-1	+	0	+	0	+	+	+	+	+
	110-3	0	+	+	0	+	+	+	0	0
	120-61	0	0	+	0	0	+	+	0	0
	194-2	+	+	0	0	0	+	+	+	+
Kelev	359-2	0	0	0	0	0	0	0	0	0
AF Street	613-2	0	+	+	+	+	+	+	+	+

[a]From Wiktor *et al.* (1980).
[b]0, No neutralization; +, neutralization.

the number of field isolates was rather small, it is impossible at present to determine whether viruses isolated from the same species of animal and/or the same
geographic area are more likely to cross-react with hybridoma antibodies in the
same way than viruses isolated from different animal species and/or distant
geographic areas.

D. Anti-NS and Anti-M Antibodies

The group of hybridomas which secrete antibodies directed against the NS
or M protein remains not well defined. The antibodies showed binding in RIA to
antigens of purified virions; however, the degree of their reactivity was only
about 30–50% of that of the antibodies secreted by anti-N or anti-G hybridomas.
Anti-NS and anti-M hybridomas failed to react with purified N or G antigens in
RIA (Table II).

Anti-NS hybridomas could be further distinguished from anti-N hybridomas in that anti-NS hybridomas stained intracytoplasmic inclusions in cells infected with rabies virus only following fixation with formalin and not following
fixation with acetone (Table II). The two groups of hybridomas are similar in
that both anti-N and anti-NS antibodies were completely devoid of virus-neutral-
izing activity and did not lyse rabies virus-infected cells in presence of
complement.

Anti-M hybridoma showed less neutralizing activity than anti-G hybridoma
(20–50 pfu, in contrast to 10,000 pfu); however, the two were equally active in
lysing rabies-infected cells in the presence of complement and equally well-
stained antigens present on the surface of live virus-infected cells.

Immunoprecipitation of NS and M antigens from rabies-infected cell extracts by use of corresponding antibody has not yet been successful, and further
characterization of anti-NS and anti-M antibodies awaits purification of their
antigens.

III. Selection of Rabies Virus Variants

A. Production of Variants in Vitro

The CVS-11 strain, which is neutralized by nine monoclonal antibodies of
our collection, was used for the selection of antigenic variants (Wiktor and Koprowski, 1980). Serial tenfold dilutions of virus were prepared and mixed with
equal volumes of medium or hybridoma antibody 101-1 diluted in medium 1/10
or 1/50. After 1 hr of incubation at 37°C, 0.1 ml virus–antibody mixture was
added to cell monolayers grown in 60-mm petri dishes. Following adsorbtion for
1 hr, 5 ml nutrient agarose containing hybridoma antibody diluted 1/20 or 1/100
were poured over cell layers. Plates were incubated at 35°C for 4 days and were

scored for the presence of rabies-virus-induced plaques, which were easily visible without staining. At the highest dilution still showing plaques, well-separated plaques were picked up by Pasteur pipettes and dispersed in 5 ml MEM containing 1×10^6 freshly trypsinized BHK-21 cells in T-25 Falcon plastic tissue culture flasks. Aliquots of 0.5 ml infected cells were transferred into wells of four-chamber Lab-Tek tissue culture slides. The T-25 flasks and Lab-Tek slides were incubated for 3 days. The presence of virus in the culture was detected through FA staining.

Several clones of virus obtained through this technique from each neutralization test were assayed for resistance to neutralization by the hybridoma antibody used for their selection. The results of a typical experiment are presented in Table XI. The titer of CVS-11 virus incubated in the presence of medium was 5×10^7 pfu/ml. Following the selecting incubation of CVS-11 virus with hybridoma antibody 101-1 diluted 1/20, the titer of virus was reduced to 5×10^{-3} pfu/ml. All of 21 virus clones surviving were found to be resistant to neutralization by antibody of hybridoma 101-1. When virus was incubated with antibody diluted 1/100, the surviving fraction of virus had an infectivity titer of 1.6×10^5 pfu/ml. The surviving progeny, six clones, was fully susceptible to neutralization by 101-1 antibody.

Eight additional hybridoma antibodies were used for the selection of variants of CVS-11 virus (Table XII). Whenever the neutralization index of hybridoma antibody was equal to or higher than 10^4, it was possible to select clones of virus which resisted neutralization by the hybridoma antibody used for their selection. It was estimated from this data that the frequency of single-epitope variants in a cloned rabies virus was approximately 1 in 10,000. This frequency was similar to that obtained for influenza virus (Gerhard and Webster, 1978).

All five variants can be differentiated from the parent CVS strain. Variants RV-101-1, RV-220-8, and RV-231-22 seem to form one distinct group on the basis of antigenic changes from parent virus recognized by four monoclonal antibodies. Variants RV-240-3 and RV-226-11 formed another group that exhibit changes recognized by two monoclonal antibodies (240-3 and 226-11).

TABLE XI

Selection of Resistant Variants of CVS Virus after Neutralization with Hybridoma 101-1[a]

Selecting treatment (dilution)	PFU/plate at virus dilution ($\log_{10}$)					
	-1	-2	-3	-4	-5	-6
None	C[b]	C	C	>100	45[c]	5
101-1 (1:20)	42(16/16)[d]	5 (5/5)	0	0	0	0
101-1 (1:100)	C	>100	16 (0/6)	0	0	0

[a]From Wiktor and Koprowski (1980).
[b]C, confluent.
[c]Total number of plaques.
[d]Number in parentheses, test of clones derived in this selection: numerator, number of virus clones *not* neutralized by hybridoma 101-1; denominator, number of clones tested.

TABLE XII

Frequency of Formation of Variants of the CVS Strain[a]

Hybridoma antibody used for selection of variants	Neutralization index (pfu $\log_{10}$)	Variants per plaque analyzed
101-1	4.3	21/21[b]
101-1	3.5	0/14
220-8	4.5	3/9
226-11	4.5	2/2
231-22	4.2	4/5
240	4.5	1/1
162	4.3	2/2
194-2	4.0	3/8
613-2	3.3	0/2

[a]From Wiktor and Koprowski (1980).
[b]Numerator, number of virus clones *not* neutralized by the hybridoma antibody used for their selection; denominator, total number of virus clones isolated.

Although the results of this analysis suggest that the variants represent single-point glycoprotein mutants of the parental virus, the data have to be confirmed in an analysis with a much larger number of hybridoma antibodies recognizing different specificities. Moreover, final proof for a selection of single-point antigenic mutants can be obtained only in a biochemical analysis of polypeptide maps and amino acid substitution of the parental strain and different variants.

B. Results of Protection Experiments in Mice

The high frequency of occurrence of rabies variants supports the assertion that they represent single-point glycoprotein mutants of parental viruses. Since they represent minor changes in the overall antigenicity of the parental glycoprotein, it was expected that immunization of mice with variant viruses would protect them against challenge with the parental virus. The results of the cross-protection experiments proved to be different from those we expected (Wiktor and Koprowski, 1980). Six-week-old ICR mice were injected with two doses of vaccine produced in BHK-21 cells infected with the respective variant representing each of the *two* groups described in Table XIII. The animals were injected intraperitoneally at one-week intervals and, 7 days after the last injection, challenged intracerebrally with dilutions of either the parental strain (CVS-11) or another variant. The following results were obtained: mice vaccinated with a variant virus were protected against the lethal infection when challenged with homologous variant but died after challenge with the parental CVS-11 strain or variant of the heterologous site. Only mice immunized with the parental CVS-11 virus were protected when challenged with either CVS-11 or with a variant virus. Variants of the same group, RV-101-1 and RV-232-2 (see Table XIII) showed cross-protection. Antibodies present in sera obtained from vaccinated mice at

TABLE XIII

Neutralization of CVS-Standard and CVS-Resistant Variants by Different Hybridoma Antibodies[a]

	Virus strains[b]					
Hybridoma	Parent CVS-11	κV-101-1	RV-220-8	RV-231-22	RV-240-3	RV-226-11
101-1	4.2	0	4.0	4.0	>4.0	>4.0
220 8	4.3	0	0	0	>4.0	>4.0
162-5	4.3	0	0	3.3	>4.0	>4.0
231-22	4.3	4.5	0	0	>4.0	>4.0
240-3	4.0	4.5	4.0	4.0	0	0
226-11	>4.0	>4.0	>4.0	>4.0	0	0
613-2	3.3	>3.0	>3.0	>3.0	>3.0	0
248-2	4.0	>4.0	>4.0	>4.0	>4.0	4.0
194-2	4.2	4.5	>4.0	4.0	>4.0	3.0

[a]From Wiktor and Koprowski (1980).
[b]pfu $\log_{10}$.

the time of challenge showed as good a neutralizing capacity of the challenge virus which caused their death as of the virus to which they were resistant.

In light of these results and because of the existence of at least seven groups of variants recognized by hybridoma antibodies among field strains of rabies, cross-protection experiments were extended to mice immunized with a standard vaccine and challenged with rabies viruses isolated from human lethal cases and shown to have either similar or different specificities to the vaccine strain. Vaccinated mice were protected against challenge with the field strain that was more closely related to the vaccine strain but were at best only partially protected against challenge with more distantly related virus (Wiktor and Koprowski, 1980).

IV. Protection of Mice by Hybridoma Antibody

Hybridoma cells (1×10^5) of clones 101-1, 110-3, and 234 were sealed in Millipore chambers, and two such chambers were implanted into the peritoneal cavity of BALB/c mice. Four days after the implantation of hybridoma cells, animals were challenged by intracerebral or foot-pad inoculation with a lethal dose of PM, ERA, or AF street virus. Mice that had received hybridoma cells which produce antibodies capable of binding in RIA to the challenge virus (Table XIV) were protected, with the exception of hybridoma 110-3, which did not protect mice infected with AF street virus, although the virus was neutralized by hybridoma 110-3 *in vitro*, as shown in Table X. The latter results as well as those obtained in cross-protection experiments (Section III.B) indicate the necessity for further investigations of the mechanism(s) involved in protection of animals and man against rabies.

TABLE XIV
Protection of Mice by Hybridoma Antibodies

Clone	Hybridoma[a] binding to virus strains			Mortality ratio of mice challenged with viruses		
	PM	ERA	AF[b]	PM	ERA	AF[b]
101-1	+	+	+		0/5	1/5
						0/3[c]
110-3	+	+	+	3/16	0/5	5/5
234	−	−	−		5/5	5/5
Control				8/8	5/5	5/5

[a]Cell implanted in Millipore chambers and placed in the peritoneal cavity.
[b]Street virus isolated from a rabid fox in France.
[c]Challenge into foot pad; all others intracerebrally.

V. Conclusions

Through the use of hybridoma techniques it is possible to distinguish between rabies viruses and rabies-related viruses either isolated in different parts of the world or maintained as laboratory strains in various laboratories. The use of antinucleocapsid antibodies permits rapid identification of viruses causing rabies in man and animals. The antigenic variations demonstrated in these results emphasize the question of careful choice of strain used for vaccination purposes in a given country.

ACKNOWLEDGMENT

This work was supported, in part, by Grant No. AI-09706 from the National Institutes of Health and Grant No. R2/181/9 from the World Health Organization.

References

Flamand, A., Wiktor, T. J., and Koprowski, H., 1980a, Use of hybridoma monoclonal antibodies in the detection of antigenic differences between rabies and rabies-related virus proteins. I. The nucleocapsid, J. Gen. Virol. (in press).
Flamand, A., Wiktor, T. J., and Koprowski, H., 1980b, Use of hybridoma monoclonal antibodies in the detection of antigenic differences between rabies and rabies-related virus proteins. II. The glycoprotein, J. Gen. Virol. (in press).

Gerhard, W., and Webster, R. G., 1978, Antigenic drift in influenza A viruses. I. Selection and characterization of antigenic variants of A/PR/8/34 (H0N1) influenza virus with monoclonal antibodies, *J. Exp. Med.* **148:**383.

Sokol, F., Stancek, D., and Koprowski, H., 1971, Structural proteins of rabies virus, *J. Virol.* **7:**241.

Wiktor, T. J., and Koprowski, H., 1978, Monoclonal antibodies against rabies virus produced by somatic cell hybridization: Detection of antigenic variants, *Proc. Natl. Acad. Sci. USA* **75:**3938.

Wiktor, T. J., and Koprowski, H., 1980, Antigenic variants of rabies virus, *J. Exp. Med.* (in press).

Wiktor, T. J., Flamand, A., and Koprowski, H., 1980, Use of monoclonal antibodies in diagnosis of rabies virus infection and differentiation of rabies and rabies-related viruses, *J. Virol. Methods* **1:** 33.

Zaides, V. M., Krotova, L. I., Selimova, L. M., Selimov, M. A., Elbert, L. B., and Zhdanov, V. M., 1979, Reevaluation of the proteins in rabies virus particles, *J. Virol.* **29:**1226.

20
Monoclonal Antibodies against Streptococcal Antigens

RICHARD A. POLIN

I. Importance of Group B Streptococci as a Pathogen in Neonates

Despite recent advancements in infant intensive care, and the introduction of broad-spectrum antimicrobial agents, generalized bacterial infections in infants less than 1 month of age remain one of the leading causes of neonatal mortality and morbidity. The lack of significant improvement during the last decade in the outlook for infected neonates is due, at least in part, to the continuing difficulty of distinguishing bacterial sepsis from several other commonly encountered diseases of neonates. Today, among infected neonates, one third to one half die, one third develop meningitis (Anthony and Okada, 1977), and up to one half of surviving children with a history of central nervous system infection later display neurological handicaps.

The bacterial pathogens most frequently recovered from infected infants are Group B streptococci (GBS) (Baker, 1979). Identification of a streptococcus as type A or type B is determined by the structure of the "C substance" cell-wall polysaccharide. Group B is further subdivided into five types (IA, IB, IC, II, and III) by identification of variations in structure of a second cell-wall polysaccharide, "S substance" (Lancefield, 1934, 1938; Lancefield and Freimer, 1966; Wilkinson and Eagon, 1971). Many of these differences are immunologically distinguishable.

To facilitate rapid diagnosis of GBS sepsis, and thus allow early initiation of treatment, many clinical microbiology laboratories now use immunological assays to detect bacteria or bacterial antigens in tissue specimens. These tests presently rely on antisera that frequently differ in quality and in background or

RICHARD A. POLIN • Department of Pediatrics, University of Pennsylvania, School of Medicine, and The Children's Hospital of Philadelphia, Philadelphia, Pennsylvania 19104.

baseline activity of the preimmune sera from the immunized animal. Recent advancements in somatic cell hybridization have permitted isolation of hybrid myeloma cell lines secreting homogeneous antibody of predetermined specificity (Köhler and Milstein, 1975). In order to produce more precise reagents for diagnosis of GBS sepsis, we have immunized mice with formalinized strains of type II and type III GBS and generated hybrid cell lines secreting type-specific anti-GBS antibody. These antibodies, harvested from cell-culture supernatants, have proven specific and useful for typing GBS. An analysis of these monoclonal antibodies comprises the substance of this chapter.

II. Production of Monoclonal Antibodies against Type II and Type III Group B Streptococcus

Vaccines of formalinized group B streptococcus were prepared from type II 18RS21/67/2 and type III D135C reference strains obtained from Dr. Rebecca Lancefield (Lancefield, 1934). Female BALB/c mice were given three immunizations of either type II or type III GBS at weekly intervals. The first injection consisted of antigen in incomplete Freund's adjuvant administered intraperitoneally. The second, diluted in saline, was given both intraperitoneally and subcutaneously. The final dose was given intravenously.

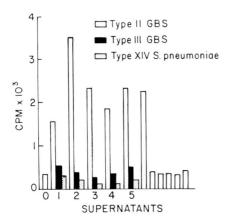

FIGURE 1. Binding of hybridoma supernatants to bacterial cell pellets detected with [^{125}I]anti-mouse Fab; mice immunized with Type II GBS. Bar graphs represent the mean of duplicate samples from a single assay. Each supernatant was tested on two additional occasions and yielded identical results. Five supernatants which did not bind to the bacteria are illustrated for comparison. (last five values on right side). 0, Control supernatant.

A polyvinyl chloride plate with 96 V-shaped microtiter cells was filled with RPMI 1640 with HEPES Buffer (20 mM) and 1% bovine serum albumin (BSA). The plates were incubated 4 hr at room temperature, the media removed, and 2 × 10^6 bacteria in formalinized saline placed into each well. The bacteria were pelleted by centrifugation (2500 rpm) and were resuspended in 50 μl of the antibody to be tested. Following a 1-hr incubation on melting ice, the plates were centrifuged (2500 rpm) and all wells washed with RPMI 1640 and 1% BSA. ^{125}I-labeled antimouse immunoglobulin (Fab-specific) was diluted in 0.5% BSA to 200,000 cpm/100 μl and 50 μl added to each well. The bacteria and radiolabeled antisera were incubated 1 hr on ice. The cells were pelleted, washed again, and the pellets counted in a gamma counter. Duplicate samples were run for all supernatants on three separate occasions. Each supernatant was tested for binding type II GBS, type III GBS, and type XIV S. *pneumoniae*. Control supernatants were obtained from actively growing cultures of SP2/0-Ag 14.

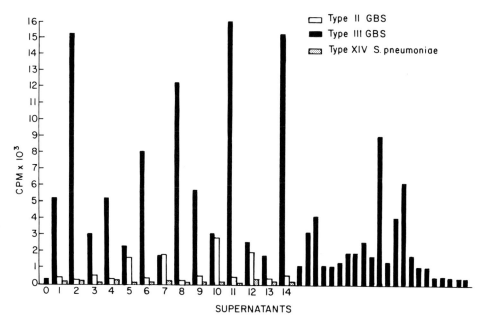

FIGURE 2. Binding of hybridoma supernatants to bacterial cell pellets detected with [^{125}I]anti-mouse Fab; mice immunized with Type III GBS: radioimmunoassay. Bar graphs represent the mean of duplicate samples from a single assay. Each supernatant was tested on two additional occasions and yielded identical results. Five supernatants which did not bind to the bacteria are illustrated for comparison (last five values on right side). Positive clones 1–14 were chosen for further analysis. 0, Control supernatant. Assay was performed as indicated in Fig. 1.

Three days after the intravenous injection, the spleen cells were removed and fusions were done according to methods reported previously (Kennett *et al.*, 1978) using plasmacytoma line Sp2/0-Ag14 (Shulman *et al.*, 1978).

Fusions with spleen cells immunized with type III GBS yielded 88 growing wells whose supernatants were tested for antibody production. Of these, 31 were producing anti-type III GBS antibody and 14 of these 31 supernatants were subjected to further analysis. Following immunization with type II GBS, 46 hybrids grew; 6 produced antibody against type II GBS and 5 of these were studied further. Of colonies cloned in agarose 100% secreted antibody identical to the originally isolated hybridoma cell line.

Figures 1 and 2 show the results of screening hybridoma supernatants from the two fusions for binding activity against the immunizing bacteria, the other GBS type, and *Streptococcus pneumoniae* type XIV. Assay of the supernatants using an enzyme immunoassay gave identical results (Table I). The supernatants exhibiting binding activity were tested for their ability to agglutinate GBS (Table II). Type III GBS were agglutinated by 6/10 of the antibodies that bound specifically to this type. None of these antibodies nor any of the anti-type II GBS antibodies agglutinated type II bacteria. The class of each of the anti-GBS antibodies was determined by immunodiffusion against class-specific reagents (Table III).

TABLE I
Binding of Hybridoma Supernatants to Bacterial Cell Pellets: Enzyme Immunoassay[a]

		Bacterial antigen		
Antibodies	N	Type III GBS	Type II GBS	Type XIV S. pneumoniae
Anti-type III GBS[b]	10[c]	10/10[e] (3+)	0	0
	4[d]	4/4 (3+)	4/4 (2+)	0
Anti-type II GBS	5	0	5/5 (3+)	0
Control	12	0	0	0

[a]A polyvinyl chloride plate with 96 V-shaped microtiter wells was filled with 1% gelatin in RPMI 1640 with 20 mM HEPES buffer (pH 7.6) and incubated 1 hr. The gelatin was removed and the following added; 2×10^8 fixed bacteria suspended in 50 μl of 0.1% gelatin in RPMI 1640, and 50 μl of the antibody solution to be tested. The bacteria and antibody were incubated 1/2 hr at room temperature then centrifuged (2500 rpm) for 5 min. The pellets were washed twice more with 0.1% gelatin in RPMI 1640, at which time 100 μl of peroxidase-labeled anti-mouse immunoglobulin (Cappel 1/1000 dilution) was added to each well. The cells and peroxidase-conjugated antisera were incubated 1/2 hr at room temperature, centrifuged, and washed three times with 0.1% gelatin in RPMI 1640. Following the last wash, 100 μl of a solution containing 10 mg orthophenylenediamine, 2 μl 30% H_2O_2 in 10 ml 0.1 M citrate buffer pH 4.5 was added to each well. The color of the well contents was recorded at the end of a 30-min incubation and graded 0–3+. Duplicate samples were run for all supernatants on three separate occasions. Each supernatant was tested for binding to type II GBS, type III GBS, and type XIV S. pneumoniae. Control supernatants were obtained from actively growing cultures of SP2/0-Ag 14. N, total number of antibodies tested; 0, negative; 1+, weakly positive; 2+, moderately positive; 3+, strongly positive.
[b]Clones resulting from immunization with type III GBS.
[c]Subgroup of mouse antibodies that bind to type III GBS, but not type II GBS.
[d]Subgroup of mouse antibodies that bind to both type II and type III GBS.
[e]Number positive/number tested.

III. Discussion

Using technology pioneered by Köhler and Milstein (1975), we have isolated and cloned hybrid myeloma cell lines secreting antibodies against specific types of group B streptococci. Each of the anti-type II streptococcal antibodies resulting from immunizations with type II GBS reacted only with type II bacteria. Four of the 14 antibodies derived following immunization with type III GBS cross-reacted with type II GBS. None of the anti-type III antibodies cross reacted with type XIV S. pneumoniae. The core antigen of type III GBS, and the capsular polysaccharide of type S. pneumoniae are immunochemically identical (Fischer et al., 1978; Lindberg et al., 1977; Kasper et al., 1978). Both cell walls consist of a trisaccharide backbone (galactose, glucosamine, glucose) in a molar ratio of 2:1:1 (Russell and Norcross, 1972). The more complex type III GBS native antigen contains a terminal sialic acid attached to each galactose end group and does not cross react with type XIV pneumococcal antisera (Baker et al., 1976; Kasper et al., 1978). In vitro, opsonic immunity to type III GBS infection correlates best with the presence of antibody to the native antigen. Infants recovering from invasive disease caused by type III GBS frequently develop

Table II
Agglutination of Bacteria by Hybridoma Supernatants[a]

| Antibodies | N | Number of supernatants agglutinating bacteria | |
		Type III GBS	Type II GBS
Type III GBS supernatants	10[b]	6	0
	4[c]	0	0
Type II GBS supernatants	5	0	0
Control	12	0	0

[a]10^6 Bacteria suspended in 25 μl PBS–1% BSA (pH 7.2) were placed in each well of a 96-well curved bottom microtiter plate (Linbro). 25 μl of the supernatants to be tested were pipetted into each well. The plates were covered, incubated 2 hr at 37°C, and checked for macroscopic agglutination. Each hybrid myeloma supernatant was tested in duplicate on two separate occasions. Bacterial agglutination was performed with three different concentrations of each supernatant (undiluted, 1/5, 1/10). Each supernatant was incubated with type II and III GBS. Control supernatants were obtained from actively growing cultures of SP2/0-Ag 14.
[b]Subgroup of mouse antibodies that bind to type III GBS, but not type II GBS.
[c]Subgroup of mouse antibodies that bind to both type II and type III GBS.

Table III
Immunoprecipitation of Hybridoma Supernatants[a]

Antibodies	N	μ	$\gamma1$	$\gamma2a$	$\gamma2b$	a	κ	λ
Type III GBS supernatants	10[b]	6	1	1			10	
	4[c]	3					4	
Type II GBS supernatants	5	5					5	

[a]Each hybrid myeloma supernatant was concentrated 10× and tested by double immunodiffusion in agar against class- and subclass-specific antibodies (Meloy Laboratories).
[b]Subgroup of mouse antibodies that bind to type III GBS but not type III GBS.
[c]Subgroup of mouse antibodies that bind to both type II and Type III GBS.

antibody to type III native antigen, and rarely develop titers to the core antigen. The lack of reactivity between anti-type III GBS hybridoma antibody and type XIV *S. pneumoniae* is suggestive evidence that the myeloma antibody is directed against the more complex type III GBS native antigen.

Precise and rapid identification of bacterial pathogens in culture or clinical specimens is of diagnostic and therapeutic importance. The most sensitive assays for detecting low numbers of bacteria are immunological in nature (latex agglutination and counterimmunoelectrophoresis). The difficulty, however, is that both of these assays rely on animal antisera which frequently vary in their sensitivity and specificity (Siegal and McCracken, 1978; Thirumoorthi and Dajani, 1979). Hybrid myeloma antibodies are monospecific, and their uniformity can be maintained by cloning the hybrid and checking the antibody produced. We have demonstrated the usefulness of hybridoma supernatants for typing GBS using an enzyme immunoassay. It seems probable that hybrid myeloma antibodies will soon replace animal antisera in most of the diagnostic tests now used to detect bacterial antigens *in vitro*.

Hybrid myeloma antibodies may also find use as therapeutic agents. Certain human infectious diseases (such as serum hepatitis) are now commonly treated with passively administered antibodies. A number of observations suggest that passively acquired antibodies can play a role in modifying the course of GBS disease; e.g., Baker and Kasper (1976) compared the serum antibody titers of a group of mothers and infants who were asymptomatically colonized with GBS with titers from a second group of women who delivered septic infants. Of mothers who delivered asymptomatic infants 76% had serum antibody titers against GBS, whereas none of the seven infected neonates or their mothers had demonstrable anti-GBS serum antibodies. Moreover, Shigeoka *et al.* (1978) reported that administration of blood containing type-specific GBS antibodies to septic infants resulted in survival of all nine infants so treated while the control group who received blood without type-specific antibody suffered a 50% mortality. Taken together, these observations suggest that passively administered anti-GBS antibodies if given in highly purified form would be expected to protect neonates from GBS sepsis.

Certain of the currently available anti-GBS hybridomas described in this chapter may therefore provide protection from GBS sepsis. Experiments are currently underway to evaluate the protective effects of these hybridoma antibodies in a murine model system. Although heterologous immunoglobulins have, in the past, been used to treat patients stricken with certain overwhelming infections, the incidence of serum sickness and/or anaphylactic reactions following treatment with such heterologous proteins severely limits this therapeutic approach. One presumes that similar adverse reactions might be seen in patients following administration of murine hybridoma antibodies. It is particularly encouraging, therefore, to note that several groups have now reported secretion of human immunoglobulin by mouse–human hybridomas (Koprowski *et al.*, 1978, Levy, this volume). We may, therefore, anticipate the development of monoclonal human antibodies for therapeutic application within the next few years.

ACKNOWLEDGMENTS

The author wishes to thank Barbara Erwins for her editorial assistance and Joseph Campos, Ph.D. and Martin Trandler for their technical assistance.
This work was supported in part by NIH grant RR-00506-17.

References

Anthony, C. J., and Okada, D. M., 1977, The emergence of group B streptococci in infections of the newborn infant, *Annu. Rev. Med.* **28:**355.

Baker, C. J., 1979, Group B streptococcal infections in neonates, *Pediatr. Rev.* **1**:5.

Baker, C. J., and Kasper, D. L., 1976, Correlation of maternal antibody deficiency with susceptibility to neonatal group B streptococcal infection, *N. Engl. J. Med.* **294**:753.

Baker, C. J., Kasper, D. L., and Davis, C. E., 1976, Immunochemical characterization of the "native" type III polysaccharide of group B streptococcus, *J. Exp. Med.* **143**:258.

Fischer, G. W., Lowell, G. H., Crumrine, M. H., and Bass, J. W., 1978, Type 14 pneumonococcal antisera is opsonic in vitro and protective in vivo for group B streptococcus type III, *Pediatr. Res.* **12**:491.

Kasper, D. L., Goroff, D. K., and Baker, C. J., 1978, Immunochemical characterization of native polysaccharides from group B streptococcus: The relationship of the type III and group B determinants, *J. Immunol.* **121**:1096.

Kennett, R. H., Denis, K. A., Tung, A., and Klinman, N. R., 1978, Hybrid plasmacytoma production: Fusions with adult spleen cells, monoclonal spleen fragments, neonatal spleen cells, and human spleen cells, *Curr. Top. Microbiol. Immunol.* **88**:77.

Köhler, G., and Milstein, C., 1975, Continuous cultures of fused cells making antibody of predefined specificity, *Nature* **256**:495.

Koprowski, H., Gerhard, W., Wiktor, T., Martinis, J., Shander, M., Croce, C. M., 1978, Anti-viral and anti-tumor antibodies produced by somatic cell hybrids, *Curr. Top. Microbiol. Immunol.* **88**:8.

Lancefield, R. C., 1934, A serological differentiation of specific types of bovine streptococci (group B), *J. Exp. Med.* **59**:441.

Lancefield, R. C., 1938, Two serological types of group B hemolytic streptococci with related but not identical type specific substances. *J. Exp. Med.* **67**:25.

Lancefield, R. C., and Freimer, E. H., 1966, Type specific polysaccharide antigens of group B streptococci, *J. Hyg. (Camb.)* **64**:91.

Lindberg, B., Lonngren, J., and Powell, D. A., 1977, Structural studies of the specific type 14 pneumococcal polysaccharide, *Carbohydr. Res.* **58**:177.

Russell, H., and Norcross, N. L., 1972, The isolation and some physiochemical and biological properties of type III antigen of group B streptococci, *J. Immunol.* **109**:90.

Shigeoka, S. O., Hall, R. T., and Hill, H. R., 1978, Blood transfusion in group B streptococcal sepsis, *Lancet* **1**:636.

Shulman, M., Wilde, C. D., and Köhler, G., 1978, A better cell life for making hybridomas secreting specific antibodies, *Nature* **276**:269.

Siegel, J.D., and McCracken Jr., G. H., 1978, Detection of group B streptococcal antigens in body fluids of neonates, *J. Pediatr.* **93**:491.

Thirumoorthi, M. C., and Dajani, A. S., 1979, Comparison of staphylococcal coagglutination, latex agglutination, and counterimmunoelectrophoresis for bacterial antigen detection, *J. Clin. Microbiol.* **9**:28.

Wilkinson, H. W., and Eagon, R. G., 1971, Type specific antigens of group B type IC streptococci, *Infect. Immunol.* **4**:596.

Appendix
Methods for Production and Characterization of Monoclonal Antibodies

Introduction

The purpose of this appendix is to provide the details of methods for the production and characterization of monoclonal antibodies that are used in several of the laboratories actively involved in the development of hybridoma technology. In a field as active as this such a compilation can be neither complete nor up to date, but it will provide the uninitiated with the basic procedures necessary to try their hand at the production of monoclonal antibodies. Many monoclonal antibodies against common antigens are already available in several laboratories, and some are even available commercially. Those who have not made hybridomas and who need such standard reagents would probably be wise to obtain the ones already available. On the other hand, there will certainly be, for a long time, the need to make monoclonal antibodies against many additional antigens.

Plasmacytoma Cell Lines

Most of the plasmacytoma cell lines used to make hybridomas and some hybridomas producing monoclonal antibodies are available from The Salk Institute, Cell Distribution Center, P.O. Box 1809, San Diego, California 92112, or Institute for Medical Research, NIGMS Cell Repository, Copewood and Davis Streets, Camden, New Jersey 08103.

The cells are generally grown in Dulbecco's Modified Eagle's Medium (DMEM) with high glucose (4.5 g/liter) or in RPMI 1640. Addition of glucose to RPMI 1640 up to 4.5 g/liter does improve growth at higher densities. Cells are maintained in stationary suspension culture at a concentration of 10^5–10^6/ml. Optimum condition of a culture to be used for fusion is high viability (>90%) with 3–8×10^5 cells/ml.

The optimal ratio of spleen cells/plasmacytoma cells may vary with the source of primary lymphocytes, immunization protocol, and the specific antigens involved. Most fusions have been done with one to a few immunizations given via various routes followed by an intravenous injection 3–5 days prior to fusion.

Fusion Protocols
Fusion by Centrifugation of Cells Suspended in Polyethylene Glycol

ROGER H. KENNETT

Materials

1. Polyethylene glycol 1000 (Baker)
   Batches vary in toxicity and fusion efficiency.
2. Hypoxanthine (H) (Sigma) 100 × stock—136 mg/100 ml
   Thymidine (T) (Sigma) 100 × stock—76 mg/100 ml
   H and T solution may be prepared together. To dissolve, add 1 N NaOH until H is dissolved. Add T and readjust pH to 9.5 with acetic acid. Filter to sterilize. Store frozen at −20°C.
   Aminopterin (Sigma or Lederle) 100 × stock—1.8 mg/100 ml
   Add NaOH to dissolve. Adjust to pH approx. 7.8. Filter to sterilize. Store −20°C.
3. Hybridoma Medium (HY)
   Dulbecco's MEM with high glucose (4.5 g/liter) with glutamine added weekly
   10% NCTC 109 (Microbiological Assoc.)
   20% serum
   0.15 mg/ml oxaloacetate (Sigma)
   0.05 mg/ml pyruvate (Sigma)
   0.2 U/ml bovine insulin (Sigma)
   Oxaloacetate, pyruvate, insulin (OPI) may be prepared as 50× stock and stored frozen in plastic bottles.
4. Serum for cultures: Fetal calf serum or heat-inactivated (56°C, 30 min) calf serum or horse serum. Serum should be tested to see if there is any

ROGER H. KENNETT • Department of Human Genetics, University of Pennsylvania, School of Medicine, Philadelphia, Pennsylvania 19104.

background binding due to antibodies in the serum. Agamma horse serum helps in this respect. Serum lots differ widely in their capacity to support cloning of plasmacytoma lines and hybridomas. They should be screened for their capacity to clone the parental plasmacytomas. Those in which the parental lines give the best cloning efficiency (up to approx. 50% with a feeder layer) will be the best for hybridoma production, which is effectively cloning of the hybrid lines.

Removal of Spleen Cells

Spleen cells for the fusion are removed 3–4 days after the mouse is immunized intravenously. The spleen is placed in a 60-mm petri dish in tissue culture medium with serum and is perfused with medium by injecting with a 26-gauge needle at several sites, thereby forcing medium into the spleen. This is continued until most of the cells are removed; the number of spleen lymphocytes recovered is usually $5–10 \times 10^7$ per organ. Care must be taken not to repeatedly draw the suspended cells up into the syringe and force them through the needle. We have also removed cells using a loose-fitting glass homogenizer with equally good viability ($>95\%$).

Fusion Method

Remove the cells to a centrifuge tube, pellet them (1000 rpm, IEC MS), remove the supernatant liquid, and suspend them in 5 ml of cold 0.17 M NH_4 Cl. Keep the tube on ice for 10 min to lyse erythrocytes, and then add 10 ml of cold medium with 20% serum. Pellet the cells, count and check viability, and mix with 10^7 of plasmacytoma cell line.

1. Wash the cells in medium free of serum by centrifugation in a round-bottomed tube (Falcon 2001).
2. Remove all the supernatant liquid by suction and loosen the pellet by tapping the tube.
3. Add 0.2 ml of 30% PEG in medium without serum. The 30% PEG is made by adding 3 ml of PEG 1000 at 41°C to 7 ml of medium without serum at 41°C. Warm pipette in flame before pipetting PEG. PEG tends to lower the pH of the medium which should be adjusted to approx. 7.6 with NaOH. After mixing the PEG solution it is kept at 37°C until used.
4. The cells are maintained in the 30% PEG for 8 min. During the 8-min period, cells are pelleted in the 30% PEG (1000 rpm, IEC MS, radius 35 cm). The centrifugation time should be 3–6 min. It is our impression that the longer the centrifugation, the more hybrids. The limitation is the toxic effect of PEG on the particular cells used. This may be monitored by phase microscopy or trypan blue exclusion. At the end of 8 min

the PEG is diluted with 5 ml of medium without serum, and then 5 ml of medium with 20% serum is added.

5. The cells, in diluted PEG, are pelleted and resuspended in 30 ml of HY culture medium with serum (Kennett *et al.,* 1978). In addition to the purine and pyrimidine bases present in the NCTC 109 medium, thymidine (16 μM) and hypoxanthine (0.1 mM) are added to the medium in which the fused cells are plated.

6. The 30 ml of cells are evenly suspended and gently distributed into 6 microplates (Linbro FB96TC), 1 drop (about 50 μl) per well. The next day an additional drop of the above medium with aminopterin (0.8 μM) is added to make hypoxanthine–aminopterin–thymidine (HAT) selective medium (Littlefield, 1964).

7. The wells are fed two additional drops of medium without aminopterin 6–7 days later; clones appear macroscopically within 2 weeks.

8. If necessary, the clones may be fed by removing most of the medium in the well and replacing it with fresh medium.

9. In most fusions clones arise in nearly all the wells of the six microplates. Viable wells are identified by screening the supernatant liquid for production of the desired antibody, and these clones are transferred to larger wells (Linbro FB16-24-TC) with not more than 0.5 ml of medium.

10. At early stages, the clones must be watched carefully so that they are not allowed to grow to too high a density nor diluted too sparsely.

11. When the cells have been transferred into four of the larger wells, they may be transferred to flasks, grown, and stocks prepared and frozen.

12. The frequency of hybrids usually requires that the cells be cloned in agarose over a feeder layer of human fibroblasts to be sure that the cells are truly clonally derived. We have often cloned the cells from the original well into two cloning plates successfully (see page 372).

13. If the reversion rate of the parental lines is not known, control cells should be fused without spleen cells and be put under selective conditions. For those cells selected against in HAT medium it is wise to grow the parental cells in the appropriate selective drug, 5-bromodeoxyuridine or 8-azaguanine, before the fusion.

14. For hard to fuse cells PEG may be increased to 50% and 5% DMSO added.

References

Kennett, R., 1979, Cell fusion, in: *Methods in Enzymology* (W. Jakoby and J. Pastan, eds.), Academic Press, New York, pp. 345–349.

Kennett, R. H., Denis, J., Tung, A., and Klinman, N., 1978, Hybrid plasmacytoma production: Fusions with adult spleen cells, monoclonal spleen fragments, neonatal spleen cells, and human spleen cells, *Curr. Top. Microbiol. Immunol.* **81**:77.

Littlefield, J. W., 1964, Selection of hybrids from matings of fibroblasts in vitro and their presumed recombinants, *Science* **145**:709.

Fusion of Cells in an Adherent Monolayer

Thomas J. McKearn

Materials

1. Spleen cells (lymph node cells) from animal immunized 2–3 days previously
2. Mutant myeloma cells from culture, e.g., P3/X63-Ag8, 45.6TG, NS1, or Sp2/0-Ag14
3. Polyethylene glycol (PEG) 1500 (Fisher)—autoclaved in 3- to 5-ml aliquots
4. Hybridoma (HY) medium with hypoxanthine–aminopterin–thymidine (HAT) additives (see Kennett protocol)
5. Heat-inactivated serum (either agamma horse or fetal calf)
6. 60-cm Falcon tissue culture dishes (Falcon # 3002)
7. 96-well Costar plates (# 3596)
8. Ficoll 400, 14% (w/v) in distilled H_2O
9. Hypaque, 32.8%, (w/v) sodium metrizoate in distilled H_2O
10. Sodium azide, 25% (w/v) stock in distilled H_2O
11. Ficoll–Hypaque mixture, 12 parts 14% Ficoll + 5 parts 32.8% sodium metrizoate + 0.1% sodium azide. Density = 1.09 g/ml
12. 3-ml plastic sterile syringe

Fusion Method

1. Sterile spleen cell suspensions are prepared in serum-free HY medium.
2. Cells are washed twice with HY medium and then resuspended to approximately the following volumes:
   a. Whole rat spleen—9 ml
   b. Whole mouse spleen—3 ml
3. 3 ml of this cell suspension is added to a sterile siliconized 10-ml glass test tube (Vacutainer tube # 4710) and underlaid with 4 ml of Ficoll–Hypaque–Azide solution using a 5-ml pipette and a mechanical pipettor (Pipet Aid, Bellco).
4. Tubes are capped and spun at 2000 × g for 15 min at 23°C.
5. While the cells are spinning prepare a 50% (v/v) solution of PEG 1500 (Fisher) by preheating a tube of sterile PEG and a second tube of HY

Thomas J. McKearn • Department of Pathology, Divisions of Research Immunology and Laboratory Medicine, University of Pennsylvania, School of Medicine, Philadelphia, Pennsylvania 19104.

medium to 56°C in a water bath. Mix the solution by drawing 5 ml of warm HY into a 10-ml pipet followed by 5 ml PEG. Rinse contents of pipet vigorously into and from a 15-ml plastic conical tube before the mixture has a chance to cool. Place the well-mixed solution in the laminar flow hood in order to cool to room temperature. If necessary, adjust pH of PEG solution to 7.0 using sterile sodium bicarbonate solution.

6. Immune cells are removed from the gradient interface and washed twice with serum-free Hy. Cell concentration is adjusted to 50×10^6/ml.

7. Mutant myeloma cells from culture are washed twice with serum-free HY (centrifuged 5 min at $250 \times g$) and adjusted to 5×10^6/ml.

8. 1 ml of immune cell suspensions is mixed with 1 ml of mutant myeloma cells in 60-mm tissue culture dish (Falcon # 3002). 3 ml of serum-free HY is then added.

9. Tissue culture dishes are placed in microtiter plate carriers (Cooke) and centrifuged at $250 \times g$ for 3 min. This results in formation of an adherent monolayer of cells on the bottom of the dish.

10. Supernatant is aspirated and the dish gently flooded with 1 ml of 50% PEG in HY. After 30 sec at room temperature, the plate is flooded with 5 ml of serum-free HY. This is aspirated and replaced with 5 ml of HY. The plate is again aspirated and flooded with 5 ml of HY containing 20% serum.

11. Petri dish is incubated overnight at 37°C in CO_2 incubator.

12. After overnight incubation, rinse cells from dishes with $5^3/4$- in. Pasteur pipette. Refill plate with 3 ml of HY with 20% serum and gently scrape plate with plunger from 3-ml sterile disposable syringe (Becton-Dickinson).

13. Spin cells into pellet in 50-ml tube at $50 \times g$ for 5 min.

14. Carefully aspirate supernatant, leaving approximately 1–2 ml of supernatant over the cell pellet.

15. Resuspend the pellet in 30–35 ml of HY containing HAT, 20% serum, and glutamine.

16. Label 96-well Costar dishes. Place 2 drops of cell suspension from 10-ml pipette into each well of 96 well Costar cluster dish (3 plates per group).

17. Return plates to humidified CO_2 incubator for 1 week.

18. After 1 week, add 2 drops of HY with 20% serum and HT to all wells and return to humidified CO_2 incubator.

19. When wells containing proliferating hybrids become acid, aspirate 50–100 μl of supernatant for antibody assay.

20. Wells positive for antibody production are transferred to 2-ml wells of 24-well Linbro plates which had been seeded 1 hr to 10 days previously with 10^7 irradiated Lewis rat thymocytes in a volume of 1 ml of HY medium with 20% serum and glutamine.

Fusion of Cells in Suspension and Outgrowth of Hybrids in Conditioned Medium

WALTER GERHARD

Materials

1. NH₄Cl (8.3 g/liter), pH 7.0.
2. Heat-inactivated fetal calf serum (FCS).
3. Dulbecco's modified phosphate-buffered saline (PBS) (GIBCO).
4. Dulbecco's Modified Eagle's Medium (DMEM) with 4.5 g glucose/liter, 2 mM glutamine, and gentamicin (50 μg/ml), Fetal calf serum and horse serum (each 75 ml/liter)
5. 50% (v/v) polyethylene glycol (PEG)-1000 freshly prepared in serum-free DMEM adjusted to pH 7

Standard Fusion Protocol

The entire procedure is performed at room temperature. The donor lymphocyte preparation is incubated for 5 min in NH₄Cl (8.3 g/liter), spun through a cushion of heat-inactivated FCS and washed once with Dulbecco's modified phosphate-buffered saline (PBS). In parallel the myeloma cells (at exponential growth phase) are spun out of their culture medium (DMEM) and are washed with PBS. The "preconditioned" myeloma culture medium is saved and diluted 1/2 in DMEM containing hypoxanthine (13.6 μg/ml), aminopterin (0.186 μg/ml), and thymidine (15.5 μg/ml) (HAT) at double strength and containing an increased concentration of FCS and agamma horse serum (each 125 ml/liter) to make the conditioned DMEM-HAT. The washed lymphocytes and myeloma cells are counted, mixed at a ratio of 7/1, and spun down together (7 min, 300 × g). The supernatant is removed except for approx. 50 μl, into which the cell pellet is resuspended by tapping the bottom of the centrifuge tube. Fusion is performed by resuspending the cell slurry in 0.5 to 1 ml of 50% (v/v) PEG-1000. After incubation for 1 min the cell suspension is gradually filled up with serum-free DMEM to approx. 30 ml, the cells are spun down, the supernatant is discarded, the cell pellet is gently resuspended by pipetting into conditioned DMEM-HAT and diluted to give a final cell concentration of 0.5 to 1.5 × 10⁶

WALTER GERHARD • Wistar Institute of Anatomy and Biology, Philadelphia, Pennsylvania 19104.

lymphocytes/ml. Aliquots of approximately 0.1 ml are added to wells of 96-well flat-bottom tissue culture plates (Flow Laboratories, Rockville, Md.) and are incubated at 37°C in humidified 8% CO_2 in air. The cultures are left undisturbed for the first 5–7 days and are then fed with approximately 0.05 to 0.1 ml DMEM-HAT. The culture fluid of individual cultures is tested in the radioimmunoassay for the presence of antibodies when microscopically visible hybrid cell colonies reach a diameter of at least 1 mm (7–14 days after fusion). Positive cultures are transferred in DMEM-HT (the same as DMEM-HAT but containing no aminopterin) into individual wells of 24-well tissue culture plates and are cloned in soft agarose as soon as the hybrid cells exhibit vigorous cell growth.

Cloning of Hybridomas
Cloning in Semisolid Agarose

Roger H. Kennett

Materials

1. Hybridoma (HY) medium—*Note:* Sera vary in their ability to support cloning of plasmacytomas and hybridomas. Screen several lots to obtain one that supports optimal cloning efficiency. Up to 50% cloning efficiency can be obtained with good serum and good agarose.
2. 2.4% agarose in 0.15 M NaCl

    2.4 g Seakem Agarose (Microbiological Assoc. and Marine Colloids, Rockland, Maine) is suspended in 0.15 M NaCl to final volume of 100 ml and autoclaved. Divide when still hot into 10-ml aliquots in 100-ml sterile bottles. *Note:* Varying cloning efficiences are obtained in different batches of agarose. Screen several at first to obtain one that gives optimum cloning.
3. Diploid human or rabbit fibroblasts for feeder layer, or conditioned culture medium from dense (approx. 10^6/ml) culture of plasmacytoma cells filtered through a 0.22-μm filter

    We have used human and rabbit fibroblasts.
4. Tissue culture tubes
5. Water bath at 41°C
6. Hybridomas with good viability—can clone with as few cells as are in a small macroscopically visible colony

Method

1. Prepare tubes with feeder cells. Pipette 2 ml of HY medium containing

---

ROGER H. KENNETT • Department of Human Genetics, University of Pennsylvania, School of Medicine, Philadelphia, Pennsylvania 19104.

5×10^4 feeder cells into each tube. Tubes are slanted so that the medium and cells come in contact with the side of the tube up to the point that 4 ml of medium would reach when the tube is upright. Alternatively the tube may be rotated so the cells attach all around the bottom up to this point. These tubes or plates may be used as soon as the cells attach or for the next few days. Prepare 2–4 tubes for each hybridoma to be cloned. Alternatively tubes may be set up containing 2 ml of medium conditioned by growth of plasmacytomas

2. Autoclave 2.4% agarose which has been stored in 10-ml aliquots. When this cools to 50–60°C, add 40 ml of medium that has been warmed to 41°C. Keep this 0.48% agarose at 41°C.

3. Vortex hybridoma cells before dispensing to assure a single-cell suspension. Add hybridoma cells to cloning tubes in 100 µl or less. For each hybridoma set up tubes with at least 2-cell concentrations (approx. 200 and 2000/tube). Contents of small well (96-well plate) may be taken up in approx. 5 drops of medium and 1 drop put in one tube, 4 in the other.

4. To each tube then add 2 ml of 0.48% agarose solution. Add to tube so it mixes well with medium containing hybridomas already in tube. Let stand upright in rack to solidify agarose. This may be facilitated by placing in refrigerator or ice bucket for a few minutes.

5. Place in CO_2 (approximately 8%) incubator. Macroscopic clones appear within 2 weeks.

6. Choose tube in which there are not too many clones and use pasteur pipette to remove clones from agarose. Dispense cells in 2 drops of medium that has been placed in well of 96-well microtiter plate. Pick approximately 20 clones from each hybridoma unless this is found to be too few to pick up positive clone. Cells which have been cloned and picked to wells will tend to grow faster than when they first appear after fusion. Test clones for antibody production and expand up to culture volume that allows freezing of several ampoules of cells for future use.

Cloning of Hybridoma Cells by Limiting Dilution in Fluid Phase

THOMAS J. MCKEARN

Materials

1. 6- to 8-week-old Lewis rat
2. Hybridoma (HY) medium
3. Selected lot of serum (agamma horse or fetal calf) chosen for its ability to support cloning
4. 96-well tissue culture dish (Costar # 3596)

Method

1. Aseptically remove thymus from 6- to 8-week-old Lewis rat and place in sterile tissue culture tube containing HY medium. Irradiate tube contents with 1200–1500 rads of gamma irradiation.
2. Prepare single-cell suspension from thymus and wash once with HY medium containing 20% serum supplement.
3. Adjust thymocyte cell concentration to 10^7/ml and place 0.1 ml of cell suspension into each well of a 96-well dish (Costar).
4. Prepare suspensions of hybridoma cells containing 500, 50, and 10 cells/ml.
5. Add 0.1 ml of hybridoma cell suspension to each well of the dishes previously seeded with thymocyte feeders. Set up one full dish for each dilution of hybridoma cells.
6. After 10–14 days inspect dishes for macroscopic clusters of hybridoma cells. Assay supernatants of wells showing growth from those dishes which show growth of hybridoma cells in less than 30% of the wells.
7. If positive for relevant antibody activity, expand the cells into 2-ml wells (Linbro).

THOMAS J. MCKEARN • Department of Pathology, Divisions of Research Immunology and Laboratory Medicine, University of Pennsylvania, School of Medicine, Philadelphia, Pennsylvania 19104.

Freezing of Hybridoma Cells

Roger H. Kennett

Hybridomas can be frozen and recovered successfully using the following procedure:

1. Freeze only cultures that are healthy in mid-log phase (approx. 6×10^5/ml).
2. Centrifuge cells and resuspend in ice-cold 5% dimethylsulfoxide (DMSO) plus 95% serum (fetal calf, calf, or horse) at 10^6–10^7/ml.
3. Put 1 ml of cell suspension into each 2-ml plastic freezing ampoule and place immediately into −70°C freezer. When frozen or after overnight at −70°C move to liquid nitrogen.
4. To reconstitute, thaw ampoule rapidly and dilute to 10 ml with HY medium. Remove sample to count and check viability and pellet cells by centrifugation. Resuspend in HY at concentration of approx. 4×10^5 viable cells/ml. Plate some in wells of 96-well microtiter plates. Some clones of hybridomas do not freeze and reconstitute as well as others. Although most will grow well in mass culture in a flask when thawed, others do not do well under those conditions but will do well in microwells. Recently thawed cells are best grown in at least 20% serum. After they are started they then can be switched to 5–10% serum.

ROGER H. KENNETT • Department of Human Genetics, University of Pennsylvania, School of Medicine, Philadelphia, Pennsylvania 19104.

Enzyme-Linked Antibody Assay with Cells Attached to Polyvinyl Chloride Plates

ROGER H. KENNETT

Materials

1. Poly-L-lysine (PLL) (Sigma, P-1886) 1 mg/100 ml of phosphate-buffered saline (PBS) pH 7.2
2. Glutaraldehyde Sigma G5882—stored frozen and diluted to 0.5% in cold PBS just prior to use
3. Bovine serum albumin (BSA)—Calbiochem 126575—must be free of peroxidase activity
   Make 0.1% solution in RPMI 1640 with 20 mM HEPES pH 7.4.
4. Orhthophenyldiamine (OPD) Sigma-P-3888.
   Substrate solution: 10 ml 0.1 M citrate buffer pH 4.5, 10 mg OPD, 4 μl H_2O_2 (30% stock). For given stock of H_2O_2 solution one should titrate the H_2O_2 added to obtain maximum activity. Too much H_2O_2 irreversibly inhibits the activity so that the reaction can be followed for only a short time, while too little H_2O_2 becomes limiting.
5. Peroxidase-conjugated anti-mouse Ig—Cappel, IgG fraction of sheep anti-mouse Ig. Each lot must be titered to determine optimal dilution with no background. We use most lots at 1/1000.
6. Multiscan (FLOW) to read optical density of microwell contents at 450 nm. This spectrophotometer reads OD of 96 wells in 1 min. Other instruments which do similar job are available.
7. Polyvinyl chloride (PVC) 96-well microtiter plates—flat-bottomed, and polystyrene flat-bottomed tissue culture plate for reading OD of solutions on Multiscan.

ROGER H. KENNETT • Department of Human Genetics, University of Pennsylvania, School of Medicine, Philadelphia, Pennsylvania 19104.

Binding of Cells to Plates

1. Add 50 μl PLL solution to wells of PVC plate—30 min.
2. Flick plate to remove PLL; aspirate any excess.
3. Prewash cells in PBS and add them to well (10⁵/well) in 50 μl PBS. Centrifuge plates 5 min at 2000 rpm in microplate carriers (Cooke).
4. Add 50 μl/well of 0.5% glutaraldehyde in cold PBS; incubate 15 min at room temperature.
5. Wash twice in PBS by immersion in PBS and flicking into sink.
6. Fill wells with 100 mM glycine in 0.1% BSA solution for 30 min at room temperature to block gluteraldehyde.
7. Wash twice in PBS by immersion-flicking. May be stored in 0.1% BSA frozen at −20°C.

Assay

1. Centrifuge antisera or supernatants 5 min in refrigerated microfuge to pellet protein aggregates.
2. Add chosen dilution of antibody solution to wells, use 25–50 μl. Incubate 2 hr at room temperature.
3. Wash 3 times in PBS by immersion and flicking.
4. Add 100 μl of peroxidase-labeled anti-mouse Ig. Incubate 2 hr at room temperature.
5. Wash 6 times in PBS by immersion and flicking.
6. Add 200 μl of substrate solution.
7. Incubate and stop reaction with 5 μl 1 M NaF.
8. Reaction may be followed up to at least 2 hr. We usually stop it at ¹/₂ hr. Read qualitatively by eye or transfer 100 μl to 96-well tissue culture plate to be read quantitatively. For positive/negative screening reading by eye is as sensitive as reading by a spectrophotometer.
9. Note that BSA and other reagents must be free of background peroxidase activity and that azide inhibits the reaction.
10. We have found this procedure to be as sensitive for screening hybridomas as the radioimmunobinding assay.
11. For other enzyme-linked procedures using other enzymes see E. Engvall and A. J. Pesce, eds., 1978, Quantitative enzyme immunoassay, *Scand. J. Immunol.* [*Suppl. 7*].
12. We have also used this assay for proteins attached to PVC plates. Many proteins will stick directly to the PVC plates (different batches of plates show different capacities to bind protein in this way) or they may be fixed in various ways such as gluteraldehyde, methanol–acetone, or as discussed in this Appendix by Slaughter *et al.*, page 385.
13. In place of PVC plates one may use polystyrene. These can be blocked and washed with a detergent solution of 0.05% TWEEN 80 in PBS.

Peroxidase-Conjugated Antiglobulin Method for Visual Detection of Cell-Surface Antigens

Zdenka L. Jonak

Materials:

1. Mylar tape, Cooke Engineering Co., catalogue number 1-220-30
2. Poly-L-lysine, Sigma, catalogue number P1886. Solution of 1 mg/ml in distilled water.
3. 3,3'-diaminobenzidine tetrahydrochloride monohydrate (DAB), Aldrich Chemical Co., catalogue number D1,240-6. Just prior to use add 12.5 mg of DAB to 25 ml of 0.05 M Tris HCl, pH 7.6, plus 0.13 M NaCl and stir at room temperature. When dissolved add H_2O_2 to 0.012% and use immediately. *Caution:* DAB is considered to be carcinogenic!
4. Osmium tetroxide (Sigma). 1.33% OsO_4 in PBS, pH 7.2. To prepare OsO_4 solution add crystals to phosphate-buffered saline and stir on ice in fume hood for 1 hr. Protect bottle from light and use parafilm to help seal the bottle. Store in refrigerator. May be used for several weeks.
5. Hydrogen peroxide (30%), J. T. Baker Chemical Co., Phillipsburg, N.J.
6. NKH buffer: 8.5 g NaCl, 0.4 g KCl per liter of 0.015 M HEPES, pH 7.4
7. NKH gelatin: NKH buffer plus 0.1% (w/v) gelatin
8. Peroxidase-conjugated immunoglobulin G (IgG) fraction of anti-mouse Ig, Cappel Laboratories. Prepare peroxidase-conjugated antiglobulin in distilled water as described in the instructions from Cappel Labs. Aliquot and store in the freezer in glass vials. Any dilutions should be done in

Zdenka L. Jonak • Wistar Institute of Anatomy and Biology, Philadelphia, Pennsylvania 19104.

NKH gelatin. It can be frozen and thawed a few times without losing activity. Determine the right concentration in your system by checking dilutions against your cells with and without specific antibody. Use highest dilution which gives no nonspecific staining. We used one half in our system.

9. 50% glycerin–0.025% gluteraldehyde prepared in NKH buffer. Store in refrigerator.

Methods

Wash slides with acid–ethanol solution (95% ethanol, 3% HCl). Cut mylar tape to cover glass microscope slide and punch 8 holes with regular paper punch. Put the tape on the slide and coat the glass area with 1 drop of poly-L-lysine solution. Store in a wet chamber for 1 hr. Just before you are going to apply the cells to the slide, throughly wash, dropwise, the glass area with NKH buffer. Remove buffer by suction.

Prepare your cells. Determine the viability of the cells by trypan blue staining. The viability of the cells is important, since the dead cells will appear in the test as solid dark brown or black cells. Wash cells in the NKH gelatin and distribute them into round-bottomed 96-well polyvinylchloride plates, or into tubes, for the antibody-binding steps. We usually use 500,000 cells in 50 μl. Add a few drops of NKH gelatin and centrifuge 1000 rpm/5 min. Withdraw the buffer by gentle suction, disperse the pellet, and add 20 μl of your antibody dilution in NKH gelatin. Incubate the cells on ice for 30 min. Disperse the pellet and twice repeat the washing. Withdraw the supernatant by gentle suction and disperse the cells. Add 20 μl of peroxidase-conjugated antiglobulin. Mix by gentle pipetting (use Eppendorf pipette with disposable tips). Incubate 15 min on ice. Add NKH gelatin, centrifuge 1000 rpm for 5 min, remove buffer by suction, and twice repeat the washing. After last wash, take 10 μl of NKH gelatin in the tip of an Eppendorf pipette and disperse the cells by pipetting. Withdraw 10 μl of cell suspension and apply on the slide.

Incubate slides in a wet chamber on ice for 15 min. The cells should be firmly attached to the poly-L-lysine. You may, alternatively, fix cells at this point with 0.05% glutaraldehyde in NKH gelatin for 15 min. This helps attach some cell types, and the fixation does not interfere with the specificity of the assay. By gentle suction remove excess of buffer and apply immediately mixture of DAB–H_2O_2. Incubate for 10 min at room temperature. Wash wells dropwise by addition of buffer and removal of buffer by suction. After washing add OsO_4 solution and incubate the slides at 4°C, in the dark, for 20 min. Remove the tape, wash the slides with NKH buffer and cover with 50% glycerin–0.025% glutaraldehyde. You can evaluate the assay immediately under a light microscope and then decide on the type of histological staining.

In a strong reaction the positive cells are observed as if they have a black ring around the cell membrane (see Kennett et al., and Bechtol et al., this volume). The strength of the reaction may vary due to the antibody titer of the sera used and also to the number and the distribution of the antigens on the cell surface.

Reference

Bross, K. J., Pangalis, G. A., Staatz, Ch. G., and Blume, K. G. 1978, Demonstration of cell surface antigens and their antibodies by the peroxidase–antiperoxidase method, *Transplantation* **25:**331.

Radioimmunoassay

Kathleen B. Bechtol

Materials

1. Buffered balanced salt solution (BBSS), pH 7.4
2. Bovine serum albumin (BSA; Sigma, Fraction V): To remove excess salts, dialyze against 10^{-4} M ethylenediaminetetraacetic acid (EDTA) and then against distilled H_2O, spin and lyophilize.
3. [^{125}I]rabbit or -goat anti-mouse immunoglobulin (Ig): Purify from whole immune serum by passing over a column of mouse Ig coupled to Sepharose 4B and elute with acid (Klinman and Aschinazi, 1971; Jensenius and Williams, 1974). Either the intact rabbit or goat Ig molecules or F(ab')$_2$ fragments can be used. The F(ab')$_2$ offers the advantage that there is no binding due to Fc receptors on the cells. For iodination of the purified anti-mouse Ig see Klinman *et al.* (1976) and iodination section of this Appendix. New preparations of anti-Ig must be tested to determine that this reagent is being used in sufficient quantity to be nonlimiting under the given assay conditions.

Method

The assay can be carried out in glass or plastic tubes (10 mm × 75 mm or 6 mm × 50 mm) or in 96-well V-bottom plastic plates. To each well add 25 µl of the various dilutions of supernatant or ascites fluid to be tested.

1. Suspend target cells at 10^6 cells/50 µl in 0.5% isotonic BSA in BBSS. Add 50 µl of the cell suspension to each tube/well. Alternatively the target antigen (viz., membrane fragments) can be attached to the plates before

Kathleen B. Bechtol • Wistar Institute of Anatomy and Biology, Philadelphia, Pennsylvania 19104.

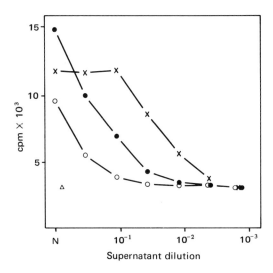

FIGURE 1. Representative indirect radioimmunoassay. Abscissa units are the dilution of culture supernatant used; N is undiluted supernatant. The ordinate units are cpm $\times$ 10^{-3} of [^{125}I]rabbit anti-mouse immunoglobulin (Ig) bound to the target cells when the supernatant added in the first binding incubation is buffer or P3/X63-Ag8, parent myeloma supernatant (Δ); two supernatants from the same clone (■,O), but containing higher (●) or lower (O) concentration of the monoclonal antibody; or supernatant from a second independent clone ($\times$). The antigen bound by antibody ($\times$) becomes limiting at high supernatant concentrations under the given assay conditions. The [^{125}I]rabbit anti-mouse Ig concentration used is nonlimiting.

the antibody is added. See description under enzyme-linked immunosorbent assay (ELISA) technique, this Appendix.

2. Mix and incubate antibody with target antigen for 1 hr on an ice-water bath (0°C) with occasional remixing.

3. Following this incubation, wash the target antigen two to four times with 0.6 ml (tube) or 0.2 ml (plates) of 0.1% BSA in BBSS at 0°C. For cells in suspension spin the tubes/plates at 500 $\times$ g for 5 to 10 min and remove supernatant by suction. For antigen attached to the plates, wash by immersion in buffer.

4. Dilute the ^{125}I-labeled anti-mouse Ig (approx. 20 μCi/μg) to 2 $\times$ 10^5 cpm/ 100 μl of 0.5% BSA in BBSS. Add 100 μl to each tube/well, mix, and incubate 1 hr at 0°C.

5. After this incubation wash as above and count the bound radioactivity in the tubes/wells in a gamma counter.

6. Results from a representative indirect radioimmunoassay are shown in Fig. 1.

References

Jensenius, J. C., and Williams, A. F., 1974, The binding of antiimmunoglobulin antibodies to rat thymocytes and thoracic duct lymphocytes, *Eur. J. Immunol.* **4**:91.

Klinman, N. R., and Aschinazi, G., 1971, The stimulation of splenic foci *in vitro*, *J. Immunol.* **106**:1338.

Klinman, N. R., Pickard, A. R., Sigal, N. L. H., Gerhardt, P. J., Metcalf, E. S., and Pierce, S. K., 1976, Assessing B cell diversification by antigen receptor and precursor cell analysis, *Ann. Immunol.* **127c**:489.

Quantitative Absorption/ Blocking Assay

Kathleen B. Bechtol

Method

1. Preincubate 0.1-ml aliquots of a constant dilution of culture supernatant or ascites fluid with serial dilutions of the preparations to be tested (viz., cell suspensions or membrane preparations from various tissues; column eluate fractions) for 1 hr at 0°C. All serum and antigen dilutions are in 0.5% BSA.
2. Centrifuge the absorption mixture at $500 \times g$ for 5 min to remove the cells plus bound antibody.
3. Centrifuge the resulting supernatant in a Beckman microfuge at $8700 \times g$ for 5 min at 4°C to remove large complexes. Remove duplicate aliquots from each absorption tube for assay of the remaining binding activity as described above.
4. Results from a representative quantitative absorption assay are shown in Fig. 2.

Note: Because individual monoclonal antibodies may be relatively slower than the average in reaching equilibrium binding, absorption incubations of several hours or overnight may be required to attain equilibrium. Caution must, therefore, be used in comparing results of absorption of different monoclonal antibodies with the same cell source (see Mason and Williams, 1980).

Kathleen B. Bechtol • Wistar Institute of Anatomy and Biology, Philadelphia, Pennsylvania 19104.

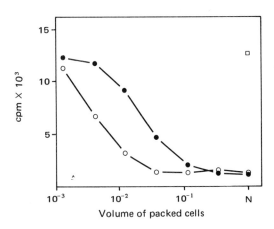

FIGURE 2. Representative quantitative absorption assay. Abscissa units are volume of packed cells used in absorption of hybridoma supernatant aliquots (constant concentration). N, taken as 1, is 0.1 ml of 1/3 packed cells incubated with 0.1 ml of supernatant for absorption. Ordinate is counts per minute of [^{125}I]rabbit anti-mouse Ig bound to the target cells following absorption with the buffer only (Δ); the target-cell type (●); or another cell preparation (O) with higher concentration of antigen per packed volume of absorbing cells.

References

Mason, D. W., Brideau, R. J., McMaster, W. R., Webb, M., White, R. A. H., and Williams, A. F., Chapter 15, this volume.

Mason, D. W., and Williams, A. F., 1980, The kinetics of antibody binding to membrane antigens in solution and at the cell surface, *Biochem. J.* **187**:1.

Morris, R. J., and Williams, A. F., 1975, Antigens on mouse and rat lymphocytes recognized by rabbit antiserum against rat brain: The quantitative analysis of a xenogeneic antiserum, *Eur. J. Immunol.* **5**:274.

Radioimmunoassay for Genetic Screening of Proteins Using Monoclonal Antibodies

C. A. SLAUGHTER, M. C. COSEO, C. ABRAMS, M. P. CANCRO, AND H. HARRIS

In the course of studies of allelic variation in human placental alkaline phosphatase an indirect binding solid-phase radioimmunassay suitable for genetic screening studies using monoclonal antibodies was developed (see Chapter 7). This assay is applicable in principle to a wide variety of enzyme and protein antigens.

The antigen may be supplied either in pure form or in a crude tissue or cell extract. It is selectively immobilized on the wells of polyvinyl microtiter plates precoated with a specific antiserum raised against it in rabbits. Binding to the solid-phase antigen of monoclonal or whole-serum antibodies from mice is then detected with a radioiodinated anti-murine immunoglobulin having broad specificity for different mouse isotypes, e.g., a rabbit anti-mouse Fab.

Protocol

1. Absorb rabbit antibodies specific for antigen to Dynatech V-bottomed polyvinyl microtiter plates using a 0.1-ml aliquot, per well, of a dilution of whole antiserum in phosphate-buffered saline (PBS), pH 7.2. Allow to stand 2 hr at room temperature.

C. A. SLAUGHTER, M. C. COSEO, C. ABRAMS, AND H. HARRIS • Department of Human Genetics, University of Pennsylvania, School of Medicine, Philadelphia, Pennsylvania 19104. M. P. CANCRO • Department of Pathology, University of Pennsylvania, School of Medicine, Philadelphia, Pennsylvania 19104.

2. Block further nonspecific absorption of proteins to plastic by filling wells with 0.5% bovine serum albumin (BSA) in 0.1 M diethanolamine buffer at pH 9.0. Allow to stand $1/2$ hr at room temperature. Wash plate by filling wells twice with PBS.

3. Specifically couple antigen to the precoated plate using 0.1 ml/well of an antigen dilution made in 0.5% BSA in PBS at pH 7.2. Incubate overnight at 4°C. Wash plate by filling wells twice with PBS.

4. Add 20-μl aliquots of unknown mouse antibody. Incubate for 6 hr at room temperature. Wash plate by filling wells twice with PBS.

5. Tag specifically bound mouse antibodies using 0.1 ml ^{125}I-labeled (15–20 μCi per μg) rabbit anti-mouse Fab diluted in 0.5% BSA in PBS at pH 7.2. Incubate overnight at 4°C.

6. Wash plate 6–8 times by filling wells under running tap. Dry. Count individual wells in gamma counter.

Special Points

Optimal Dilution of Antiserum for Coating Plastic

The antigen-binding capacity of the plastic depends on the dilution of the antiserum used to precoat it. There exists an optimal dilution above and below which antigen-binding capacity declines. Optimal dilutions are usually very high; for example, in the placental alkaline phosphatase (ALP) system, the working dilution of the current batch of rabbit anti-placental ALP antiserum is 1/16,000.

pH Dependence of Protein Absorption to Plastic

Different proteins may adsorb optimally at different pH values. It is our experience that the antigen-binding capacity of plastic precoated with specific antiserum is relatively insensitive to the pH during precoating. This step is therefore carried out at neutral pH. However, BSA blocks nonspecific sticking of proteins most effectively when adsorbed to the plastic at alkaline pH (e.g., pH 9.0). All antigen–antibody interactions are, of course, carried out at physiological pH. The ionic strength also effects the amount of protein binding to the polyvinyl chloride (PVC) plates.

Antigen Concentration

Antigen is supplied in at least twofold excess of the quantity required to saturate the precoated wells. In the placental ALP system, 500 ng/well are used.

Controls for Binding by Mouse Antibodies

In all assays with monoclonal antibodies an optimal dilution of whole-mouse antiserum specific for the antigen is used to verify the presence of expected levels of each test antigen in the system. The background level of binding of each different antibody is also measured in "no antigen" controls. This is especially important, since background levels of binding may vary considerably between different monoclonal antibodies (Chapter 7, Section III.B). The specificity of the assay system should be verified for each new monoclonal antibody by comparing the level by binding pure antigen with the level of binding to previously unpurified antigen (Chapter 7, Section III.A).

Concentration of Labeled Second Antibody

Each fresh batch of iodinated second antibody, standardized by radioactivity, is tested in a series of dilutions against a standard mouse antiserum using the normal assay protocol. A working concentration is chosen to give a useful range of counts bound.

Binding Hybridoma Antibodies to Polyvinyl Chloride Microtiter Dishes

Thomas J. McKearn

Introduction

Monoclonal antibodies vary in terms of the optimal conditions under which they will bind spontaneously to polyvinyl chloride dishes. We have found that the ionic strength and pH of the buffer used for adsorption to plastic are extremely important variables in this binding reaction. Under optimal conditions, substantial amounts of hybridoma antibody can be bound to the plates even if one starts with unpurified hybridoma supernatant grown in the presence of 10–20% agamma horse or fetal calf serum.

Materials

1. 96-well V-bottom polyvinyl chloride microtiter dishes (lots of dishes vary in their suitability for this assay)
2. 2 M NaCl solution
3. 0.2 M buffer (phosphate or borate) at the following pHs: 5, 6, 7, 8, 9
4. Hybridoma supernatant
5. ^{125}I-labeled anti-mouse (or rat) Ig
6. 1% (w/v) bovine serum albumin (BSA) solution in phosphate-buffered saline (PBS)

Thomas J. McKearn • Department of Pathology, Divisions of Research Immunology and Laboratory Medicine, University of Pennsylvania, School of Medicine, Philadelphia, Pennsylvania 19104.

Method

1. One must first establish the pH and ionic strength optima for binding a particular hybridoma antibody to the flexible plate. First, wet the plate with tap water, and then flick off the water.
2. Each row of plates receives 50 μl of distilled H_2O, and the first column receives an additional 50 μl of 2 M NaCl. The concentration of NaCl is then titrated across the plate using a multichannel 50 μl Eppendorf pipette.
3. Each well then receives 50 μl of a 1:100 dilution of hybridoma supernatant. Diluent varies as a function of the row into which the solution will be placed, e.g.,

    Row A—1:100 dilution of hybridoma in 0.04 M PO_4 buffer pH 6.0
    Row B—1:100 dilution of hybridoma in 0.04 M PO_4 buffer pH 7.0
    Row C—1:100 dilution of hybridoma in 0.04 M borate buffer pH 8.0
4. Hence a pH and ionic strength grid will have been established on the plate for each protein. The proteins are allowed to adsorb to the plates for either 4 hr at room temperature or overnight at 4°C.
5. Plates are then washed once in tap water and the wells filled with 1% BSA solution and allowed to incubate for 1 hr at room temperature.
6. Plates are then washed four to five times under tap water and are ready for assay using ^{125}I-labeled anti-mouse (or rat) Ig sera.
7. After 4-hr incubation at room temperature, aspirate well contents, wash five times with tap water, dry the plates, cut and count the bound counts (see Table I).
8. This titration will give the optimal pH and ionic strength for binding. The optimal dilution of hybridoma supernatant should be determined as a second step.

As one alternative to using hybridoma supernatants, one can prepare 50% saturated ammonium sulfate precipitates from the hybridoma supernatants.

TABLE I
Binding of Hybridoma Antibody to Polyvinylchloride Dish[a]

pH	Concentration of NaCl added to 0.02 M buffer					
	1.0 M	0.5 M	0.25 M	0.125 M	0.06 M	0
6.0	248	1210	1135	1119	1080	1788
7.0	285	908	813	828	730	987
8.0	236	1987	2087	2133	2245	3056
8.6	217	1496	1309	1455	1588	2199

[a] 1:80 Dilutions of hybridoma supernatant D4,68 grown in 20% fetal calf serum were added to each well of the dish at the pH and additional NaCl concentrations shown. After blocking the remaining sites on the plate with 1% bovine serum albumin (BSA), 15,000 cpm of [^{125}I]rabbit anti-rat immunoglobulin was added. Optimal binding occurred at pH 8.0 with 0.02 M buffer and no additional NaCl. BSA background, 140.

Such precipitates should be reconstituted with a minimal volume of PBS and dialyzed against two changes of PBS. The optimal buffer pH and ionic strength conditions for ammonium sulfate precipitated proteins are essentially the same as for the hybridoma antibodies used as supernatants.

We have used such immobilized hybridomas to determine antibody class of the hybridoma by adding radiolabeled monospecific antiimmunoglobulin antisera and have also used the immobilized immunoglobulins in solid-phase idiotype assays.

Microcytotoxicity Assay

ROGER H. KENNETT

Materials

1. Microtiter plates, Falcon 3034 or other microcytoxicity plate
2. 0.1% bovine serum albumin (BSA) in RPMI 1640 pH 7.4 with 20 mM HEPES
3. Rabbit serum as complement (C′) source. Obtain several rabbit sera and test for toxicity to cells to be used and for C′ activity. Rabbit sera containing C′ activity which has been screened to obtain lots which are nontoxic to mouse or human lymphocytes can be obtained from Cederlane Laboratories Ltd. (supplied in U.S. by Accurate Chemical Co., Hicksville, N.Y.). Lots of serum vary considerably in their ability to support cytolysis, so care must be taken to obtain a lot which gives optimal cytolysis. Sublytic amounts of heterospecific antibody probably contribute to the efficiency with which the serum supports lysis (Kennett *et al.*, 1975)
4. Hamilton syringes with multiple dispenser for aliquoting 1-μl and 5-μl amounts into microwells
5. TB solution—trypan blue 0.4% in phosphate-buffered saline (PBS) with 0.05% methyl *p*-hydroxybenzoate added as preservative, pH 7.2

Procedure

1. Aliquot supernatants to be tested in 1- to 5-μl amounts in microwells.
2. Wash cells in 0.1% BSA and suspend to approximately 2000 cells/μl.
3. Add 1 μl cells to be tested to each well and incubate with the antibodies for ½ hr at room temperature.
4. Add 5 μl of rabbit serum which gives optimal lysis with control antibody

ROGER H. KENNETT • Department of Human Genetics, University of Pennsylvania, School of Medicine, Philadelphia, Pennsylvania 19104.

and no lysis when added without additional antibodies. Incubate at room temperature for 1 hr.

5. Read percent cells killed with microscope. Assay may be done with cells prelabeled with fluorescein diacetate as in Bodmer *et al.* (1967), which requires a fluorescent microscope to detect labeled live cells. To read by trypan blue exclusion add 1–2 μl of TB solution. Observe under 100 × (10 × 10) magnification and estimate percent dead cells that are labeled with blue dye compared to live cells, which are not labeled because their membrane remains intact.

6. Since only some classes of antibody fix C′ and cytolysis may depend on antigen density and/or distribution, only certain monoclonal antibodies are cytolytic. Those that are not cytolytic may often be treated with the proper dilution of a second antibody—rabbit anti-mouse Ig—and then C′ to obtain cytolytic activity (W. Bodmer and P. Goodfellow, personal communication).

References

Bodmer, W., Tripp, M., and Bodmer, J., 1967, Application of fluorochromatic cytotoxicity assay to human leukocyte typing, in: *Histocompatibility Testing 1979* (E. S. Cortoni, P. L. Maltior, and R. M. Tosi, eds.), Munksgaard, Copenhagen, pp. 341–350.

Kennett, R. J., Fairbrother, T., Hampshire, B., and Bodmer, W., 1975, An analysis of the specificity of cytotoxic antibodies in normal rabbit sera used as complement source, *Tissue Antigens* **6**:80.

^{51}Cr Release Cytotoxicity Assay

THOMAS J. MCKEARN

Materials

1. Mouse or rat spleen or lymph node cells
2. Concanavalin A (Con A) (Pharmacia)
3. Hybridoma (HY) medium; Dulbecco's Modified Eagle's Medium (DMEM) with 0.01 M HEPES buffer
4. Selected lot of agamma horse or fetal calf serum
5. Sodium chromate (^{51}Cr—New England Nuclear)
6. 96-well round-bottom polystyrene microtiter dish (Linbro)
7. Selected batches of rabbit complement

Method

1. Prepare Con A blast cells by incubation of $1-2 \times 10^6$ cell/ml in HY medium containing 2–5% serum and 1–2.5 g/ml of Con A. Generally, blast cells are harvested from culture one day 3, although with certain strain combinations blasts can be harvested on day 2 or 4.
2. Viable blast cells are separated on a Ficoll–Hypaque–Azide gradient according to the method of Davidson and Parish (1975), which is outlined in the accompanying protocol for polyethylene glycol (PEG) fusion in tissue culture dishes.
3. Blast cell are labeled with ^{51}Cr by incubating $2-5 \times 10^6$ cells with 200 μCi ^{51}Cr (New England Nuclear) in a total volume of not more than 0.5 ml of DMEM with 2% serum. This mixture is incubated at 37°C for 1 hr with occasional mixing.
4. Cells are washed once with warm DMEM with 2% serum and allowed to incubate at room temperature for 15–20 min before being washed twice with DMEM. This room-temperature incubation allows release of

THOMAS J. MCKEARN • Department of Pathology, Divisions of Research Immunology and Laboratory Medicine, University of Pennsylvania, School of Medicine, Philadelphia, Pennsylvania 19104.

"loosely bound" ^{51}Cr and therefore results in lower background release in the assay.

5. An aliquot of cells is counted and the total counts of the cell suspension adjusted to approx. 5000–6000 cpm/50 μl (usually 8–10 × 10^3 blasts/50 μl).

6. 50 μl of hybridoma supernatant is added to each well of a 96-well round-bottom polystyrene microtiter dish (Linbro). 50 μl of ^{51}Cr-labeled cells is then added and the plates incubated at room temperature for 60–90 min.

7. Plates are then centrifuged at 150 × g for 5 min and the supernatant "flicked off." 100 μl of fresh DMEM is added and the centrifugation step repeated.

8. After "flicking" off the wash solution, 50 μl of a 1 : 8 to 1 : 16 dilution of carefully selected agar-absorbed rabbit serum is added as a complement source.

9. Plates are incubated at 37°C for 45–60 min.

10. 50 μl of fresh DMEM is then added and the plates centrifuged as before.

11. Following centrifugation, 50 μl of supernatant is withdrawn from each well and counted in a gamma scintillation counter.

12. Controls required for this assay include:
    a. Spontaneous release; i.e., ^{51}Cr release obtained from cells that have not been exposed to antibody and/or complement.
    b. Nonspecific release; i.e., ^{51}Cr release obtained from cells exposed to P3/X63-Ag8 or other parental myleoma supernatant *and* complement.
    c. Maximum release; i.e., ^{51}Cr release obtained from cells exposed to a known cytolytic antibody and complement.

In general, spontaneous release should be approximately 3–6% of the maximum release, nonspecific release should account for an additional 6–10% of the maximum release value and the maximum release value calculated in this fashion should be 60–90% of the number of counts released by repeated freeze–thawing of the ^{51}Cr-labeled cells.

The single most critical factor in optimizing the sensitivity of this assay is the complement source. We have found only 5–10% of the fresh rabbit sera tested give both low nonspecific ^{51}Cr release and still support lysis of blast cells at high dilutions of hybridoma antibody.

Nonstimulated lymphoid cells (e.g., lymph node cells) can also be used as ^{51}Cr-labeled targets. However, they take up much less ^{51}Cr isotope per cell and, in our experience, are much less susceptible to lysis by IgG2 antibodies.

Reference

Davidson, W. F., and Parish, C. R., 1975, A procedure for removing red cells and dead cells from lymphoid cell suspensions, *J. Immunol. Methods* **7**:291.

Immunoprecipitation with Monoclonal Antibodies

LOIS A. LAMPSON

Uses

An important use of monoclonal antibody is to serve as a tool for the simple, rapid isolation of individual molecules from complex starting material. This can be done most conveniently through solid-phase immunoadsorption, with the monoclonal antibody either covalently bound to Sepharose or noncovalently absorbed to *Staphylococcus aureus* (SA). The procedure below uses SA as an immunoadsorbant for the isolation of histocompatibility antigens, which are present in a high concentration in the membranes of human B-cell lines. Other antigens which are present in smaller quantities or which are of different molecular composition may require modifications of this method to precipitate the antigen–monoclonal antibody complex from solution.

Preparation of ^{125}I-Labeled Membrane Extracts

Below is a common procedure for radioiodination of cell membranes. The advantages are that only external membrane proteins are labeled, and it is easy to follow the extraction and immunoprecipitation by following gamma counts. The disadvantage is that not all surface proteins are accessible to iodination, either because they lack tyrosine or because they are physically blocked (Hubbard and Cohn, 1972). As an alternative, cells may be labeled biosynthetically. Both [^{14}C]amino acids and [^{35}S]methionine are commonly used, following a procedure similar to that given below for biosynthetic labeling of antibody.

LOIS A. LAMPSON • Department of Anatomy, University of Pennsylvania, School of Medicine, Philadelphia, Pennsylvania 19104.

In a fume hood, 45×10^6 viable cells, suspended to 0.5 ml in Dulbecco's phosphate-buffered saline (DPBS)* are mixed with 0.1 ml of 1 M phosphate buffer, pH 7.2; 0.2 ml of lactoperoxidase (Sigma L-2005) at 1 mg/ml in PBS,[†] 1 mCi of [^{125}I]-NaI in 20 µl of 0.1 N NaOH; and, finally, 25 µl of freshly prepared H_2O_2 solution (10 µl of 30% H_2O_2 added to 10 ml cold PBS). The mixture is left at room temperature for 5 min. Fresh aliquots of lactoperoxidase and freshly prepared H_2O_2 solution are then added. After an additional 5 min, the cells are washed three times in DPBS, and resuspended in 0.5 ml cold PBS. To prepare detergent extract, 0.5 ml of cold NP-40 (Particle Data Lab, Elmhurst, Ill.) solution [1% NP40 in PBS with 1 mM phenylmethane sulfonyl fluoride (PMSF)] is then added, the cells are resuspended vigorously, and kept on ice for 1/2 hr. The extract is kept cold from this point on. Extracts are cleared by spinning once at $2000 \times g$ for 15 min, and once at $25,000 \times g$ for 2 hr.

Preparation of SA

SA binds to immunoglobulin molecules of some, but not all, classes and subclasses (Goding, 1978). Since a given monoclonal antibody will consist of only a single subclass, it is desirable to make the immunoprecipitation class-independent. To do this, Formalin-fixed Cowan strain I SA (purchased from New England Enzyme Center, Boston, Ma.) is precoated with anti-mouse immunoglobulin. Rabbit anti-mouse κ serum (Litton Bionetics) and goat anti-mouse κ serum have both been used. In either case, the SA is washed 3 times in washing buffer (WB): PBS pH 8.6, 0.1% BSA, 0.02% NaN3, 0.5% NP40, 0.1% SDS. The washed SA is brought to a 10% suspension in whole antiserum. After 1/2 hour at room temperature the SA is washed 6–8 times with WB and kept refrigerated as a 10% suspension in WB until use. The SA with anti-κ attached has been used successfully after refrigeration for up to 2 weeks.

Immunoprecipitation

Precoated SA suspension is pelleted for 2 min in an Eppendorf centrifuge (Brinkmann), and the pellet is resuspended to 10% in spent culture medium. (In this procedure, spent culture medium is used as the source of monoclonal antibody; the antibody is not purified or concentrated.) After 40 min at room temperature, the SA is washed twice, and resuspended to 10% in WB. This results in preparation of a sandwich, with the monoclonal antibody bound to the SA through an antiimmunoglobulin antibody bridge. Finally, 0.3 ml of this SA preparation is added to 0.3 ml of ^{125}I-labeled extract, which represents the extract from 15×10^6 human B cells, and incubated overnight at 4°C. The SA is washed $3\times$ in WB, and the pellet is resuspended in 100 µl WB + 50 µl sample buffer (0.0625 M Tris HCl (ph 8.6), 10% glycerol, 5% 2-ME. 3% SDS, 0.001%

---

*Dulbecco's PBS: 8 g/liter NaCl, 0.29 g/liter KCl, 0.29 g/liter KH_2PO_4, 1.16 g/liter Na_2HPO_4, 0.19 g/liter $CaCl_2$, 0.19 g/liter $MgCl_2 \cdot 6H_2O$.
[†]PBS: 0.15 M NaCl, 0.02 M phosphate, pH 7.3.

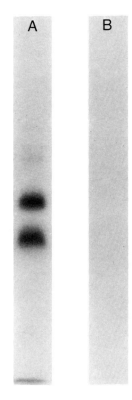

FIGURE 3. SDS-PAGE analysis of material immunoprecipitated by monoclonal antibody to human Ia-like molecule. Cells from a human B-cell line were externally labelled with ^{125}I and the membranes were solubilized with NP40. Antibody L203 was used to precipitate its antigen from the labelled extract. The precipitate was solubilized in 2-ME/SDS and electrophoresed on a 10% acrylamide gel under reducing conditions. Banding patterns are shown of material precipitated by antibody L203 (A) and by MOPC21 (B).

bromophenol blue). This mixture is heated to 100°C for 2 min, to release the antibodies and antigen from the SA. The mixture is pelleted once more, and 25 µl of the supernatant is applied to each lane of a 10% acrylamide gel.

Example

Immunoprecipitation of human Ia-like molecules is shown in Fig. 3. A human B-cell line was labeled with ^{125}I as described above. In this assay, the extract was not precleared, and unpurified spent hybridoma medium was used as the source of monoclonal antibody. Lane A shows the two chains of the human Ia-like molecule precipitated by monoclonal antibody L203. Lane B is a control using spent culture medium from the mouse plasmacytoma-derived cell line P3/X63-Ag8, which secretes the monoclonal antibody MOPC21. MOPC21 does not bind to human cells, and no bands are seen in lane B.

References

Goding, J. W., 1978, The use of staphylococcal protein A as an immunological reagent, *J. Immunol. Methods* **20**:241–251.

Hubbard, J. L., and Cohn, Z. A., 1972, The enzymatic iodination of the red cell membrane, *J. Cell. Biol.* **55**:390–405.

Binding Inhibition Using Biosynthetically Labeled Monoclonal Antibody

Lois A. Lampson

Uses

Binding inhibition studies provide a simple way of asking whether different monoclonal antibodies recognize unrelated antigenic determinants. When dealing with antibodies to a complex immunogen, such as a whole cell, this assay must be used in conjunction with other types of analysis. On the one hand, antibodies to two different determinants on a single molecule may not cross-inhibit each other. On the other hand, antibodies to different cell surface molecules may cross-inhibit each other if the molecules are juxtaposed on the membrane. A rapid binding inhibition assay for analysis of monoclonal antibodies to cell-surface molecules is described below.

Labeling the Antibody with [^{14}C]Leucine

Hybridoma cells are grown as usual, with these changes in their medium: The medium is leucine-free, no serum is added, and 50 μl of [^{14}C]leucine (355 mCi/mmole, 0.1 mCi/ml, New England Nuclear) is added per milliliter of medium. Ten million cells are grown in 1 ml of labeling medium overnight or longer. Under these conditions, the predominant secreted biosynthetically/labeled protein is the monoclonal antibody.

To collect the antibody, the cells are spun as usual, the supernatant medium

Lois A. Lampson • Department of Anatomy, University of Pennsylvania, School of Medicine, Philadelphia, Pennsylvania 19104.

is collected, and 2% BSA is added to a final concentration of 0.1%. Free [^{14}C]leucine can be quickly removed as follows: Sephadex G-25 fine in phosphate buffered saline (PBS) is placed into the barrel of a 5-ml syringe that has been blocked at the end with a bit of nylon wool. The syringe barrel is placed in a tube and centrifuged briefly (2 min at 1000 × g) to remove excess buffer. Packed volume of G-25 should be about 5 ml. Then 1 ml of culture supernatant is placed at the top of the syringe, and the syringe is centrifuged for 2 min in a clean tube. The labeled antibody is collected from the tube; [^{14}C]leucine is retained by the Sepharose.

Binding Inhibition

This procedure is for use with glutaraldehyde-fixed target cells and is based on a binding assay that has been described previously (Lampson *et al.*, 1977). The buffer used throughout is 5% serum (for example, fetal calf serum or horse serum) in PBS.

Serial dilutions of unlabeled antibody to be used as inhibitor are dispensed into a 96-well, V-bottomed microtiter plate so that there is 25 μl of diluted antibody in each well. The antibody is in the form of unpurified, unconcentrated spent medium from hybridoma culture. Then 10 μl of buffer containing 250,000 target cells that have been fixed for 5 min in 0.1% glutaraldehyde are added to each well, the plate is agitated, and then left at room temperature for 1½ hr. A constant volume of biosynthetically labeled antibody is then added to each well, the plate is agitated, and left at room temperature for an additional 2 hr. The cells are washed three times by spinning the plate, flicking off the supernatant, and resuspending the cells in fresh buffer. Finally, the cells from each well are resuspended in 100 μl buffer and added to 2 ml of Aquasol (New England Nuclear) for scintillation counting. Counts from wells to which no inhibitor was added are taken as a baseline, and inhibition is measured as reduction of the amount of biosynthetically labeled antibody bound (Fig. 4).

Example

An illustration of this assay is given in Fig. 4. The four monoclonal antibodies used as inhibitors were raised against the human B-cell line 8866. One of the antibodies, L203, was also labeled biosynthetically. As expected, unlabeled L203 inhibits the binding of [^{14}C]leucine-L203. In addition, a second antibody, L243, inhibits, but two other antibodies, L227 and L368, do not inhibit. The results of this assay were complemented by immunoprecipitation and absorption studies: L203 and L243 precipitate the same form of human Ia-like molecule, L227 precipitates a second form of human Ia-like molecule, and L368 precipitates HLA-A, B, C,-like molecules.

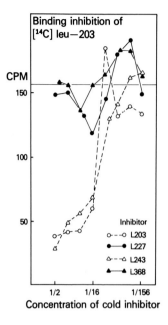

FIGURE 4. Binding inhibition assay. 25 μl of serial dilutions of (unlabeled) antibody was incubated with 2.5 × 10⁵ 8866 target cells for 1½ hr at room temperature. 10 μl of biosynthetically labeled antibody, [¹⁴C]leucine-L203, was then added, and the cells were incubated for a further 2 hr. The target cells were then washed and transferred to vials of scintillant for counting. Inhibition of [¹⁴C]leucine-L203 by four different monoclonal antibodies to human histocompatibility antigens is shown. Baseline: mean of 8 values obtained when no inhibiting antibody was present.

Reference

Lampson, L. A., Royston, I., and Levy, R., 1977, Homogeneous antibodies directed against human cell surface antigens: I. The mouse spleen fragment culture response to T and B cell lines derived from the same individual, *J. Supramol. Struct.* **6**:441.

Protein Iodination Suitable for Labeling Hybridoma Antibodies

DENNIS M. KLINMAN AND J. C. HOWARD

Materials

1. Saturated solution of L-tyrosine in phosphate-buffered saline (PBS)
2. Purified immunoglobulin in PBS (1–1.5 mg/ml)
3. Chloramine-T (0.30 mg/ml in 0.5 M phosphate buffer, pH 7.2)
4. Carrier-free ^{125}I (l mCi/10 μl)
5. Amberlite IRA 400 (Fisher)
6. 9-in. disposable Pasteur pipette
7. 1% (w/v) bovine serum albumin (BSA) in PBS

Method

1. Draw one of the following solutions into each of three 1-ml disposable syringes fitted with 21 g × 1¹/₂-in. needles:
   a. 50 μl protein
   b. 30 μl Chloramine -T
   c. 100 μl tyrosine solution
   Note: Chloramine-T solution must be prepared immediately before use.
2. At $t = 0$ sec add (in order) to the V-bottom vial containing ^{125}I:
   a. Protein
   b. Chloramine-T
   and mix well.

DENNIS M. KLINMAN AND J. C. HOWARD • Department of Pathology, University of Pennsylvania, School of Medicine, Philadelphia, Pennsylvania 19104.

3. At $t = 15$ sec, add $100\,\mu l$ of saturated tyrosine solution and mix well.

4. Draw contents of vial into syringe, empty solution onto column of Amberlite in Pasteur pipette, and wash with 1% BSA in PBS.

5. Collect effluent and determine proportion of ^{125}I bound to protein. The Amberlite column serves as an ion-exchange resin and effectively removes all of the non-protein-bound iodine from the reaction mixture, thereby making dialysis of the reaction mixture unneccessary.

6. *Note:* The stated concentration of Chloramine-T has been reduced by 50% without affecting the amount of iodine incorporated but with an improvement in the antibody activity retained. To what extent the concentration of the reagent can be reduced without affecting the amount of label incorporated has not yet been determined and warrants further analysis.

Method for Growing Hybridomas in Rats or Mice

Materials

1. Young adult mice or rats
2. Pristane (2,6,10,14-tetramethylpentadecane, Aldrich)
3. Antilymphocyte serum (ALS) (Microbiological Associates)

Method for Interspecies Hybridomas (Rat × Mouse)

1. For ascites production, inject mice intraperitoneally with 0.5 ml of pristane. Rats receive 1.0 ml of pristane. Pristane-primed animals are then rested 3 weeks to 2 months.
2. On days −4 and −3 relative to transfer of interspecies hybridomas, inject recipient animals with antilymphocyte serum. Although the dose may vary somewhat with the batch of serum, we have used the following:
   a. Mice: 40–50 μl
   b. Rats: 0.25–1.0 ml
   Injection is given intraperitoneally for those animals who will receive subcutaneous tumor. Conversely, ALS is given subcutaneously to those animals who will receive intraperitoneal tumor.
3. On day of tumor transfer, recipient animals receive total body irradiation (600–800 rads) followed 6–8 hr later by syngeneic bone marrow (1–2 × 10^7 cells/recipient). In the case of murine donors, the bone marrow is treated with monoclonal anti-Thy-1.2 plus guinea pig complement.

THOMAS J. MCKEARN • Department of Pathology, Divisions of Research Immunology and Laboratory Medicine, University of Pennsylvania, Philadelphia, Pennsylvania 19104.

4. Hybridoma cells in Dulbecco's Modified Eagle's Medium (DMEM) are injected either subcutaneously between scapulae (0.1–0.5 ml) or intraperitoneally. Numbers of cells required for tumor growth can vary considerably. In general, one should not give less than 1×10^7 cells from culture when first attempting to grow these tumors.

5. Subcutaneous tumors will become palpable within 10–14 days and serum containing a high concentration of antibody can be collected several times. Ascites fluid may develop over a longer period of time.

In general, we have had better success in growing hybridoma cells from culture first as solid tumors which then are adapted to growth as ascites tumors. One can anticipate that a mouse will give 10–20 ml of ascites fluid while a rat will produce 60–100 ml of fluid.

Method for Intraspecies Hybridomas

For growth of mouse × mouse hybridomas in mice or rat × rat hybridomas in rats the above procedures may be followed with exclusion of steps 2 and 3.

Isolation of Monoclonal Antibodies from Supernatant by (NH$_4$)$_2$SO$_4$ Precipitation

Zdenka L. Jonak

Introduction

Large volumes of cell-culture supernatant containing monoclonal antibodies are not convenient for storage. Such supernatants may also contain serum components which eventually destroy antibody activity if stored unfrozen for long periods of time. Precipitation by (NH$_4$)$_2$SO$_4$ allows one to obtain the antibodies in a much smaller volume without significant loss of activity.

Materials

To prepare a saturated solution of (NH$_4$)$_2$SO$_4$ (Baker) add crystals to distilled water. Add approximately 1000 g per liter and stir at room temperature for 8 hr. When most of the salt is dissolved allow the solution to stand at 5°C overnight. Adjust the pH to 7.0–7.1 with 30% (w/v) NaOH.

Method

1. Use 50% saturation to precipitate the monoclonal antibodies from tissue-culture medium. Add 1 vol of saturated (NH$_4$)$_2$SO$_4$ solution to 1 vol of

Zdenka L. Jonak • Wistar Institute of Anatomy and Biology, Philadelphia, Pennsylvania 19104.

medium. Mix immediately by swirling and allow the precipitation to occur for 1 hr. The whole procedure is carried out on ice.

2. The precipitate is collected by centrifugation at $48,000 \times g$ for 30 min. After centrifugation the supernatant is discarded and the precipitate dissolved in a minimal amount of distilled water. Dialyze the solution against several changes of the desired buffer and test for antibody titer. Distribute the sample into small freezing vials and keep it at $-70°C$.

Reference

Heide, K., and Schwics, H. G., 1973, Salt fractionation of immunoglobulins, in: *Handbook of Experimental Immunology* (D. M. Weir, ed.), Blackwell, Oxford, pp. 6.1–6.11.

Characterization of Hybridoma Immunoglobulins by Sodium Dodecylsulfate–Polyacrylamide Gel Electrophoresis

J. B. HAAS AND ROGER H. KENNETT

The following procedure is useful for initial characterization of the immuno-globulin (Ig) chains produced by hybrid myelomas. For those hybrids made with an Ig-producing line it usually allows discrimination of two light chains and will distinguish between γ and μ heavy chains. (See Chapters 4 and 10, and Figs. 1 and 4 for examples.) Further characterization of the subclass of IgG or class of L chain can be done with conventional immunodiffusion of dense hybridoma supernatant against antisera reacting with specific Ig chains (Research Products International).

Labeling Immunoglobulins with [³⁵S]Methionine

Materials

1. RPMI-1640 Select-Amine Kit (Grand Island Biological Co.). Prepare sterile methionine-deficient RPMI-1640. Store at 4°C. Prepare sterile 10 mM methionine. Store at 4°C.
2. L-[³⁵S]methionine solution 600-1400 Ci/mM (Amersham)

J. B. HAAS AND ROGER H. KENNETT • Department of Human Genetics, University of Pennsylvania, School of Medicine, Philadelphia, Pennsylvania 19104.

3. Fetal calf serum. Different batches should be tested as the specific serum batch and concentration affect the relative amounts of Ig and other proteins synthesized and secreted by the cell. Store at −20°C.
4. Glutamine (Sigma) 100× stock—3 g/100 ml. Store at −20°C.
5. Trichloroacetic acid (Baker Chemical Co.) 10% (w/v) in distilled water. Stable at room temperature.
6. 25 mm 0.2 μm microporous filters (Amicon)
7. Filter holder (Hoeffer)

Method

1. A sterile suspension of 2×10^6 log phase cells are washed once in methionine-deficient RPMI-1640.
2. Cells are resuspended in 5 ml of methionine-deficient RPMI-1640 containing 30 mg/ml glutamine and 5% fetal calf serum.
3. 250 μCi [^{35}S]methionine are added to the cell suspension and cells are incubated 18 hr in a 5% CO_2 incubator.
4. 20 min before harvesting supernatant 0.1 ml 10 mM methionine is added.
5. Supernatant is collected and stored at −20°C.

To Check Incorporation of Label

1. Place 5 μl of sample in 1 ml ice cold 10% trichloroacetic acid.
2. Incubate on ice for 10 min.
3. Pour sample over filter, followed by a small amount of 95% ethanol to facilitate drying.
4. Allow filter to completely dry before placing in 5 ml of scintillation fluid.
5. Vortex briefly and count on beta scintillation counter.

SDS-PAGE

Materials

1. Gel buffer 11A

   Tris (hydroxymethyl) aminomethane (Bio Rad): 36.3 g
   Hydrochloric acid lN (Baker): 48.0 ml

Dissolve tris in HCl and dilute to 100 ml with distilled water, pH 8.9. Store at 4°C.

2. Gel buffer 11B

   Tris: 5.7 g
   Phosphoric acid 1 M (Fisher): 25.6 ml

   Dissolve tris in phosphoric acid and dilute to 100 ml with distilled water, pH 6.7. Store at 4°C.

3. Acrylamide (Bio Rad) 30% (w/v) in distilled water. Store at 4°C.
4. TEMED (N,N,N',N'-tetramethylethlenediamide) (Bio Rad). Store at 4°C.
5. DATD (N,N'-diallyltartardiamide) (Bio Rad). Store at 4°C.
6. SDS (sodium dodecyl sulfate) (Bio Rad) 10% (w/v) in distilled water. Stable at room temperature.
7. APS (ammonium persulfate) (Bio Rad) 10% (w/v) in distilled water. Good for 1 week when stored at 4°C.
8. 2× SDS sample buffer

   Tris: 7.57 g
   Glycerol (Mallinckrodt): 100.0 g
   SDS: 23.0 g
   β-Mercaptoethanol (Sigma): 50.0 ml

   Dilute to 500 ml with distilled water, and add 1 g Coomassie Brilliant Blue R250 (Bio Rad).

9. Electrode buffer

   Tris: 6.0 g
   Glycine (Sigma): 28.8 g
   SDS (20%): 10.0 ml

   Dissolve tris and glycine in 1500 ml of distilled water. Add SDS and dilute to 2 liters with distilled water. Stable at room temperature.

10. Stain

    Coomassie Brilliant Blue R250: 2.0 g
    Methanol (Baker): water (50/50, v/v): 1000.0 ml

    Prior to use, add 7 ml glacial acetic acid (Baker) to 93 ml of stain. Stable at room temperature.

11. Destaining solution

    Methanol: 500.0 ml
    Distilled water: 500.0 ml
    Glacial acetic acid: 100.0 ml

    Stable at room temperature.

12. Slab gel electrophoresis apparatus (Hoeffer).
13. Gel slab dryer (Bio Rad).
14. Cronex MRF 31 single side emulsion X-ray film (Picker Corp. Medical Products Division).

Slab Gel Preparation

Acrylamide 30%	6.6 ml
Buffer 11A	2.5 ml
SDS 10%	0.1 ml
Distilled water	4.7 ml
DATD 10%	0.230 ml
TEMED	0.005 ml
APS 10%	0.05 ml

Combine all ingredients except APS. Degas solution for 2 min, or until air bubbles cease rising to the surface. Add APS, swirl solution, and pour the gel, leaving enough room (about 1.5 cm) at the top for the stacking gel. Layer distilled water on top of the gel and let set 1 hr.

Stacking Gel Preparation

Acrylamide 30%	2.0 ml
Buffer 11B	1.25 ml
SDS	0.1 ml
Distilled water	6.13 ml
DATD 10%	0.230 ml
TEMED	0.005 ml
APS 10%	0.150 ml

Combine all ingredients except APS. Degas the gel solution. Drain water completely from the top of the slab gel. Insert comb about 75 mm above slab gel. Add APS, swirl solution, and pour the gel. Let set 45 min. Remove comb and drain any excess ungelled solution from the wells and rinse with electrode buffer before adding sample.

Sample Preparation

1. Mix sample with an equal volume of 2× SDS sample buffer. Approximately 80,000 cpm will be visible after 18–24 hr exposure to x-ray film.
2. Place in a boiling water bath for 2–3 min.
3. Centrifuge for 5 min in a microfuge (Beckman).

Running the Gel

1. Remove buffer from the wells of the stacking gel and place samples in wells.

2. Carefully layer electrode buffer on top of each sample, taking care that the samples do not spill over into adjacent wells.
3. Pour electrode buffer in the top of the apparatus and in the housing.
4. Run gel at constant current, 5 mA per gel for 15 min. Increase current to 12 mA per gel for the remainder of the run. Current should be turned off when blue dye front is about 2 cm from the bottom of the gel.
5. Separate the glass plates by inserting a spatula between the gel and the glass plate, and gently applying pressure while turning the spatula.
6. Remove gel from glass plate by forcing water from a syringe through a 3-in. 22-gauge needle between the plate and the gel.
7. Stain for 30 min; destain 1 hr or more.
8. Gel is dried onto filter paper on slab gel dryer for 1 hr.
9. Expose gel to x-ray film. Store at −20°C until ready to develop.

References

Heine, J. W., Honess, R. W., Cassai, E., and Roizman, B., 1974, Proteins specified by herpes simplex virus XII the virion polypeptide of Type I strains, *J. Virol.* **14:**640.

Maizel, Jr., J. V., 1971, Gel electrophoresis of proteins, in: *Methods in Virology*, Vol. 5 (K. Maramorosch and H. Koprowski, eds.), Academic Press, New York, pp. 179–246.

Sarmiento, M., Haffey, M., and Spear, P. G., 1979, Membrane proteins specified by herpes simplex viruses. III. Role of glycoprotein VP7 (B2) in virion infectivity, *J. Virol.* **29:**1149.

The Calculation of Antigen–Antibody Binding Constants by Radioimmunoassay

Mark E. Frankel

A standard method for the characterization of the interaction between an antibody molecule and the complementary antigen is the determination of binding constants for that reaction. Numerous methods for the determination of these values have been published (for review see Day, 1972). In the past, affinity measurements of the antibody–antigen reaction have yielded average affinity constants for the sum total of all reactions. Monoclonal hybridoma antibodies will allow the determination of binding constants for individual antibody–antigen reactions.

This section is a short description of several methods for the determination of binding constants, including an adaptation of the solid-phase radioimmunoassay (RIA) used in many laboratories for the analysis of the antibody specificity.

Consider the equilibrium between an antibody A with valence n and a ligand P with valence s:

$$A + P \rightleftharpoons AP \tag{1}$$

The equilibrium constant K for this interaction is

$$K = n[A]_{bound}/n[A]_{free} \, (s[P]_{total} - n[A]_{bound}) \tag{2}$$

and the Scatchard relationship (Scatchard, 1949) is

$$[A]_{bound}/[A]_{free}[P]_{total} = ([A]_{bound}/[P]_{total})nK \tag{3}$$

Mark E. Frankel • Wistar Institute of Anatomy and Biology, Philadelphia, Pennsylvania 19104.

Various arrangements of this equation can be used for the calculation of binding constants. The data used to determine these constants determine the form of equation (3) to be used.

Equilibrium Dialysis

Equilibrium dialysis is often used to determine binding constants for antibodies to antigen. In this technique a membrane permeable to one component but not the other is used. The nonpermeable component is placed on one side of the membrane and the concentration of the freely permeable component is determined on both sides of the membrane after equilibrium has been reached. This method has been most frequently used for the determination of antihapten binding constants using radiolabeled antigen and membranes permeable to the hapten but not the antibody.

One of three forms of equation (3) are generally used to determine binding constants from such data.

The Scatchard Equation

The ligand form of the Scatchard equation (3) is

$$[P]_{bound}/[P]_{free}[A]_{total} = (nK - [P]_{bound}/[A]_{total})\,Ks \qquad (4)$$

For univalent antigens this equation can be used to calculate K. A plot of $[P]_{bound}/[P]_{free}[A]_{total}$ vs. $[P]_{bound}/[A]_{total}$ will have a slope of $-K$. (For a detailed treatment of such data, see Karush, 1957.)

Briefly, $[P]_{bound}$ and $[P]_{free}$ are measured at constant antibody concentration in equilibrium dialysis with a membrane permeable to antigen (hapten) only.

The Sips Equation

Equation (3) can be rewritten as

$$[A]_{bound} / (s[P]_{total} - n[A]_{bound}) = ([A]_{total} - [A]_{bound})K \qquad (5)$$

One may assume that the right-hand side of equation (5) is an exponential (Sips, 1948; Karush, 1962):

$$\log\left[\,[A]_{bound} / (s[P]_{total} - n[A]_{bound})\,\right] = \alpha\log K + \alpha \log [A]_{free} \qquad (6)$$

Similarly, from equation (4):

$$\log[[P]_{bound} / (n[A]_{total} - s[P]_{bound})] = \alpha \log K + \alpha \log [P]_{free} \qquad (7)$$

A plot of $\log [P]_{free}$ vs. $\log [P]_{bound} / (n[A]_{total} - s[P]_{bound})$ will give K as $1 / [P]_{free}$ when $[P]_{bound} = n[A]_{total}/2$ and the slope α is termed the heterogeneity index, which for monoclonal antibodies should be 1.0 (for example, see Schwartz et al., 1978).

Equation (6) can also be used if the antibody molecule is sufficiently smaller than the antigen. Thus for the reaction between antibodies and influenza virus particles a membrane permeable to antibody but not virus can be used and the concentration of antibody free and bound determined at constant virus concentration and increasing antibody concentration (Fazekas de St. Groth and Webster, 1963).

The Langmuir Equation

Equation (4) can be rewritten

$$[P]_{bound}/nK([P]_{free}[A]_{total}) + (s[P]_{bound}/n[A]_{total}) = 1$$

and

$$(1/nK[P]_{free}) + s/n = [A]_{total}/[P]_{bound} \qquad (8)$$

For univalent antigen a plot of $1/[P]_{free}$ vs. $[A]_{total}/[P]_{bound}$ will have a slope $= 1/nK$ (see Eisen and Karush, 1949).

Precipitation of Bound Antigen

Equation (4) can also be used directly for the interaction of antibody and univalent antigen by Farr precipitation of the antibody with ammonium sulfate after equilibrium has been reached. With radiolabeled antigen, the $[P]_{free}$ and $[P]_{bound}$ can then be determined (see Schwartz et al., 1978).

Radioimmunoassay

The use of equilibrium dialysis or precipitation for the determination of binding constants requires that at least one component of the system be monovalent; with antihapten antibodies this is no problem. However, when multivalent antigen is used, univalent Fab' fragments of antibody must be used (see Mamet-

Bratley, 1966). Also, for hybridoma antibodies specific for protein antigens, discriminatory membranes are often unavailable.

A general method for screening hybridoma cultures for specific activity is the solid-phase RIA in which antigen is adsorbed to the bottom of 96-well flexible polyvinyl microtiter plates. Antibody reactivity is then determined by a two-step incubation first with hybridoma-culture fluid and then with a radiolabeled antiantibody. We have developed a treatment of binding data from this assay which allows the determination of binding constants (Frankel and Gerhard, 1979). Equation (3) has been rewritten as:

$$[A]_{bound}/([A]_{total} - [A]_{bound}) = sK[P]_{total} - nK[A]_{bound}$$

In this case, a plot of $[A]_{bound}/([A]_{total} - [A]_{bound})$ vs. $[A]_{bound}$ will have a slope of $-nK$, or $-2K$ for bivalent antibody. It is not necessary to know the antigen concentration as long as it is kept constant throughout the experiment. In practice, the binding of hybridoma to antigen is then determined by incubating different dilutions of antibody with wells of constant amounts of antigen. After appropriate incubations and washing procedures the wells are developed with purified [^{125}I]rabbit anti-mouse $F(ab')_2$ antibody. The amount of bound antibody in each well is then determined by extrapolation of the radioactivity bound to a standard curve of antibody of known concentration. The total amount of antibody per well is determined by a binding curve done simultaneously, using increasing antigen concentration. Antibody concentration is then determined as the maximum antibody bound at maximum antigen concentration.

Although neither s nor $[P]_{total}$ is known, the quantity $(s[P]_{total})$ can be approximated from the Y intercept of the Scatchard plot which equals $(sK[P]_{total})$. Thus equation (6) can be used to calculate α, the heterogeneity constant.

The Thermodynamic Parameters of the Interaction Between Hybridoma Antibody and Influenza Virus

The RIA procedure described above has the advantage that large numbers of samples can be analyzed simultaneously. Therefore, the calculation of parameters such as enthalpy is facilitated. The van't Hoff relationship

$$\ln K = (\Delta S/R) - (\Delta H/RT) \tag{10}$$

allows calculation of the enthalpy of an interaction by plotting $\ln K$ as a function of l/T. The slope is then $\Delta H/R$.

The results from such a calculation for the interaction of the hemagglutinin specific hybridoma H2/6A5 with the influenza virus A/PR/8/34(HON1) are shown in Table II. The heterogeneity constant α has been calculated from a

TABLE II
Thermodynamic Parameters of the Interaction of H2/6A5 and A/PR/8/34(H0N1)

$T°(C)$	$(1/T_{abs}) \times 10^3$	K
4.0	3.61	$2.49 \times 10^{10} M^{-1}$
17.0	3.45	$4.96 \times 10^9 M^{-1}$
27.0	3.33	$1.81 \times 10^9 M^{-1}$
37.0	3.23	$5.78 \times 10^8 M^{-1}$
43.5	3.16	$2.20 \times 10^8 M^{-1}$
32.0	3.23	$5.78 \times 10^8 M^{-1}$
43.5	3.16	$2.20 \times 10^8 M^{-1}$

$$K^0 = 2.13 \pm 0.1 \times 10^9 M^{-1}$$
$$a = 1.16 \pm 1.16$$
$$F^0 = 12.6 \text{ kcal/mole}$$
$$H^0 = -20.3 \text{ kcal/mole}$$
$$S^0 = -25.8 \text{ E.U./mole}$$

treatment of the binding data at 27°C in the Sips form [equation (6)]. This procedure for calculation of binding constants has the advantage of allowing the data shown in Table 1 to be assembled from one experiment.

Affinity or Avidity?

The affinity (K_i) of an interaction of antibody and antigen is a thermodynamic parameter determined by the average association constant between antibody and antigen. Multivalence of both components will affect the observed binding constants. Furthermore, it is quite possible that the presentation of antigen in a solid-phase RIA may alter the binding constant. Therefore, the treatment of RIA binding data by Scatchard analysis results in the calculation of avidity constants. The specificity of hybridoma antibodies is routinely determined by binding in an RIA [or alternatively enzyme-linked immunosorbent assays (ELISA)]. The effective interaction that is being monitored by screening assays is avidity and thus, the determination of avidity constants by the same method should be appropriate.

References

Day, E. D., *Advanced Immunochemistry,* 1972, Williams & Wilkins, Baltimore, MD.
Eisen, H. N., and Karush, F., 1949, The interaction of purified antibody with homologous hapten. Antibody valence and binding constant, *J. Am. Chem. Soc.* **71:**363–364.

Fazekas de St. Groth, S., and Webster, R. G., 1963, The neutralization of animal viruses. IV. Parameters of the influenza virus–antibody system, *J. Immunol.* **90:**151–164.

Frankel, M. E., and Gerhard, W., 1979, The rapid determination of binding constants for antiviral antibodies by a radioimmunoassay. An analysis of the interaction between hybridoma proteins and influenza virus, *Mol. Immunol.* **16:**101–106.

Karush, F., 1957, The interaction of purified anti -β-lactoside antibody with haptens, *J. Am. Chem. Soc.* **79:**3380–3384.

Karush, F., 1962, Immunologic specificity and molecular structure, *Adv. Immunol.* **2:**1–40.

Mamet-Bratley, M. D., 1966, Evidence concerning homogeneity of the combining sites of purified antibody, Immunochemistry **3:**155–162.

Scatchard, D., 1949, The attraction of proteins for small molecules and ions, *Ann. NY Acad. Sci.* **51:**660–672.

Schwartz, M., Lancet, D., Mozes, E., and Sela, M., 1978, Affinity and avidity of antibodies to the random polymer (T.G.)-A-L and a related ordered synthetic polypeptide, *Immunochemistry* **15:**477–481.

Sips, R., 1948, On the structure of a catalyst surface, *J. Chem. Phys.* **16:**490.

References to Other Methods

References to other methods useful for the detection and characterization of monoclonal antibodies are listed below. These include both methods that have been specifically applied to the use of antibodies produced by hybridomas or methods that are potentially useful in that context.

Braun, D. G., Hild, K., and Ziegler, A., 1979, Resolution of immunoglobulin patterns by analytical Isoelectric focusing, in: *Immunological Methods* (I. Lefkovits and B. Pernis, eds.), Academic, New York, pp. 107–121.

Brodsky, F. M., Parham, P., Barnstable, C. J., Crumpton, M. J., and Bodmer, W. F., 1979, Monoclonal antibodies for analysis of the HLA system, *Immunol. Rev.* **47**:3.

Coffino, P., Laskov, R., and Scharff, M. D., 1970, Immunoglobulin production: Method for quantitatively detecting variant myeloma cells, *Science* **167**:186.

Elwing, H., Nilsson, L., and Ouchterlony, O., 1977, A simple spot technique for thin layer immunoassays (TIA) on plastic surfaces, *J. Immunol. Methods* **17**:131.

Juy, D., Legrain, P., Cazenave, P., and Buttin, G., 1979, A new rapid rosette-forming cell micromethod for the detection of antibody-synthesizing hybridomas, *J. Immunol. Methods* **30**:269.

Köhler, G., Hengartner, H., and Shulman, M. J., 1978, Immunoglobulin production by lymphocyte hybridomas, *Eur. J. Immunol.* **8**:82.

Parks, D. R., Bryan, V. M., Oi, V. T., and Herzenberg, L. A., 1979, Antigen-specific identification and cloning of hybridomas with a fluorescence-activated cell sorter, *Proc. Natl. Acad. Sci. USA* **76**:1962.

Schlach, W., and Braun, D. G., 1979, Isolation of monoclonal antibody by preparative isoelectric focusing in horizontal layers of Sephadex G-75, in: *Immunological Methods* (I. Lefkovits and B. Pernis, eds.), Academic, New York, pp. 123–130.

Schneide, M. D., and Eisenbar, G. S., 1979, Transfer plate radioassay using cell monolayers to detect anti-cell surface antibodies synthesized by lymphocyte hybridomas, *J. Immunol. Methods* **29**:331.

Sharon, J., Morrison, S. L., and Kabat, E. A., 1979, Detection of specific hybridoma clones by replica immunoadsorption of their secreted antibodies, *Proc. Natl. Acad. Sci. USA* **76**:1420.

Stähli, C., Staehelin, T., Miggiano, V., Schmidt, J., and Häring, P., 1980, High frequencies of antigen-specific hybridomas: Dependence on immunization parameters and prediction by spleen cell analysis, *J. Immunol. Methods* **32**:297.

Sunderland, C. A., McMaster, W. R., and Williams, A., 1979, Purification with monoclonal antibody of a predominant leukocyte-common antigen and glycoprotein from rat thymocytes, *Eur. J. Immunol.* **9**:155.

Williams, A. F., 1977, Differentiation antigens of the lymphocyte cell surface, *Contemp. Top. Mol. Immunol.* **6:**83.

Ziegler, A., and Kohler, G., 1979, Isotachophoresis of immunoglobulins, in: *Immunological Methods* (I. Lefkovitz and B. Pernis, eds.), Academic, New York, pp. 131–136.

Index

This index includes references to topics in Chapters 1–20. It does not include references to methods described in detail in the Appendix, pages 361–419.